S0-AYU-908

THERAPEUTIC RECREATION SERVICE

Principles and Practices
Third Edition

Richard Kraus, Ed.D.

Department of Recreation and Leisure Studies,
Temple University

wcb
Wm. C. Brown Publishers
Dubuque, Iowa

Copyright © 1983 by CBS College Publishing.

Copyright © 1973 by W. B. Saunders Company; 1978 by Saunders College Publishing/Holt, Rinehart and Winston.

Copyright © 1989 by Wm. C. Brown Publishers. All rights reserved

Library of Congress Catalog Card Number: 82–24059

ISBN 0–697–06145–0

No part of this publication may be reproduced, stored in a retrieval system, or transmitted, in any form or by any means, electronic, mechanical, photocopying, recording, or otherwise, without the prior written permission of the publisher.

Printed in the United States of America by Wm. C. Brown Publishers 2460 Kerper Boulevard, Dubuque, IA 52001

10 9 8 7 6 5 4 3 2

Preface

In this third edition of *Therapeutic Recreation Service: Principles and Practices*, the author seeks to present the reader with a fully up-to-date, comprehensive introduction to the field of recreation service for special populations. In so doing, major emphasis has been given to a number of important trends that emerged during the 1960's and 1970's and became a reality in the early 1980's.

First, the steady growth of therapeutic recreation means that it is no longer a relatively minor field of professional service. Many more institutions and community agencies today recognize the value of recreation for the disabled and use it in varied ways to enrich their lives and overcome their handicaps. The gap between institutions and community-based programs has increasingly been bridged, as a result of cooperative programming, leisure counseling and education, and the strong thrust toward mainstreaming of the disabled in American and Canadian society.

Second, the field itself has become much more highly professionalized. Years ago, the conceptual base for therapeutic recreation service was extremely limited, and there were few programs of professional preparation. Today, there are numerous well-staffed college and university curricula preparing specialists in this field. With an expanded body of literature and research, stronger standards and credentialing processes for practitioners, and active professional organizations on national, state and provincial levels, therapeutic recreation has developed a much more solid base than it had in the past.

Closely linked to this development has been the shift from a casual, diversional approach to programming to a much more purposeful, sophisticated and systematic approach. In part, this has been due to the need to demonstrate accountability by showing the values and outcomes of therapeutic recreation service during a "tight-money" era in which all forms of human and social services have come under increasingly severe scrutiny. It is also due to the rapid coming-of-age of a relatively young and untested professional discipline, and to the contributions made by a number of professional leaders and scholars in the field. As a consequence, therapeutic recreation's cutting edge today is marked by a strong emphasis on the scientific assessment of patients' or clients' functional abilities and needs, by the establishment of sharply defined behavioral objectives and treatment plans, by activity and task analysis, by systems-based programming and modification of activities, and by other sophisticated techniques within a clinical, treatment-based model of service.

At the same time, there is a clear recognition that many disabled individuals are not in need of therapy as such, but rather require appropriate recreational opportunities as a basic life need or as part of community-living experiences. Many programs for special populations, in senior centers, schools for the retarded, penal and correctional institutions or municipal agencies, are not staffed by therapeutic recreation professionals and can not be regarded as therapy in a strict sense.

This text therefore strongly endorses the contemporary philosophy of therapeutic recreation which was developed by the National Therapeutic Recreation Society and widely disseminated in 1982. This multi-model approach identifies three broad purposes of therapeutic recreation: therapy, leisure education and recreational participation. Depending on the needs of the population being served and the organization's goals and resources, any or all of these purposes may be met.

In addition to describing all three functions of therapeutic recreation, the text presents a general understanding of the meaning, history and background of therapeutic recreation service as a professional discipline, examines its application to five major categories of disability and presents guidelines for programming, leadership, evaluation and research. It does not go as fully into the specific processes of patient or client assessment, treatment-plan development and activity analysis as other texts by such authors as Gunn and Peterson, Wehman and Schleien, or Sherrill. The reader is urged to use these sources for advanced study in such areas.

While this text presents a considerable amount of factual material describing actual programs and leadership techniques, it is also concerned with giving a broad picture of therapeutic recreation service from a humanistic perspective. Certainly, it is possible to computerize therapeutic recreation program planning and to reduce the needs of a patient or client to a list of desired behavioral changes. However, it is also important to deal with people as people and to be deeply concerned with human relationships and emotions. The individual who seeks to work with the disabled must realize that despite the very positive picture that has generally been presented about programs and services for special populations in our society, the real lives of the disabled have been extremely barren until very recently. Historically, the mentally and physically disabled have been shunned, ignored or shamefully abused. Even today, there are far too many human beings being "warehoused" with little attempt at rehabilitation or other meaningful services in our mental hospitals, prisons and nursing homes, or living as derelict "bag" men and women on our city streets. For every physically disabled person who is living up to his or her real capability as a human being, there are probably dozens who are not permitted and helped to reach their own potential.

Yet, for all its negatives, the story of the disabled in our society is also an inspiring and encouraging one. Again and again, we see handicapped persons struggling courageously to overcome their limitations. The blind who ski swiftly down mountainsides or the paraplegic or other seriously physically disabled individuals who crawl painfully up them; the quadriplegics who paint laboriously with brushes attached to their foreheads; the alcoholics who rehabilitate their ravaged bodies to compete in Olympics; the mentally retarded who struggle to survive in often-hostile community environments—all are superb examples of indomitable human spirit.

The place of recreation and leisure in the lives of the disabled is critical. For all humans, recreation can provide a strong sense of identity, self-affirmation, pleasure, acceptance by others and creative expression. For the disabled, it becomes all the more important because these values are so difficult to attain, and other channels of expression are so frequently cut off. While such outcomes are not easily obtained by the handicapped, with persistence and sound professional leadership, they can be achieved.

Every effort has been made to bring this text up to date by citing numerous new references from such sources as *Therapeutic Recreation Journal, Parks and Recreation, Journal of Physical Education and Recreation* and other leading texts and professional reports. New trends in therapeutic recreation service have been identified and thoroughly described.

A number of the organizations whose programs were described in previous editions provided new descriptions of their services and structure. These include the Clinical Center of the National Institutes of Health in Bethesda, Maryland; the Athens, Ohio, Mental Health Center; the Mt. Sinai Hospital Center in New York; the Penetanguishene Mental Health Centre and the Ontario Crippled Children's Centre in Canada; and a number of other institutional programs. Other agencies which contributed fresh descriptions included the Recreation Center for the Handicapped in San Francisco; Camp Courage in Brainerd, Minnesota; and two municipal park and recreation departments, in Des Moines, Iowa, and Miami, Florida.

The author wishes to stress that although he has included a number of references to therapeutic recreation agencies and programs in Canada, several of which were obtained with the assistance of William Knott, a leading official with a special responsibility for research in the Ministry of Culture and Recreation in Ontario, Canada, he has certainly not covered this subject adequately. While Canadian educators and students will find this text helpful, they should also examine their own literature and professional practices fully in any contemporary study of therapeutic recreation in Canada.

Appreciation is expressed to Ann Durante and Susan Singer of Friends Hospital, Philadelphia, for their assistance.

Others whose assistance should be acknowledged include Professor Jerry Jordan and Professor William Dayton, of the Department of Recreation and Leisure Studies of Temple University, and Cara Albom, a graduate student in that department. The work of numerous other college and university educators and authors specializing in this field was invaluable in preparing this third edition, and the author has quoted liberally from such sources. Finally, this Preface should give credit to individuals like Janet Pomeroy, director of the outstanding Recreation Center for the Handicapped in San Francisco, and to thousands of others like her, who have literally dedicated themselves to helping the disabled achieve fuller and more rewarding lives—through recreation service. In a real sense, *they* are the authors of this text.

Richard Kraus
Temple University, 1983

Contents

CHAPTER 7
Recreation for the Mentally Retarded and Learning-Disabled   **228**

CHAPTER 8
Recreation for the Physically Disabled   **263**

CHAPTER 9
Recreation and the Aged   **290**

CHAPTER 10
Programs and the Socially Deviant   **331**

CHAPTER 11
Community Services for the Disabled

CHAPTER 12
Evaluation and Research in Therapeutic Recreation

APPENDIX A
Selected Films on Recreation and Related Services for the Disabled

APPENDIX B
List of Organizations

APPENDIX C
Professional Standards

APPENDIX D
Equipment and Supply Sources

Bibliography

Author Index

Subject Index

Therapeutic Recreation Service: Past and Present

From a relatively minor area within recreation service only ten or 15 years ago, therapeutic recreation service has become a major field.

A decade ago, few students were specializing in programming for the disabled; today therapeutic recreation majors often comprise a majority of all recreation students.

State and national professional organizations today have strong sections concerned with therapeutic recreation services; programs for the registration and certification of specialists in this area have been developed.

Increasingly, federal and state laws have promoted awareness of the special needs of the ill and disabled and have provided a strong base for their development and support.

Special populations of all sorts are now being involved in recreation programs where none existed in the past. Leisure involvement is being perceived as an important means of mainstreaming the disabled.

EXAMPLES OF THERAPEUTIC RECREATION PROGRAMS

There are dozens of examples of innovative and effective programs serving the mentally and physically disabled.

In a large state-sponsored school for retarded children and youth, extensive programs of sports, hobbies, social activities, art and music are provided. In a community-based mental health center, clients are involved in a variety of individual and group social activities and projects, many of which they plan and carry out themselves. Elderly residents in a nursing home enjoy hobbies, discussion groups, crafts, entertainment, bingo and group singing. Orthopedically disabled children attend a summer day camp sponsored by a community's recreation and park department, with facilities and equipment specially designed for their use.

Growing numbers of paraplegics and amputees today take part in vigorous wheelchair sports, including national and international tournaments. Teen-age patients from a state psychiatric hospital meet the challenge of white-water canoeing or high-risk Outward Bound camp programs. In prisons and correctional institutions, there is increased emphasis on leisure education and counseling to help discharged inmates make a constructive transition to community life.

In thousands of similar settings throughout the United States and Canada today, groups of children, youth and adults with varied kinds of disability are being provided with specially planned and directed *therapeutic recreation service*. Since World War II, this field has become a key area of specialization within the broad field of professional recreation.

MEANING OF THERAPEUTIC RECREATION SERVICE

Exactly what does this term mean? How did it come into being? What are the goals of therapeutic recreation service? Who provides it, and what does it consist of? It is the purpose of this textbook to answer these questions.

Value of Recreation for All

As Chapter 2 points out in detail, recreation provides important health-related benefits for all human beings. With increased amounts of leisure available to most individuals today, recreation offers the opportunity for physical participation, emotional release, social involvement and creative expression essential for healthy adjustment. Gray comments that tension, boredom and frustration in daily living contribute to emotional disorders for millions of individuals, who are troubled by feelings of alienation and depression. Often, such stresses lead to destructive, pleasure-seeking habits such as alcohol or drug abuse or pathological risk-taking.

For many individuals, creative and satisfying leisure activities represent a positive means of *maintaining* sound mental health and *preventing* disability. Gray writes, "As therapists, recreation personnel have a role in curing the sick, but as devotees of the recreation movement, we all have a role in developing a society that will help keep people well."[1]

Thus, all recreation must be seen as therapeutic. Without question, it is a health-related area of human service, and contributes directly to personal well-being. However, in a more specific sense, the term *therapeutic recreation service* is used to describe recreation programs and experiences that are provided for individuals who have special impairments that limit their involvement. Such persons usually have intensified needs for constructive and satisfying recreational outlets but are often unable to enjoy the programs and services that are provided for the general public. Specially designed programs must be developed, both to contribute to disabled persons' recovery and rehabilitation and to enrich their lives.

---

[1]David E. Gray: "Exploring Inner Space." *Parks and Recreation,* December 1972, p. 19.

Other Descriptive Terms

In the past, several other descriptive terms were applied to this field of service, including (a) *hospital recreation;* (b) *medical recreation;* and (c) *recreation for the ill and handicapped.* For a variety of reasons these terms are no longer fully appropriate.

Hospital recreation implies that recipients of service are patients in a residential treatment center. However, therapeutic recreation programs may also be provided in the community at special schools, sheltered workshops, or social clubs.

Medical recreation suggests that programs must be carried on under direct medical supervision. Obviously, many individuals with mental or social disabilities may require specially designed recreation programs; however, these programs frequently do not require medical supervision.

Recreation for the ill and handicapped is no longer widely used today because of its emphasis on the term "handicapped." Many individuals have impairments or disabilities but they need not be significantly handicapped. It is the task of therapeutic recreation service, along with other rehabilitative services, to minimize the functional limitations of those it serves. For this reason the term *disability* has become more widely accepted than the term *handicap.*

Recreation for special populations is the way authorities such as Stein and Sessoms have described the field. This description is particularly useful when it includes such special groups as the socially or economically disadvantaged, alcoholics or drug abusers, or the aging—who may not suffer from an obvious disability, but who may require special services.

Use of Term "Therapy"

In some settings the term *recreation therapy* has been used to describe the field. For example, in a manual describing programs offered by its physical medicine and rehabilitation service, the Veterans' Administration states

---

Recreational therapy is a professional and integral part of Physical Medicine and Rehabilitation Service . . . The role of recreation in patient treatment becomes greatly expanded in the rehabilitation of long-term, chronically ill, and psychiatric patients. Recreation helps the patient accept and utilize constructively a prolonged period of hospitalization. Recreation activities develop interpersonal relationships, resocialization, relieve anxieties and tensions, and promote the patient's ability to more fully participate in society.[2]

Many state mental health systems and other hospital networks may designate their recreation leaders as *recreation therapists* in job descriptions under Civil Service

---

[2]*Manual on Physical Medicine and Rehabilitation Service.* Washington, D.C., Veterans' Administration, Manual M-2, July 1966, pp. 4–6.

codes. However, this title has not been fully accepted throughout the field. Some authorities have questioned whether the field should be defined as a therapy designed to cure specific illnesses, comparable to physical or occupational therapy. Knudson writes

---

"Is recreation therapy?" Since the word therapy has different meanings for different people, the answer requires a distinction. If therapy is defined as prescribed or medically guided participation of the team mobilized for a potential therapeutic attack on illness, then most assuredly recreation is frequently therapy. But recreation cannot be labeled as therapy in the sense of a precise cure for a specific ailment.[3]

During the past decade there has been pressure to make recreation a scientifically based form of treatment. Today, a strong case can be made that recreation is a legitimate form of therapy. It utilizes system-based program planning, patient assessment, activity analysis, and careful techniques for documenting outcomes. However, many authorities continue to stress that the chief value of recreation lies in its ability to meet overall human needs, rather than in its specific therapeutic benefits.

Use of Term "Therapeutic"

The term *therapeutic recreation service* has become increasingly widely accepted since the early 1960's. For example, the Public Health Service's definition is

---

Therapeutic recreation is the specific use of recreational activity in the care, treatment and rehabilitation of ill, handicapped and aged persons with a directed program.[4]

Some authors stress that therapeutic recreation is an ongoing process. Sherrill, for example, refers to it as

---

. . . a process which utilizes recreation services for purposive intervention in some physical, emotional, and/or social behavior to bring about a desired change in that behavior and to promote the growth and development of the individual.[5]

---

[3]A. B. C. Knudson: "Concepts of Recreation in Rehabilitation." In *The Doctors and Recreation in the Hospital Setting*. Raleigh, North Carolina Recreation Commission, Bulletin No. 30, 1962, p. 40.
[4]*Health Resource Statistics—1968*. Washington, D.C., Public Health Service, 1968, p. 185.
[5]Claudine Sherrill: *Adapted Physical Education and Recreation: A Multi-Disciplinary Approach*. Dubuque, Iowa, Wm. C. Brown, 1981, p. 45.

DEFINITION OF THERAPEUTIC
RECREATION SERVICE

This text defines therapeutic recreation service as a professionally directed service that provides recreational and related activities specially designed to meet the needs of individuals suffering from some significant degree of illness or disability. It seeks to help these participants help themselves, through referral, counseling, instruction, or actual program involvement. It may be geared to achieving specific therapeutic outcomes through prescriptive programming, or may be more broadly diversional in nature, or may combine both emphases. It may be provided in an institution, where its primary purpose is to contribute to the process of overall recovery and to facilitate a successful return to the community. It may also be a continuing service intended to enrich the quality of the lives of those with permanent disabilities by providing important psychological, physical and social benefits.

Therapeutic recreation may be a carefully prescribed and structured activity administered by an institution or agency, or it may involve a much more informal program which attracts disabled persons living in the community who come voluntarily for self-directed involvement. Therapeutic recreation may be provided for disabled persons only, or may mainstream the disabled by integrating them with the nondisabled.

PHILOSOPHY OF THERAPEUTIC
RECREATION SERVICE

A 1982 statement by the National Therapeutic Recreation Society suggests that the primary purpose of therapeutic recreation is to help patients or clients to eliminate leisure barriers, develop leisure skills and attitudes, and make the most of their leisure.

The society identifies three services that should be offered as part of a comprehensive approach to therapeutic recreation: *therapy, leisure education* and *recreational participation.* Therapeutic recreation specialists should be prepared

---

. . . to provide all three services. The decision as to where and when each of the services would be provided would be based on the assessment of client need. Different individuals have a variety of different needs related to leisure utilization. For some clients, improvement of a functional behavior or problem (physical, mental, social or emotional) is a necessary prerequisite to meaningful leisure experiences. For others, acquiring leisure skills, knowledge, and ability is a priority need. For others, special recreation participation opportunities are necessary, based on place of residence or because assistance or adapted activities are required.[6]

---

[6]*Statement of Philosophy of Therapeutic Recreation Service.* Arlington, Virginia, National Therapeutic Recreation Society, 1982.

Some individuals may need all three services. Others may require only leisure education or opportunities for participation. All three services must be viewed as interdependent and should be offered as part of a total service rather than as independent entities.

O'Morrow identifies two broad approaches to therapeutic recreation service, *clinical* and *nonclinical:*

The clinical approach focuses on the use of recreation in the treatment of illness or disability. The nonclinical approach centers on the broader conception of recreation: the subjective enjoyment and enrichment of the patient's living experience.[7]

This distinction is somewhat arbitrary, because most agencies and therapeutic recreation specialists seek both to meet the general human needs of patients or clients for healthy and satisfying recreation experience and to use recreation as a specific treatment technique.

GOALS OF THERAPEUTIC RECREATION

To illustrate the broad range of purposes for carrying on therapeutic recreation programs, an excellent statement of goals was developed by the Veterans' Administration. It would apply to programs operated by many chronic disease or psychiatric hospitals:

1. To facilitate the patient's adjustment to hospital life and to make him more receptive to treatment.
2. To facilitate the patient's early physical, mental and social rehabilitation, recovery and discharge.
3. To assist in minimizing the risk of unnecessary readmission, by aiding in the patient's transition to his community, following discharge.
4. To improve his morale and sustain it at a high level.
5. To encourage the formation of habits and attitudes which will permit his confident participation in normal activities.
6. To compensate for his disabilities and limitations while inspiring him to fulfill his potentialities.
7. To channel his aggressive drives into appropriate outlets.
8. To encourage his desire to remove or overcome the physical or mental barriers that stand between him and a normal life.
9. To stimulate new or dormant interests and talents, as well as to reestablish old ones.[8]

[7]Gerald S. O'Morrow: *Therapeutic Recreation: A Helping Profession.* Reston, Virginia, Reston, 1976, p. 123.
[8]C. C. Bream, Jr.: "Rehabilitative Recreation in V.A. Hospitals." *Recreation,* May 1964, pp. 224–225.

In a somewhat similar listing of the functions of therapeutic recreation in a general hospital serving a broad range of community health needs, West suggests that the following objectives would prevail:

1. To provide for patients through recreation an outlet for the stress and emotional frustration created by illness, disability and the inability to participate in normal activities.
2. To overcome social isolation, boredom, and loneliness while away from family and friends.
3. To provide functional activities that will aid the patients' social and psychological adjustment and physical independence.
4. To provide activities, diversional in nature, that will offer the opportunity for the constructive use of hospital leisure time.
5. To educate and counsel the patient in the use of activities that can be used after discharge as a continuation of the therapeutic regimen, or to support health maintenance.
6. To assist all health care professionals in the planning and administering of optimal and comprehensive health care for the entire community.[9]

To accomplish such goals, therapeutic recreation specialists must be prepared to play a variety of significant roles that go far beyond the direct leadership of recreation activities.

ROLES OF THERAPEUTIC RECREATION SPECIALISTS

Therapeutic recreation specialists are *not* concerned solely with providing recreational activities for ill and disabled persons in institutional or community settings. Today, they may also serve as counselors, community educators, advocates and organizers, researchers and consultants, members of treatment teams and in a variety of other roles.

These diversified functions were not always available to therapeutic recreation specialists. O'Morrow points out that when he first entered the field in a state psychiatric institution, he was reprimanded for suggesting a counseling service. His role, the superintendent made clear, "was to be in the institution, not out in the community surveying recreation resources and following up ex-patients as to what they were doing during their nonworking hours." The range of services he provided was limited to administration, activity programming, leadership and coordination of services with other professional disciplines.[10]

Today, this situation has changed markedly. Therapeutic recreation specialists in most settings are encouraged to assist in diagnosis and rehabilitation team plan-

---

[9]Ray E. West: "Therapeutic Recreation Service as a Component of Optimal Health Care in a General Hospital Setting." *Therapeutic Recreation Journal*, Third Quarter, 1979, p. 9.

[10]O'Morrow, *op. cit.*, p. 124.

ning. They are often expected to provide counseling, referral and other forms of personal assistance with respect to developing community programs and cooperative arrangements among public and private agencies. In many situations, the emphasis is not so much on *providing activities* as on developing a *social climate* or living situation in which the patient or disabled client can function with satisfaction and increasing social capability.

Even when the professional's task is primarily to lead activities, that role may involve many different duties, as Nesbitt describes:

Therapeutic recreation specialists perform many roles and functions in the course of a week, during a work day, within any given hour. They move quickly and easily from role to role. In a short period of time a therapeutic recreation specialist will set up a day room for the evening . . . arrange for a large group of patients to participate in a community recreation program . . . set up a special party for a small group of patients not yet ready to go into the community or act on their own . . . and sit down for one-to-one counseling with a patient having problems socializing with other people. . . . The therapeutic recreation specialist performs many roles — therapist, administrator, supervisor, leader and consultant among others . . .[11]

Therapeutic recreation includes a wide variety of social situations and deals with an extremely broad range of disabilities or levels of impairment. For example, specialists who work primarily as program leaders may be employed in any of the following types of situations:

Varied Types of Group Settings

1. Community recreation programs (operated by either voluntary agencies or public recreation and park departments) in which mildly disabled individuals mingle and take part in activities with the nondisabled in a fully integrated way.

2. Community recreation programs in which disabled individuals with somewhat more severe levels of disability—such as an orthopedically disabled child with limited mobility—may take part in some activities that are integrated with the nondisabled and may also be involved in some activities or groups that are designed specifically for groups of disabled individuals.

3. Community recreation situations in which the only participation by physically or mentally disabled individuals is within specially organized, segregated groups, and they do *not* mingle with other participants.

4. Institutions in which the recreation specialist may be primarily responsible for providing mass activities seen chiefly as diversional leisure-time programs, with little direct therapeutic purpose, such as films, entertainment, informal games and sports, or bingo.

---

[11]John A. Nesbitt: "The Mission of Therapeutic Recreation Specialists: To Help and to Champion the Handicapped." *Therapeutic Recreation Journal*, Fourth Quarter, 1970, pp. 2–4, 41–42.

5. Settings in which the leader may provide program activities and services that are designed to meet the needs of individuals or of groups of patients, based on deliberately prescribed programs that are carefully evaluated.

6. Situations in which the recreation specialist may provide programs that operate on several levels, such as (a) prescribed individual or small-group activities of an instructional or carefully structured nature; (b) large-group activities that patient groups are required or urged to attend, but in which their actual participation is more or less voluntary; or (c) programs that participants may choose freely.

The Recreation Leader as Therapeutic Agent

In working with patients or clients, the recreation specialist frequently transcends the role of activity leader and becomes instead a therapeutic agent. Collingwood describes this function as one in which " . . . a 'helper' (counselor, teacher, parent, recreational therapist) attempts to better the 'helpee's' (client, patient, student, child) lot in life and help him to live his life more effectively."[12]

In assuming this helping role, Buscaglia points out, it is essential that the therapeutic agent learn to interact positively with disabled individuals. He suggests a number of useful guidelines for such interaction:

1. Remember that each person who is disabled is different; no matter what label is attached to them, they are still totally unique individuals.

2. Remember that disabled people are human beings first and individuals with a disability second. They have the same right to the fullest possible self-actualization that others have — at their own rate, in their own way, and using their own strengths and gifts.

3. Remember that disabled persons have exactly the same needs that you have — to love and be loved, to learn, to share, to grow and to experience, in the same world you live in.

4. Remember that the disabled have the same right as you to fall, to fail, to cry, to curse, to hope, to despair. To protect them from these experiences is to keep them from life.

5. Remember that only those who are disabled can show or tell you *what is possible for them*. We who love them must be attentive, attuned observers.

6. Remember that the disabled must do for themselves. We can be present to reinforce, encourage, hope and help, and to provide alternatives, tools and possibilities — but only they can put these things into action.

7. Remember that persons with disabilities, no matter how disabled, have a limitless potential for becoming — not what *we* want them to become, but what is within *them* to become.

8. Remember that all persons with disabilities have the right to honesty about themselves and their condition. To be dishonest with them is a disservice; honesty forms the only solid base upon which all growth can take place. And for them to change, develop and grow, *you* must also be free to learn, change, develop and experience along with them.[13]

---

[12]Thomas Collingwood: "The Recreation Leader as a Therapeutic Agent." *Therapeutic Recreation Journal,* Fourth Quarter, 1972, p. 147.
[13]Leo Buscaglia: *The Disabled and Their Parents: A Counseling Challenge.* Thorofare, New Jersey, Charles B. Slack, 1975.

Collingwood stresses that empathy, respect, genuineness, concreteness, immediacy and confrontation are key interpersonal elements in helping relationships. After establishing a strong feeling of rapport and trust, the recreation specialist is more effective as a therapeutic agent. Systematic human relations training can help recreation specialists to assume this critical role.

Community Organizer

On an entirely different level, the therapeutic recreation specialist may be employed by community agencies not to provide direct service, but to act in a promotional, advisory or organizational role, assisting and encouraging other groups to provide recreation for the disabled as part of a multi-service approach. In Canada, for example, a study of recreation programs for the disabled in the province of Alberta indicated that specialists working for municipal recreation and park departments could assist voluntary agencies to provide such programs by doing the following:

Providing or adapting facilities for use by the disabled

Helping set up community recreation programs in cooperation with institutional recreation authorities

Assisting in the provision of transportation services

Sponsoring leadership training seminars or workshops

Helping to bring about a greater public awareness and appreciation of the recreation needs of the disabled

Sponsoring demonstration projects[14]

In a reversal of this situation, therapeutic recreation specialists employed within institutions may play an influential role in community education and organization to help discharged patients become successfully integrated in community social and recreation programs. These specialists may provide consultation and referral services, make appearances before community organizations, help design special facilities, educate the lay public about the needs of the disabled or organize other types of special programs and services.

Consumer Advocate

In recent years, many therapeutic recreation specialists have moved from a position of "institutional lethargy"—ignoring the social and cultural injustices com-

---

[14]*A Report on the Survey of Recreation Services for the Disabled in Alberta.* Edmonton, Alberta, Department of Recreation, Parks and Wildlife, 1975, p. 28.

monly perpetrated against the disabled in society—to the more positive and aggressive position of consumer advocate.

However, the disabled must be given the opportunity to speak out on their own, to define their own needs and goals. Therapeutic recreation specialists should recognize this principle and help the disabled themselves to become more knowledgeable consumers of leisure services and to work more effectively within the sociopolitical system. For example, an activities director in a large nursing home has consistently helped residents plan current events seminars. She invites political candidates to address them during election campaigns and helps residents to vote on election day for candidates who support older citizens.

Edginton and Compton point out that the consumer advocate's role may include acting in the following capacities: (a) initiator, planner, strategist or organizer; (b) investigator or ombudsman; (c) mediator, arbitrator or negotiator; (d) lobbyist; (e) counselor; (f) technician or resource specialist; (g) educator; and (h) critic, analyst or evaluator. They conclude:

The development of stronger advocate and consumer roles within parks, recreation and leisure services for and with special populations is long overdue. Higher levels of advocacy and consumerism will yield more efficient, relevant and quantitative services to our special populations.[15]

Recreation professionals must join with professionals in other human service fields and with interested citizens to promote public consciousness of the needs of the disabled. In a recent address on the needs of the mentally retarded in the 1980's, the President of the American Association on Mental Deficiency (AAMD), M. Carl Haywood, stressed the need for all disciplines to contribute to the development of public policies in this area:

. . . many public policies are constructed without even casual information derived from the professional opinions of those who work with and on mental retardation. Laws are made for various reasons, only one of which is the direct personal welfare of citizens who are directly affected by those laws. I propose that the AAMD make stronger alliances with other professional and volunteer organizations for the purpose of exerting direct influence on the formation and modification of public policy on the basis of our combined best professional understanding.[16]

Team Member

In addition to their relationships with patients or clients and with the public, therapeutic recreation specialists must also develop effective working relationships

---

[15]Christopher R. Edginton and David M. Compton: "Consumerism and Advocacy: A Conceptual Framework for the Therapeutic Recreator." *Therapeutic Recreation Journal,* First Quarter, 1975, p. 31.
[16]M. Carl Haywood: "Reducing Social Vulnerability Is the Challenge of the Eighties." *Journal of Mental Retardation,* August 1981, p. 190.

with individuals in a wide variety of other professional disciplines. The recreation worker must be able to relate closely to occupational therapists, physical therapists, doctors, vocational counselors, social service personnel, mental health aides and ward personnel, nurses and volunteers.

In some hospitals therapeutic recreation specialists are regarded in a narrow and superficial light, but in many others they have full access to all medical files and case histories and play an important role in case presentation and analysis. Within the community as well, therapeutic recreation specialists are likely to have close contact with the parents or relatives of disabled individuals, with administrators and supervisors of community recreation programs and with social workers, vocational counselors and school teachers.

AGENCIES PROVIDING THERAPEUTIC RECREATION SERVICE

Therapeutic recreation service is carried on in many types of agencies. The following are the major types of institutions and programs, both residential and nonresidential.

Hospitals of All Types

These include hospitals under various sponsorships, such as Veterans' Administration, military, public health, state, county, municipal, voluntary, sectarian and proprietary hospitals. They serve many types of patients: general, psychiatric, pediatric, chronic disease, geriatric and others. Some are long-term hospitals, while others involve short patient stays.

Nursing Homes

Nursing homes generally are described as extended-care facilities for ill or disabled aged persons who can no longer function in the community or with their own families. However, middle-aged persons who have suffered heart attacks, strokes or other trauma and who cannot live independently may also be residents of nursing homes.

Schools or Residential Centers for Those with Specific Disability

There are thousands of such institutions throughout the country that house, either permanently or for a period of years, the physically disabled (blind, deaf, orthopedically or neurologically impaired) or the mentally retarded or emotionally disturbed. As in the case of hospitals, they operate under a wide variety of auspices: voluntary agency, sectarian, municipal, county- or state-sponsored.

Special Schools or Treatment Centers for the Socially Deviant

These include adult penal institutions, such as prisons, jails or other detention centers, as well as work camps, reformatories and special schools for youth who have been committed by the courts for delinquent behavior. They may also include special schools or shelters for emotionally disturbed children and youth or those from broken families or families incapable of providing adequate care. In some cases, these include custodial treatment centers for alcoholics or drug addicts, particularly when such individuals have been involved in delinquent or criminal behavior. In other situations, alcoholics and drug abusers may be treated during the acute phase of their dependency in special units of general or psychiatric hospitals and rehabilitation centers and, after that, in after-care centers or other sheltered community-based facilities.

Homes for Aged Persons

There are increasing numbers of residential centers for aged persons who cannot live independently or with their families but do not require intensive nursing or medical care and can meet some of their own needs independently. These centers may include municipal, county or state homes for the elderly, residential centers sponsored by sectarian agencies or service organizations or even low-income housing projects with special units for the aged.

Centers for Physical Medicine and Rehabilitation

These are treatment centers for those who have suffered serious physical disability but are no longer under treatment for the acute phase of their illness or injury and are being given varied forms of physical, psychological, vocational and social rehabilitation to facilitate their return to their families and community life.

Programs Operated by Public Recreation and Park Departments

Such agencies have traditionally concentrated their efforts on serving the non-disabled population of all ages with recreational activities and facilities. However, in recent years many have initiated programs to serve the disabled—particularly the mentally retarded and physically handicapped.

Programs of Voluntary Agencies

A number of national organizations have been established to promote services for specific groups of handicapped children, youth or adults, such as the blind, deaf, cerebral palsied, physically handicapped or mentally retarded. Usually operating through county or local chapters, many of these organizations sponsor recreation programs specially designed to meet the needs of the disabled. In addition, many other voluntary agencies, such as the Young Women's Christian Association or the Boys' Clubs of America, may operate one or more programs for the disabled. Other organizations play a national role in providing special types of activity for disabled participants, such as wheelchair sports or Special Olympics.

After-Care Centers and Sheltered Workshops

Particularly in the fields of mental illness, mental retardation and drug addiction, many organizations have established after-care centers, sheltered workshops, drop-in centers and similar facilities to provide multi-service programs to meet the needs of those who have been institutionalized and who need assistance adjusting to the demands of community life. Such programs frequently include recreational and social activities.

It is the function of all these different types of agencies or institutions to provide therapeutic recreation service to meet the needs of the physically, mentally and socially disabled in our society.

APPROPRIATE DESIGNATION AS "THERAPEUTIC" RECREATION

Because of the broad range of settings in which disabled persons are served, it may be inappropriate to designate *all* such programs as forms of therapeutic recreation service. This issue was raised in a dialogue that appeared in the *Therapeutic Recreation Journal* in 1977 and 1978. Witt suggested that the term "therapeutic" was inappropriate when it was used to describe community programs designed for individuals who required specially modified leisure services, but did not need therapy as such. He went on to point out that " . . . a label that implies special skills and services may discourage communities that cannot hire a 'therapeutic recreator' from extending their efforts to disabled individuals."[17]

In response, Gary M. Robb, then President of the National Therapeutic Society, agreed that in many situations within the community disabled individuals were capable of taking part in regular programs through "normal channels" and did not

---

[17]Peter A. Witt: "Therapeutic Recreation: An Out-moded Model." *Therapeutic Recreation Journal*, Second Quarter, 1977, pp. 31–41.

require the services of a fully qualified therapeutic recreator. However, Robb went on to point out that the therapeutic recreation field is still primarily represented by those working with institutionalized clients and patients, and that it does not seem probable that this will change substantially in the near future. He concluded:

Within the institutional structure and . . . for individuals still requiring therapeutic intervention within the community, "therapy" is still the essential ingredient. These situations and interventions do require an individual with special skills and the ability to render special services. Therefore, by and large, the term "therapeutic recreation" is not misused . . .[18]

NUMBERS AND TYPES OF DISABLED PERSONS

There have been many attempts to measure the number of disabled or handicapped persons in the United States. During the mid-1970's, statistics compiled by the Bureau of Outdoor Recreation and the National Center for Health Statistics indicated that there were approximately 68 million persons in the United States with limiting or disabling conditions. This figure included the subcategories of disability listed in Table 1–1.

In another tabulation of the disabled, Sherrill reported on the number of hand-

Table 1–1   Categories of Disability in United States in mid-1970's[19]

11.7 million physically disabled (including half a million people in wheelchairs; 3 million who use crutches, canes, braces or walkers; plus mobility-impaired elderly, amputees and those people with illness such as chronic arthritis, severe cardiovascular disorders, and cerebral palsy)

12.5 million temporarily injured (broken limb, injury to back or spine, severe burns, etc.)

2.4 million deaf, and 11 million hearing-impaired

1.3 million blind, and 8.2 million visually impaired

6.8 million mentally disabled (mentally retarded, severely emotionally disturbed, brain damaged, severely learning-disabled)

1.7 million homebound (chronic health disorders, wasting diseases like multiple sclerosis)

2.1 million institutionalized (mentally disturbed, mentally retarded, terminal illness)

7.6 million suffering from heart conditions

18.3 million arthritics

14.5 million with severe respiratory ailments, such as bronchial asthma

[18]Gary M. Robb: Letter to the Editor. *Therapeutic Recreation Journal*, First Quarter, 1978, p. 6.
[19]Terri Schultz: "The Handicapped, A Minority Demanding Its Rights." *The New York Times*, February 13, 1977, p. 8-E. See also *Trends for the Handicapped*. Washington, D.C., National Park Service and National Society for Park Resources, 1974, p. 4.

Table 1-2   Report of Handicapped Children Receiving Special Education and Related Services as Reported by State Agencies under Public Law 94-142 and Public Law 89-313 During School Year 1978-1979[20]

	P.L. 94-142	P.L. 89-313	Combined
Mentally retarded	801,813	114,260	916,073
Hard of hearing	38,300	3,592	41,892
Deaf	20,597	23,884	44,481
Speech-impaired	1,208,812	6,185	1,214,997
Visually handicapped	22,965	9,611	32,576
Emotionally disturbed	269,629	31,729	301,358
Orthopedically impaired	62,375	7,906	70,281
Other health-impaired	101,465	4,155	105,620
Learning-disabled	1,141,202	13,289	1,154,491
Deaf-blind	1,524	825	2,349
Multi-handicapped	40,372	10,044	50,416
Total	3,709,054	225,480	3,934,534

Note: P.L. 94-142 figures include handicapped children and youth served by public schools. P.L. 89-313 figures include persons served by residential and other state-supported schools.

icapped children and youth receiving special education and related services under federal laws during the 1978-1979 school year (Table 1-2).

It is extremely difficult to give a precise number of persons with disabling conditions, partly because the severity of impairment varies considerably within each condition and partly because many persons fall into more than one category. Different government or voluntary agencies tend to come up with widely varying statistics; for example, the number of persons with some type of cardiovascular or blood vessel disease has been reported to be as high as 25 million, in contrast to the figure of 7.6 million cited in Table 1-1. In addition, although it was reported that 2.1 million persons were institutionalized in a given year, the Statistical Abstracts of the United States indicate that there are over 5 million admissions to mental hospitals or outpatient psychiatric clinics in a given year, along with several hundred thousand persons cared for annually in institutions for the mentally retarded or other related health facilities.

In some categories of disability, only a percentage of the population is in need of specially designed recreation services; in others, all the individuals suffering from a particular disability are limited to the degree that they cannot function independently.

In addition to the figures cited, there are other major population categories that include persons who have serious impairments and might require specially planned and guided recreation programs. These include those suffering from alcoholism (estimated at 10 million), drug abusers (1.5 million) and individuals in correctional or penal institutions. In many cases, individuals suffer from multiple disabilities. For example, in a high percentage of cases in which there is a serious physical dis-

---

[20]Sherrill, *op. cit.*, p. 31.

ability, the individual may have severe psychological problems stemming from or related to the other disability.

Although a relatively high proportion of those with acute mental illness or social disability are institutionalized, many such persons live in the community. Similarly, the majority of persons with physical disabilities or mental retardation are not institutionalized, as later chapters will show. It should be noted that although this chapter has given figures only for disabled persons in the United States, the statistics would be roughly comparable in Canada, in proportion to its smaller population.

Summing up, although there are varied estimates of the total number of disabled persons, as well as differences in the extent to which such persons may require specialized services, the figures are obviously extremely high. If one were to include also those who fall into the category of being special populations because they are severely socioeconomically disadvantaged, or because they are confined in correctional institutions, the numbers would become even more imposing.

For all such individuals, leisure becomes a critically important area of self-enrichment. The need for creative and enjoyable recreational outlets tends to be far greater among the disabled than among the nondisabled because their other areas of life experience are often so limited. But at the same time their leisure opportunities tend to be constricted and barren for many reasons.

ACTIVITIES IN THERAPEUTIC RECREATION SERVICE

The most obvious service provided by therapeutic recreation specialists in institutional and community settings is planning, organizing and carrying out a well-rounded program of recreational activities. Normally, these might include such program elements as the following:

Social activities: parties, cards, discussion groups, bingo, clubs and informal game room or lounge programs.

Sports and active games: dual sports, such as golf, tennis, badminton, bowling, shuffleboard and horseshoes; team sports, such as basketball, volleyball and softball; and individual activities, such as skating, swimming and archery.

Entertainment: professional entertainment or programs presented by community theater groups, bands, orchestras or dance clubs; watching television, listening to radio and listening to records; films; and patient talent shows.

Hobbies: various types of collections, such as stamps, coins or matchbooks; creative writing; ham radio; construction activities; bird-watching; and cooking.

Arts and crafts: drawing, painting and sculpture; ceramics, leathercraft, weaving, print-making, jewelry work and macramé.

Performing arts: dramatics, instrumental music (learning to play instruments or taking part in bands or orchestras), choral music, ballet and modern dance.

Service activities: in a large hospital, being on the staff of a hospital radio station or newspaper or assisting with the recreation program.

Outdoor recreation: swimming and other water sports, picnicking, camping, nature study and group travel.

Motor activities: gymnastics, stunts and tumbling and other motor learning activities, particularly of a developmental nature, especially for the retarded or those with perceptual motor problems.

Special events: barbecues, carnivals, holiday celebrations, scavenger hunts, treasure hunts or progressive contests.

In all settings, such activities may be approached purely as diversions which provide pleasure and self-enrichment. They may also be presented as part of a deliberate plan to achieve therapeutic objectives for patients or clients—physical recovery and restoration of function, effective social participation or other areas of behavioral or emotional need.

Other Therapeutic Modalities

Therapeutic recreation specialists also may be called upon to provide or assist in the leadership of other forms of activity therapy.

Typically, *A.D.L.* (activities of daily living) has become an important part of many treatment programs. Patients or clients may become involved in shopping, cooking their own meals, home maintenance or planning trips that help prepare them for the demands of independent living.

In nursing homes, where there may be many disoriented older patients, therapeutic recreation specialists are likely to be called upon to provide programs in *sensory training, remotivation* and *reality orientation.* In working with disturbed or dependent youth, alcoholics or drug abusers, *behavior modification* or *reality therapy* techniques may become an integral part of the activity program.

In other treatment settings, therapeutic recreation specialists may be expected to assist with *health* or *vocational counseling,* or to conduct *group therapy* meetings. Often, they may help lead sessions concerned with *dance therapy, art therapy* or similar activities.

Thus far, this chapter has provided an overview of current practices, settings, concepts and professional roles in therapeutic recreation service. For a fuller picture of the field, it is helpful to review its historical background and more recent developments.

HISTORY OF THERAPEUTIC RECREATION SERVICE

No major comprehensive analysis of the history of therapeutic recreation service has yet been written, although there have been many references to the use of varied forms of activity therapy in medical and nursing literature. Undoubtedly prehistoric man discovered for himself certain crude forms of treatment for his ills.

Krusen writes that at some time prior to the Paleolithic Age, probably before the year 7000 B.C.,

---

... the first primitive man who crawled into the sunshine to receive benefit of its warmth and vitalizing effect unwittingly started the practice of heliotherapy; the first man who bathed a wound in some woodland stream unknowingly instituted the practice of hydrotherapy; and the first man who rubbed a bruised muscle unconsciously introduced massage.[21]

In most primitive societies, the approach to the treatment of illness was based on magical belief in the supernatural. Prehistoric man believed that everything in nature was alive with invisible forces and possessed supernatural powers. Disease was caused by evil spirits that entered the body; many techniques were used to drive out these demons. Primitive man often sacrificed animals or human victims to heal the ill. He wore amulets to guard against evil spirits, and medicine men or witch doctors carried out detailed rituals intended to cure victims of disease.

Often, art, music, dancing and chanting were used in this healing process. Among the American Indian tribes of the Southwest, medicine men conducted an elaborate ceremony that went on for days in a special medicine hut. They chanted, used herbs and incense, and made sand paintings with colored sand and crushed minerals—all as part of a highly secret process intended to cure the diseased.

In a sense, such elaborate rituals carried on by primitive and prehistoric man represented an early form of therapeutic recreation service. They demonstrate a fundamental truth—that many forms of illness are psychosomatic rather than organic—and that many forms of treatment that have no medical base can be highly effective.

Therapeutic Recreation in Pre-Christian Societies

History has recorded a number of references to the early use of therapeutic recreation in ancient societies. For example, in ancient China varied forms of medical gymnastics and massage were used as far back as 3000 B.C. These included free exercises that were combined with breathing, sitting, kneeling, lying and standing positions. They were based on the view that bodily inactivity led to disease and were intended to prolong human life. The Chinese healing arts often included such magical practices as making sacrificial offerings and frightening evil spirits by beating gongs and shooting off firecrackers. Avedon states that an ancient Chinese surgeon is reported to have used recreational activities for a variety of purposes. "In one instance he operated on a poisoned arrow wound in the arm of General Kuan Kung, while encouraging the General to use the unaffected hand in a table game."[22]

---

[21]Frank H. Krusen: *Physical Medicine.* Philadelphia, W. B. Saunders Co., 1941, p. 9.
[22]K. C. Wong, et al.: *History of Chinese Medicine.* Tientsin, China, Tientsin Press, 1932, p. 37.

As early as 2000 B.C., Egyptian temples were established to treat the mentally ill by providing games and other pastimes. Priests were said to have been aware that healing was promoted by the beauty of the temple and its surrounding gardens and the songs and dances of temple maidens. One source reports that

Patients . . . were required to walk in the beautiful gardens which surrounded the temples, or to row on the majestic Nile. . . . Dances, concerts, and comic representations were planned for them. . . .[23]

Similarly, in the Indian province of Kashmir during the second century B.C., a physician named Charaka is said to have advocated the use of toys and games to divert patients and promote their recovery. Dock and Stewart describe Indian "professional musicians and storytellers who cheered and diverted patients by singing and by reciting poetry."[24]

In ancient Greece, the use of recreation became a more highly recognized technique in the treatment of the ill. The Greeks named their health temples asclepions, after the highly revered god of healing, Asklepios. One of these temples was at Epidaurus and was similar to a fashionable modern health resort. The temple was an architectural masterpiece built on a high hill with an outstanding view. Under medical supervision, patients enjoyed scenic walks and exercise and massage in a gymnasium, diet, bathing in mineral waters, an outdoor theater and an extended program of treatment similar to that in a modern spa.

Hippocrates, known as "the father of medicine" in ancient Greece, was said to have written a number of treatises on the use of exercise to prevent disability and obesity, and other Greek writers, such as Aristotle and Plato, stressed the importance of exercise in maintaining sound health.

The Romans developed an elaborate system of therapeutic exercise under the leadership of the pioneer physician Galen, who lived in the second century A.D. He developed and classified exercises that improved muscle tone, such as digging, diving, carrying weights and rope-climbing, as well as others involving sparring, punching, tumbling, ball play and other movements. The Roman baths represented a remarkable advance in treatment approaches. The Baths of Caracalla in ancient Rome were tremendously expensive:

. . . covering acres of land, they accommodated thousands of persons in the most grandiose manner. The spacious interior had high arched ceilings and was beautifully ornamented with marble and exquisite inlaid mosaics. There were auditoria, gymnasia, reading rooms, patios with cool foundations, soft music, and swimming pools to delight the patrons and provide diversional therapy.[25]

[23]W. A. F. Browne: *What Asylums Were, Are, and Ought to Be.* Edinburgh, A. and C. Black, 1837, pp. 141–142.
[24]Lavinia L. Dock and Isabel M. Stewart: *A Short History of Nursing.* New York, G. P. Putnam and Sons, 1938, p. 26.
[25]Josephine A. Dolan: *The History of Nursing.* Philadelphia, W. B. Saunders Co., 1969, p. 59.

Therapeutic Recreation in the Middle Ages

Following the fall of the Roman Empire, the treatment of the mentally ill, mentally retarded, crippled or other disabled persons tended to be extremely cruel and punitive.

It was thought that persons who suffered from such disabilities had been cursed by the gods. The mentally ill in particular tended to be treated like animals, chained and manacled, beaten and tortured to drive out their madness or subjected to such devices as revolving beds or whirling cages to calm them.

In England, a typical example of institutional care for the mentally ill was found in Bedlam (the name is derived from Bethlem and was the popular name for the Hospital of St. Mary of Bethlehem in Lambeth, England), built originally as a priory and used to house the insane as early as 1402. As its name has come to suggest, it was a place of uproar and confusion, as well as cruel treatment. As late as 1815, the "lunatics" were placed on view before the public; the revenue from exhibiting the inmates on Sunday for one penny per visitor netted hundreds of pounds a year. Erikson writes,

Like strange animals the mad . . . entertained, performing dance and acrobatics . . . in the popular mind, (they) were creatures apart. They lived outside of the human social order, and thus belonged truly to nature. A madhouse was like a zoo, and the antics of the inmates afforded the public a bizarre diversion.[26]

Most institutions during the Middle Ages and well into the Renaissance period served chiefly to confine the seriously ill or disabled and did little to uplift the spirits of patients. In a few hospitals, such as St. Catherine of Siena or St. John's Hospital in Bruges, beautiful frescoes or paintings were displayed to provide diversion and improve the morale of the plague sufferers or lepers who were receiving care. However, well into the eighteenth century, most hospitals were dark, dismal and lacking in rehabilitative services.

In terms of physical care, there was general disapproval of games and sports during the early Middle Ages; however, beginning in the fourteenth century, there was a renewed interest in the early Greek and Roman cultures, including their sports and exercises. In 1569, Mercurialis wrote the first modern text on therapeutic exercise, *De Arte Gymnastica*, outlining principles for the use of gymnastics from a medical perspective. A number of other authorities, including Hoffman, Tissot and Ling, over the next three centuries promoted forms of adapted sports, gymnastics, massage and therapeutic exercise, contributing ultimately to the development of both occupational therapy and physical therapy.

---

[26]Joan M. Erikson: *Activity, Recovery and Growth: The Communal Role of Planned Activities.* New York, W. W. Norton, 1976, p. 20.

Therapeutic Recreation in the Eighteenth and Nineteenth Centuries

Early in this period, most hospitals provided little real care; often they were little more than prisons. Dolan describes Newgate Prison of East Granby, Connecticut; this institution, with a pathetic history of torture, was the first colonial prison in Connecticut:

Prisoners were not segregated according to sex, type of crime or mental condition; the mentally ill and mentally retarded shared quarters with the most vicious criminal. Screams were heard for quite a distance from the dungeons to which all inmates had to descend every night.[27]

In general, there was little concern for the poor, ill or disabled. However, in a number of hospitals which served the mentally ill, medical pioneers began to introduce new and innovative services. Dr. Benjamin Rush, a leading American physician who was on the staff of the Pennsylvania Hospital in Philadelphia in the 1780's, and who was shocked by the lack of care there for the "lunatics," fought for better hospital conditions. Dolan writes,

---

. . . he called attention to the need for diversional therapy for psychiatric patients; for suitable companions to listen sympathetically to patients . . . for a plan for recreation and amusement; for personnel to direct these activities; and, lastly, to separate the mentally ill from those who were convalescing. . . .[28]

By the early 1800's, therapeutic recreation had been introduced in a number of hospitals—particularly those serving psychiatric patients. In a description of the York Retreat, an English mental hospital in 1819, physicians were urged to involve patients in "regular employment" and "bodily exercise," and to interest them in activities that would confront them with reality and involve their emotions:

. . . every effort should be made to divert the mind of melancholiacs by bodily exercise, walks, conversations, reading, and other recreations. Those who manage the insane should sedulously endeavor to gain their confidence and esteem, to arrest their attention and fix it on objects opposed to their delusions. . . .[29]

---

[27]Dolan, op. cit., p. 176.
[28]Ibid., p. 159.
[29]"Description of the York Retreat, 1819." Taken from Biennial Report for 1950–52, Calfornia State Department of Mental Hygiene.

A major step was taken in the 1830's and 1840's, when so-called insane asylums were established. In general, there had been little public concern for the poor, ill or disabled in society before this time. Erikson points out that the homeless were sheltered, whenever possible, in a neighboring household, and that "almshouses" were founded only as a last resort to serve orphans and destitute, blind, crippled or otherwise helpless children and adults.[30] Gradually, however, the new idea of providing safe and humane care for society's dependents and deviants came into being. For the first time, asylums provided a place of stability and safety where the mentally ill could find refuge as well as a regular daily routine and physical care.

In these institutions, which were generally isolated from the community, mentally ill patients were also segregated from criminals, paupers and those with other forms of illness. For the first time, insanity was regarded as a form of illness rather than a divine curse or a crime, and medical practitioners sought to treat it rationally. The conviction grew that occupations of various kinds would be helpful in overcoming mental illness and restoring rational functioning. In many hospitals in America and abroad, such activities as checkers, chess, backgammon, bowling, swinging, gardening, reading and writing were provided. Mental patients were permitted to dance, to play or listen to music, to take part in outdoor sports and to use "airing courts," rocking horses and a variety of other equipment.

One of the best examples of therapeutic recreation in a psychiatric setting was found in the Brattleboro, Vermont, Retreat, founded in 1836 as the Vermont Asylum for the Insane. An early description of this hospital made clear that "due provision has been made for the exercise, amusement, and employment of the patients." In addition to gardening and farming, there were many pastimes:

Battle-door, chess, draughts, and the like amusements will be afforded. The females will be employed in knitting, needlework, painting, etc. Carriages will be provided for the daily riding of the patients in suitable weather, and they will also take daily walks with nurses and attendants. A small and select library . . . and several periodicals will be furnished for the purpose. . . .[31]

In addition to mental hospitals, other forms of treatment or custodial institutions gradually came into being in the United States during this period. Institutions were provided for the deaf in 1817, the blind in 1832, the mentally retarded in 1850, the crippled in 1867 and the epileptic in 1890. In addition, many destitute, widowed, orphaned and sometimes crippled, blind or retarded individuals continued to be sheltered in poorhouses, or county farms; some such facilities exist even today.

In many of these institutions, diversional activities began to be provided. Particularly in mental hospitals, exercise was recommended for general health, occupational activities provided a regular daily routine and sense of accomplishment and the specific diagnosis of the patient's illness and therapeutic needs was used as

---

[30]Erikson, *op. cit.*, p. 8.
[31]Ardis Stevens: "Recreation in Community Mental Health." *Therapeutic Recreation Journal*, First Quarter, 1971, p. 14.

the basis for planning recreational activities. As medical services improved for wounded servicemen in military hospitals, a strong impetus was given to recreation by the great nursing pioneer, Florence Nightingale. In her 1873 text on nursing, she urged nurses to pay attention not only to the patient's body but also to his mind and morale. She urged that music and conversation be encouraged, that beautiful objects be placed in patient wards, that the family be encouraged to visit and that patients keep small pets. Florence Nightingale was the first to introduce innovations such as furnished classrooms and instruction for soldiers, reading rooms, day rooms and recreation huts that have become an accepted part of military life. Under her leadership, so-called bedside occupations were introduced in military hospitals to cheer up injured soldiers.

Gradually, new forms of occupational and physical therapy were refined. In mental hospitals, there was less reliance on custodial seclusion, physical restraints and sedatives and a growing understanding that patients should be occupied—both with practical work-connected tasks and with physical, mental and social activities that contributed to their recovery. By the early 1900's, a rationale had been well established for activity therapy programs, and many hospitals were making use of them, although they were not recognized as areas of special professional expertise until the 1920's.

Erikson points out that it was not until 1908, at the Chicago School of Civics and Philanthropy, that the first courses were offered in such activities as handicrafts, exercise and play techniques for nurses and attendants who worked specifically with mental patients. Before this, the little training that was offered in the leadership of "occupations" made no distinctions among patients:

Any and all occupational work was presumed to be therapeutically applicable to a range of illnesses, whether mental or physical. By 1911, however, mental hospitals were beginning to offer occupational training to nurses who planned to work specifically with mental patients.[32]

Increasingly, there was an awareness of the therapeutic value of activity—that is, occupations *other than work*. While America had always been strongly committed to the Protestant work ethic, with little respect for play and recreation, at the end of the nineteenth and the beginning of the twentieth centuries there was an increasing concern about the growing amounts of leisure available to all classes in society. Educators and psychologists explored the value of play in child development and of recreation as a restorative for adult workers. The playground movement swept the country, and settlement houses and voluntary agencies like the YMCA, YWCA and Boy and Girl Scouts began to provide comprehensive recreation programs for children and youth.

Without question, this changing attitude toward play and leisure helped to make recreation in treatment centers acceptable *as* recreation, and not solely as a form of unpaid work. Before long, recreation was to be seen as a significant aspect

---

[32]Erikson, *op. cit.*, p. 18.

of hospital and institutional care for several categories of ill and disabled individuals.

The United States in the Twentieth Century

Soon after the entrance of the United States into World War I, the Red Cross began to provide recreation programs in hospital wards and convalescent homes. Recreation leaders were employed in a growing number of military and veterans' hospitals during the 1920's. It became more widely recognized that recreation—among other innovative rehabilitative techniques—was of value in reducing the length of the patient's stay in the hospital and the extent and duration of his disability.

Gradually, federal laws, such as the Federal Vocational Rehabilitation Act of 1920, the Social Security Act of 1936 and the Barden-La Follette Act of 1942, provided for improved rehabilitation services for both children and adults in the United States.

Typically, during the 1920's public school systems began to offer special classes for disabled children and special transportation. By 1929, there were a number of special public schools for the blind. During the 1920's and 1930's, the custodial approach to caring for disabled children in institutions shifted to a stronger emphasis on reeducating and reintegrating them into community life.

Various forms of rehabilitative services came into being. More and more, recreation emerged as one of these services. As an example, at the Lincoln State School Colony in Illinois a recreation department was established in June 1929, in order to " . . . conduct a program of activities, consistent with the interests and abilities of mentally handicapped children . . . to serve as a substitute for former repressive measures of control." More and more state and private institutions began to develop extensive recreation programs.

A number of national organizations took the lead in developing such services. For example, the Association for the Aid of Crippled Children began as early as 1900 to provide services for disabled children in their homes, in schools and in hospitals. It operated camps and summer programs for the disabled and brought occupational therapy and similar therapies into the homes of crippled children as a demonstration service and a means of parental education.

The growing recognition of the need for recreation for the disabled was demonstrated in the so-called Bill of Rights for the Handicapped that was drawn up at the White House Conference on Child Health and Protection in 1932. This statement called for

> . . . a life on which his handicap casts no shadow, but which is full day by day with those things which make it worth while, with comradeship, love, work, play, laughter and tears — a life in which those things bring continually increasing growth, richness, a release of energies and joy of achievement.[33]

---

[33]*The Handicapped Child, Report of the White House Conference on Child Health and Protection.* New York, D. Appleton-Century, 1933, p. 3.

During this period, public concern about the disabled continued to grow steadily. Programs of rehabilitation were greatly strengthened through federal Social Security legislation along with workmen's compensation acts, public assistance laws and other government efforts to support health care on the local level. O'Morrow points out that recreation became an increasingly important part of this overall trend, particularly in military hospitals:

> During the 1920's and 1930's, individuals with varied backgrounds and representing various disciplines directed programs in hospitals, institutions, and special centers and schools. World War II found Red Cross personnel and volunteers providing recreation services. Also, military personnel with an education or interest in physical education or recreation were assigned to hospitals and reconditioning units.[34]

It was in 1938 that the term "therapeutic recreation" was first utilized by the federal Works Progress Administration. The term included all activities, regardless of type, which were intended to serve "disabled, maladjusted, or other institutionalized persons."

During World War II, there was a marked acceleration in the hospital recreation movement. Red Cross recreation personnel increased to a total of 1809 by the end of the war. Later, recreation became a permanent part of peacetime Red Cross services to the armed forces. In 1945, the Veterans' Administration founded a Hospital Social Service Division, including Recreation Service along with Canteen, Library, Chaplaincy and Voluntary Services; recreation personnel were assigned to all hospitals.

Therapeutic activities were refined in many long-term rehabilitation centers and convalescent programs, with adapted sports and modified games for amputees, paraplegics and those with other major disabilities. Adams, Daniel and Rullman point out that in the United States and other countries that had suffered major casualties in World War II, there was a new determination to give veterans with service-connected disabilities the opportunity for full physical, social and economic rehabilitation. In a review of the development of wheelchair sports, they write,

> As part of the vast rehabilitation program, sports were suddenly seen by some as an important aid to rehabilitating the disabled veterans. The program of wheelchair sports began at various Veterans Administration Hospitals throughout the United States. . . . More and more disabled men joined into the new wheelchair sport until finally several complete teams were officially organized. Thus basketball became the first organized wheelchair sport in history. . . . As the interest in the sport grew, the range of disabilities of the participants also increased. Added to the list of war-injured were those paraplegic because of polio, amputees, and other orthopedically disabled individuals.[35]

The National Wheelchair Basketball Association (NWBA), founded in 1949, and later the National Wheelchair Athletic Association (NWAA) encouraged thousands

---

[34]O'Morrow, *op. cit.*, p. 102.
[35]Ronald C. Adams, Alfred N. Daniel and Lee Rullman: *Games, Sports and Exercises for the Physically Handicapped.* Philadelphia, Lea and Febiger, 1972, p. 18.

of physically disabled individuals of both sexes to enjoy sports. The Special Olympics program, established by the Joseph P. Kennedy, Jr. Foundation in 1968, provided year-round training and competition for the mentally retarded in various sports, along with seasonal competition at local, district, state and higher levels.

New organizations or sections of existing organizations were also formed to promote recreation for the ill and disabled. Each of these focused primarily on program needs within medical settings; they included the Hospital Recreation Section of the American Recreation Society (1948); the National Association of Recreation Therapists (1953); and the Recreational Therapy Section of the American Association for Health, Physical Education and Recreation (1952). These are discussed more fully in Chapter 3.

A number of major federal agencies, chiefly within the former Department of Health, Education and Welfare, initiated programs to provide enriched vocational, educational and recreational opportunities for children, youth and adults of all types—the mentally retarded, the physically disabled, the mentally ill, drug abusers, the aged and others. With funding under major federal laws passed during the 1950's through the 1970's, assistance was given to professional training, research and direct community services in therapeutic recreation. In general, such aid has not been directed to supporting on-going programs but rather to short-term demonstration or special project grants designed to encourage stronger local efforts. However, particularly in the field of mental retardation and aging, substantial on-going assistance has been given to direct program service. Medicare, for example, has reimbursed thousands of expanded programs of activity therapy programs in nursing homes and related health care facilities.

After World War II, therapeutic recreation service was increasingly recognized throughout the United States and Canada as an important rehabilitative discipline.

Growth of Organized Therapeutic Recreation Programs

Although there has been no comprehensive survey of all forms of institutions or agencies providing therapeutic recreation service, there are several surveys that give a general picture of growth in this field during the past three decades.

1959 REPORT ON RECREATION IN HOSPITALS

At the request of the Council for the Advancement of Hospital Recreation, the National Recreation Association sponsored a national study of hospital recreation. This study gave a picture of the types of hospitals which provided recreation service, the personnel employed, the activities offered and similar information.[36]

---

[36]John E. Silson, Elliott M. Cohen and Beatrice H. Hill: *Recreation in Hospitals: Report of a Study of Organized Recreation Programs in Hospitals and the Personnel Conducting Them.* New York, National Recreation Association, 1959, pp. 22–23.

Overall, it found that 42.4 percent of the 3507 hospitals that responded to the survey had organized recreation programs. Larger hospitals tended to have organized programs, while smaller ones did not; similarly, chronic-disease or long-term institutions tended to provide recreation, whereas acute-treatment, short-term hospitals did not. Many hospitals had swimming pools, gymnasiums, auditoriums, special recreation rooms or even athletic fields; wards, solariums and day rooms were also used frequently for recreation. The most popular activities were passive or mental activities, such as reading, radio-listening, television-watching and movie-viewing, although arts and crafts, social and musical activities and games and sports were also popular.

SURVEY OF COMMUNITY RECREATION SPONSORSHIP

A number of other studies were carried out during the 1960's and 1970's to determine the extent to which recreation was provided to special populations, both in institutions and in communities at large. In 1964, the National Recreation Association and the National Association for Retarded Children assisted Marson in carrying out a survey of 2000 community recreation departments to determine what community services were being provided for the mentally or physically disabled.[37] The 427 responding agencies indicated that they provided either recreation facilities or programs for the disabled.

Of 202 departments that responded to a follow-up survey requesting fuller information, 139 recreation directors reported that the mentally retarded were served separately in such facilities as playgrounds, community recreation centers, parks, swimming pools and day camps. In 164 cases, the physically handicapped were served separately in similar facilities. Only about one third of the responding communities provided transportation assistance to disabled participants. Many special programs were supported by fees or contributions from parents or interested community groups rather than by public funds.

NATIONAL SURVEY OF SENIOR CENTERS

In 1969, the Institute for Interdisciplinary Studies of the American Rehabilitation Foundation published the report of a national study of senior centers.[38] This survey was funded by the Administration on Aging of the U.S. Department of Health, Education and Welfare. Anderson reported findings from 1002 senior centers on such topics as the clientele served, types of programs and other services, budgets, facilities, staffing and relations with other community social or health agencies.

---

[37]Ruth Marson: In Morton Thompson: "The Status of Recreation for the Handicapped, as Related to Community and Voluntary Agencies." *Therapeutic Recreation Journal*, Vol. III, No. 9, 1969, pp. 20–23.
[38]Nancy N. Anderson: *Senior Centers: Information from a National Survey*. Minneapolis, Institute for Interdisciplinary Studies, American Rehabilitation Foundation, 1969.

Anderson found that despite the widespread attention recently given to the need to develop social and recreation programs for older Americans, these programs tended to be quite limited. It was apparent that even if their active memberships averaged as high as 150 to 200 members each, less than 1 per cent of the population in this age group throughout the country was actually served by senior centers. Fewer than half of the centers reported having full-time directors.

RECREATION SERVICE TO DISABLED CHILDREN

In 1971, Berryman, Logan and Lander of the New York University School of Education published a comprehensive report on recreation services for disabled children in a sampling of large metropolitan areas throughout the United States.[39] The findings were based on a three-year study financed by the Children's Bureau of the U.S. Department of Health, Education and Welfare. Of several thousand potential sponsors of recreation services for disabled children and youth, approximately 600 agencies and organizations were intensively studied; 88 per cent provided some form of recreation to disabled children and youth.

RECREATION SERVING SPECIAL POPULATIONS IN MAJOR CITIES

In 1972, the Community Council of Greater New York studied administrative problems and practices in recreation and park departments; 80 cities with populations of 150,000 or more were sampled.[40] Forty-five cities (56.2 per cent) participated in the study. A high proportion of these cities provided one or more forms of recreation service for community residents with physical, mental or social disabilities.

Examples of such programs offered by large cities included day camps for the mentally retarded, busing programs for the physically disabled, a "meals on wheels" program for the homebound, physical development and social activities programs for various disabled groups, after-care programs for discharged mental patients and many similar types of activities.

A similar study, co-sponsored by Temple University and the Heritage Conservation and Recreation Service of the U.S. Department of the Interior, found there had been a marked expansion of such services.[41] Table 1–3 indicates the level of services for several special populations in 1979.

---

[39]Doris L. Berryman, Annette Logan and Dorothy Lander: *Enhancement of Recreation Service to Disabled Children.* New York, New York University School of Education, Report of Children's Bureau Project, 1971.
[40]Richard Kraus: *Urban Parks and Recreation: Challenge of the 1970's.* New York, Community Council of Greater New York, 1972, pp. 28–29, 81–82.
[41]Richard Kraus: *New Directions in Urban Parks and Recreation: A Trends Analysis Report.* Philadelphia, Temple University and Heritage, Conservation and Recreation Service, 1980.

Table 1-3   **Municipal Recreation and Park Departments Reporting Programs for Special Populations in 1979**

Category Served	Percentage of Cities Reporting Programs
Antidelinquency programs	32
Drug addiction programs	19
Youth employment programs	75
Programs for aging persons	90
Programs for homebound persons	16
Programs for physically handicapped	90
Programs for mentally retarded	84
Programs for discharged or nonhospitalized mental patients	13

THERAPEUTIC RECREATION IN CANADA

In 1974, Peter Witt reported on a study he had made of federal, provincial, local government and voluntary agency services for the disabled throughout Canada. With the assistance of a grant from Recreation Canada, part of the federal Department of National Health and Welfare, he examined in particular intergovernmental and interagency relationships and programs. In general, he found that support for therapeutic recreation service had grown. The federal government, for example, had begun to spend millions of dollars through "local initiatives" programs to stimulate local services for the disabled. Provinces like Ontario and Alberta had employed full-time provincial consultants to promote and help coordinate recreation for special populations on the local level. On the national level, major voluntary health organizations, like the Canadian Association for the Mentally Retarded, the Canadian Rehabilitation Council for the Disabled and the Canadian Mental Health Association, had taken positive steps to promote fuller recreation services for the disabled throughout the nation.

However, in a detailed examination of special programs for the disabled on the municipal level (cities, towns, boroughs or other government authorities), Witt found that the picture was less favorable. Questionnaires were sent to 2382 local government agencies; 663 (28 per cent) replied. Witt summarized his findings:

A total of 145 out of 663 communities (21.9 per cent) indicated that they offered, co-sponsored, or provided facilities or money to serve one or more of six specific disability groups mentioned in the survey: the blind, the deaf, the mentally retarded, the physically handicapped, individuals with learning disabilities, and individuals with psychiatric problems.[42]

---

[42]Peter A. Witt: *Status of Recreation Services for the Handicapped.* University of Ottawa and Recreation Canada, Department of National Health and Welfare, 1974, p. 65.

In another survey of institutions serving groups with similar types of disability, Witt found a somewhat more positive picture. Of 422 responding institutions, 235 (55 per cent) reported offering recreation services; 189 (45 per cent) reported that they did not. Finally, in a survey of voluntary community agencies throughout Canada, it was found that 102 of 196 responding agencies (52 per cent) provided some form of recreation service for the disabled. Witt came to the conclusion that there was a wide range of concern on all levels that needed to be transferred into more effective action and made a number of recommendations for improved coordination, communication and training to strengthen therapeutic recreation service in Canada.

THE CURRENT STATUS OF RECREATION SERVICE FOR SPECIAL POPULATIONS

Based on the available evidence, it is apparent that although there has been a considerable growth in the provision of therapeutic recreation service in both the United States and Canada, programs need to be much more fully developed if they are to meet total community needs.

At the end of the 1970's, John Nesbitt estimated that the percentage of the nation's disabled population receiving special recreation services had risen from about 3 to 5 per cent during the previous decade to about 10 per cent. There were, he wrote,

---

... hundreds of recreation programs and services pioneered by recreation and park departments at the local and federal levels, by voluntary health agencies that provided summer camping as well as year-round recreation services, by youth-serving agencies such as the Boy Scouts of America and the YMCA, by advocate organizations such as Special Olympics, and consumer groups such as the wheelchair athletic associations.[43]

Nesbitt predicted the 1980's would see dramatic growth in recreation services for the disabled, based on new developments in consumerism, civil rights, advocacy, public attitudes and federal support. Today, he pointed out, recreation administrators, museum executives and park directors no longer respond negatively to requests for service for the handicapped; they are eager to serve special populations. This shift, Nesbitt concluded, is due in part to growing humanism and public acceptance of the disabled and in part to court decisions, consumer demand, advocacy and supporting legislation.

---

[43]John A. Nesbitt: "The 1980's: Recreation a Reality for All." In *Education Unlimited*. Boothwyn, Pennsylvania, Educational Resources Center, June 1979, p. 2.

Attitudes of Community Recreation Professionals

Further growth is partly dependent on the extent to which therapeutic recreation specialists and community recreation and park administrators cooperate with each other. For example, in 1969 Richard Stracke reported the findings of a survey of 500 community recreation administrators in 40 states.[44] His report showed that only 18 per cent of the administrators had frequently worked or cooperated with therapeutic recreation specialists.

A 1977 follow-up study showed there had been a marked positive shift over the previous eight years in community recreation administrators' views and practices regarding therapeutic recreation. Nolan applied Stracke's questionnaire to a similar sample of community recreation professionals, and found that a significant positive change had occurred in such areas as (a) employment of therapeutic recreation specialists on community agency staffs; (b) increase in the number of handicapped persons from local hospitals, institutions or similar agencies who use community facilities on a group basis; (c) more frequent consultation between community recreation personnel and therapeutic recreation professionals in nearby institutions; (d) decrease in the number of administrators who felt that the recreation needs of the handicapped were markedly different from those of other people; and (e) greater awareness of the need for services for special populations within the community.[45]

PROMOTING THERAPEUTIC RECREATION SERVICE

How can therapeutic recreation service be promoted in both institutional and community settings? The most important step is to develop community support for programs serving the disabled.

Arousing Public Concern

Most people are unaware of the needs of the disabled population until those needs are brought to their attention. Recent budget cuts have resulted in inadequate programs in state institutions for the mentally retarded. After newspapers and television have shown neglected children and adults in filthy, crowded wards, the public's concern has compelled immediate state action to restore needed funds.

---

[44]Richard Stracke: "The Role of the Therapeutic Recreator in Relation to the Community Recreator." *Therapeutic Recreation Journal*, First Quarter, 1969, pp. 26–29.
[45]Kathleen Nolan: "A Comparison of Two Surveys Concerning the Relationship Between the Therapeutic Recreator and the Community Recreator." *Therapeutic Recreation Journal*, First Quarter, 1978, pp. 40–49.

However, such efforts to arouse public concern and support must not be keyed only to crisis situations. There must be a fuller recognition of the needs of the mentally and physically disabled of all ages in all settings. Every effort must be made to help those living in the community to lose their fear or resentment of the disabled and to accept them as human beings. In past centuries, the crippled and deformed or mentally ill were shut up in custodial institutions—away from the public eye or conscience. Today, however, we have accepted the principle of total rehabilitation and involvement in community life for the disabled, whenever possible.

We often fail to live up to this principle by denying full support to programs serving the disabled in our communities. For example, hundreds of thousands of mentally disturbed men and women, who would in the past have been treated in state-supported or other psychiatric institutions, today live in the community. This change is due to the establishment of community mental health centers and the deliberate effort to reduce hospitalization of the mentally ill. Yet it has become increasingly clear that great numbers of these individuals simply exist on the fringes of our lives. Without adequate treatment or care, they live in grim welfare hotels or on drug-maintenance programs. Often, *no* recreation or social programs are provided for such clients, whereas in institutions they would be receiving substantial amounts of rehabilitative service—including activity programming.

Frequently, attempts to establish community-based sheltered living environments for the mentally retarded or psychiatric outpatients are vigorously resisted by neighborhood residents. Thus, there continues to be an important need to improve public attitudes concerning the disabled. The United Nations initiated a major effort in this direction in 1981 during the International Year of Disabled Persons. Over 250 organizations became affiliated with the U.S. Council for the International Year of Disabled Persons, including a number of recreation and sports organizations. Thousands of communities and corporate groups joined together to further long-term national goals in the following areas for individuals with disabling conditions:

. . . expanded educational opportunities, improved access to housing, buildings, and transportation; greater opportunities for employment; broader recreational, social and cultural activities; expanded and strengthened rehabilitation programs and facilities; purposeful application of biomedical research aimed at conquering major disabling conditions . . . and expanded international exchange of information and experience.[46]

Special efforts were made to help the public become aware of innovative programs serving the disabled, or about their unique achievements in sports, outdoor recreation and dance. Later chapters will show the truly amazing physical and mental accomplishments of many severely disabled individuals. Only as the public

---

[46]Julian Stein: "The International Year of Disabled Persons: Meeting the Challenge Through Partnerships." *The Easterner* (Journal of the Eastern District Association of the American Alliance for Health, Physical Education, Recreation and Dance), September 1981, p. 1.

comes to realize the full potential of handicapped individuals of all ages will we begin to shed the prejudices toward the disabled that have for so long limited their development.

Developing More Effective Programs

There is a critical need to develop more effective models of therapeutic recreation service as well as to improve communication with related disciplines, such as medicine, social work and vocational education.

In many cases major professional organizations have developed entirely new programs and services for the disabled. For example, the American Alliance for Health, Physical Education, Recreation and Dance (AAHPERD), which has traditionally been concerned primarily with the needs of children and youth in schools and colleges, has moved vigorously into the field of serving the aged. In 1975, the Older Americans Act was amended to broaden the definition of social service to include "services designed to enable older persons to attain and maintain physical and mental well-being through programs of regular activity and exercise." Since then, the National Association for Human Development, in cooperation with the President's Council on Physical Fitness and Sport, under a grant from the Administration on Aging, has initiated a national program of exercise for people over the age of 60. AAHPERD has made a strong effort to link exercise programs with nutritional services being provided at hundreds of agencies funded by Title VII of the Older Americans Act. In addition, AAHPERD has encouraged research, demonstration programs and conferences in the area of geriatric fitness—an excellent example of organizations moving vigorously into new programs serving special populations. More recently, the Alliance has initiated or encouraged numerous other physical education programs designed for the physically handicapped or mentally retarded.

In many states, new professional relationships have been developed to promote and improve therapeutic recreation services. In some cases, municipal departments in neighboring communities or counties have joined together to co-sponsor programs for the disabled. In other cases, local government has funded voluntary agencies providing model therapeutic recreation programs.

New Emphasis on Accountability

Overall, the trend is to gear recreation programs to meet significant psychosocial, vocational or other rehabilitative needs of patients and clients. The increased emphasis on needs assessments, activity analysis and careful monitoring of outcomes has given many programs a higher level of support by other staff.

Jewell comments that therapeutic recreation programs today can no longer justify their existence in "broad, esoteric philosophical statements that profess attainment of a loosely defined set of goals." Nor can they operate as independent services; instead they must become members of the treatment team in the fullest sense,

... facilitating desirable behavior. Namely, goals, objectives and procedures must be specified for each resident in the form of a treatment plan. In addition, each plan must be evaluated periodically in the form of a treatment plan review.[47]

Closely linked to this shift in emphasis is the growing effort to have therapeutic recreation service in institutions gain fuller recognition as a method of treatment that requires significant fiscal support and that can be reimbursable just as physical therapy and occupational therapy are reimbursable. Harsanyi points out that in the past most therapeutic recreation programs in rehabilitative agencies were not billed directly as separate patient services. Instead, they were calculated into the institution's total budget as a routine service to be covered under the daily fee paid by patients and clients. She writes,

Needless to say, this system puts the provision of therapeutic recreation at the mercy of each institution's administrator or governing body. If they believe therapeutic recreation is important, they will see to it that an adequate percentage will go to support it. If not, they can always find an excuse why there is not enough money in the till for staff and materials for therapeutic recreation.[48]

However, in a growing number of hospitals, therapeutic recreation is being provided as an active treatment service that is charged to third-party payers, such as Medicaid or patients' insurance plans. In order to qualify for third-party payment, therapeutic recreation must be carefully planned, executed and documented, and (a) be provided under an individualized diagnostic plan; (b) be expected to improve the patient's condition or used for diagnosis; and (c) be supervised and evaluated by a physician. Ingber and West have described a number of the important conditions affecting such programs (see pp. 154–155).

IMPROVING THE LEVEL OF
PROFESSIONAL PRACTICE

There is an important need to develop more professionally qualified practitioners in the field of therapeutic recreation service.

Higher Education Curricula

Many colleges and universities throughout the United States and Canada today offer majors in therapeutic recreation service. However, the content of such pro-

---

[47]David L. Jewell: "Documentation: Shibboleth for Professionalism." *Therapeutic Recreation Journal*, First Quarter, 1980, p. 23.
[48]Suzanne Harsanyi: "Practice and Promise of Therapeutic Recreation." *Journal of Physical Education and Recreation*, April 1979, p. 52.

grams varies widely, as do faculty qualifications, the opportunities for meaningful clinical experiences and field placements and the standards of training. The National Council on Accreditation and the National Therapeutic Recreation Society have been active in formulating needed guidelines for upgrading curricula in this field, and recently issued a revised set of standards for baccalaureate programs in therapeutic recreation service. However, as Chapter 3 points out, only a limited number of college and university departments have sought to meet accreditation standards; there is a strong need to strengthen the programs of many others.

Employment Standards in Therapeutic Recreation

Two closely related problems are the need to upgrade Civil Service or other employment requirements in this field and to eliminate unqualified personnel from professional-level recreation positions. The National Therapeutic Recreation Society's (NTRS) national registration plan has helped to solve the problem by approving several thousand qualified practitioners. Recently, the NTRS registration plan has become linked to the national accreditation process. States are beginning to require new applicants for registration to have degrees from accredited colleges and universities. Although controversial and not yet widely accepted, this degree requirement is a strong push toward upgrading the qualifications of those entering the therapeutic recreation field.

Continuing education represents another means of strengthening the performance of practitioners working with special populations. In some cases, continuing education may be provided by professional societies or colleges and universities. In others, it may be part of community-based training programs designed for the local staff.

STRENGTHENING WORKING RELATIONSHIPS BETWEEN COMMUNITY PERSONNEL AND THERAPEUTIC RECREATION SPECIALISTS

In the past, when almost all therapeutic recreation service was carried on in hospitals or other residential institutions, the need to improve the relationship between community recreation personnel and therapeutic recreation specialists was not as acute as it is today. However, with the trend toward providing a variety of rehabilitation services within communities themselves, the relationship has become more crucial. As legislation and public awareness continue to spotlight the needs of the great majority of disabled individuals who live within the community rather than in institutions, interagency cooperation in the community will become increasingly critical.

Throughout the United States and Canada, most state or provincial recreation and park societies have branches concerned with therapeutic recreation service. At present, many municipal, county and township recreation and park agencies not only provide services for the disabled, or cooperate with other organizations that do, but also employ qualified therapeutic recreation specialists to head their own programs. Similarly, community recreation professionals in voluntary agencies, such as the YMCA, the YWCA, the YM-YWHA, the Boys Clubs and Girls Clubs, the Boy Scouts and Girl Scouts and hundreds of similar organizations, have accepted a fuller responsibility for working with the disabled.

Increasingly, *community-based* personnel will be expected to have a solid understanding of therapeutic practice, and *therapeutic* personnel to be more and more knowledgeable about community needs.

EXPANDING GOVERNMENT SUPPORT OF THERAPEUTIC RECREATION SERVICE

Inevitably, it is more difficult and expensive to serve the disabled child, youth or adult than it is to serve nondisabled persons. Specially trained staff members, modified facilities and special transportation arrangements mean that the cost of providing therapeutic recreation is high. Although many voluntary community organizations, service clubs, private donors and foundations have contributed to the financial support of community-based recreation programs, this is often not enough.

Both the federal and state governments have contributed significantly to local therapeutic recreation programs in the United States. Typically, states have established demonstration programs, formed task forces to examine the need and develop state-wide recommendations, supported research and provided financial aid to meet the needs of disabled persons.

In Canada, similar needs exist, and provincial governments have been active in assisting local municipal and voluntary agencies in upgrading therapeutic recreation services. In 1975, a study of therapeutic recreation in the Province of Alberta identified the following ways in which agencies thought that the provincial or national government could be helpful to them:

Provide lists and access to written materials on recreation in the agency setting

Sponsor leadership training seminars or workshops

Help develop University or Community College curricula

Aid in the provision of transportation services

Sponsor research or demonstration projects

Provide money for provision of facilities specifically for the disabled or for adapting existing facilities or to support special programs or provide needed equipment[49]

---

[49]*Report on the Survey of Recreation Services for the Disabled in Alberta, op. cit.,* p. 46.

The federal government in the United States has been particularly active in funding therapeutic recreation service for the mentally retarded, the physically handicapped and, more recently, aged persons. Federal legislation has included numerous specific programs of financial support for recreation programs serving the retarded. The Division of Educational Services of the Bureau of Education for the Handicapped of the United States Office of Education provided substantial assistance to state-related schools to enhance services to the disabled. The Division of Mental Retardation of the Rehabilitation Services Administration supported numerous recreation programs, including daytime activity centers for mentally retarded adults. The Division of Training Programs of the Bureau of Education for the Handicapped initiated a program, authorized by Public Law 90–170, for the training of physical educators and recreation personnel to work with mentally retarded and other disabled children.

In November 1976, Congress enacted Public Law 94–142, the Education for All Handicapped Children Act, which resulted in dramatically increased services to the disabled, including physical and occupational therapy and recreation, which were identified as important "related services" for the disabled. This law, which came about as a consequence of pressure from parents' organizations and lawsuits seeking to force local educational agencies to provide a free and appropriate education for the disabled, will place much greater pressure on school boards, administrators and teachers to upgrade their services for impaired children and youth. These laws, coupled with changes in the Federal Register establishing "physical education and recreation as an integral part of programs for the education of handicapped children," make it clear that service for the disabled will continue to be sharply expanded in school programs.

Other Examples of Support

Various grants have been given to universities to help fund research on the role of play in the lives of the disabled, demonstration programs, comprehensive state planning for the disabled, information centers on recreation for the disabled and a number of special university programs designed to train adapted physical education and therapeutic recreation personnel (see Chapter 3).

The U.S. Administration on Aging has given substantial support to university departments preparing administrative personnel for multi-service centers, consultants and researchers concerned with gerontology and geriatrics. Each year, substantial sums have been awarded to the states to support a network of senior centers serving aging populations.

In May 1976, the federal Department of Health, Education and Welfare issued guidelines stating that otherwise qualified disabled individuals might not be excluded from participation in any programs or activities receiving federal aid. Such policies were greatly strengthened by Section 504 of the Rehabilitation Act of 1973 (P.L. 93–112). Often called the "Nondiscrimination Clause," Section 504 states,

> . . . No otherwise qualified handicapped individual . . . shall, solely by reason of his handicap, be excluded from participation in, be denied the benefits of, or be subjected to discrimination under any program or activity receiving Federal financial assistance.

Sherrill points out that schools and colleges which conduct interscholastic athletics and extra class activities must provide full opportunities for the disabled to participate in the "least restrictive environments." Similarly, athletic events in public places receiving federal funds must be accessible to all spectators, including those in wheelchairs.[50] Gradually, more and more physical education departments are offering classes, intramurals and club activities for disabled students in a wide range of areas—including traditional physical fitness activities, movement education, rhythms, dance, games, swimming and other sports and outdoor pursuits. Linked to this trend has been the widespread modification of pools, locker rooms, gyms and other facilities to give access to the handicapped. Competitive sports for the disabled have also been developed.[51]

This progress has been paralleled in the recreation and park field, where greater numbers of disabled persons have sought to take part in programs formerly closed to them. Numerous conferences have been held in the United States and Canada to promote the elimination of architectural barriers that prevent the disabled from using recreation and park facilities. Among other government agencies in the United States, the National Park Service has established a Division of Special Programs and Populations. Its primary function is to develop

> . . . a comprehensive and system-wide plan for access to ensure that parks provide, as a matter of routine, full spectrum visitor services. The Division is addressing such issues as: historic site accessibility, wilderness area experiences, expansion of interpretive programs to enable deaf and blind individuals to participate . . . and accessible transportation systems to and within park areas.[52]

STATES AND PROVINCES

Numerous states and provinces have carried out planning studies to determine the recreational needs of disabled persons and to support demonstration projects and ongoing programs to involve them in the full range of leisure activities.

In the late 1970's, for example, the Pennsylvania Department of Welfare's Office of Mental Retardation asked the Pennsylvania Recreation and Park Society to appoint a steering committee to promote recreation for disabled individuals. Based on the steering committee's recommendations, the Office of Mental Retarda-

---

[50]Sherrill, *op. cit.*, p. 33.
[51]Peter M. Aufsesser: "Adapted Physical Education: A Look Ahead, A Look Back." *Journal of Physical Education and Recreation*, June 1981, p. 29.
[52]*Brochure of National Park Service, Division of Special Programs and Populations.* Washington, D.C., U.S. Department of Interior, 1981.

tion wrote manuals and developed pilot community-based programs and personnel-training programs to promote therapeutic recreation throughout the state.

In the province of Alberta, an Advisory Board on Recreation for the Disabled was established to help coordinate various provincial agencies, associations and individuals working within the therapeutic recreation field. With funding from various government sources and the Western Canada Lottery Foundation, this advisory board has provided information on recreation programming for the disabled, evaluated programs, public information and advocacy efforts, and researched and coordinated programs with other national and provincial organizations.

ROLE OF CITIES

In the United States, a national study of urban recreation in the late 1970's revealed that there were major gaps in programming for special populations. The study concluded that while the recreation needs of handicapped individuals were gaining more recognition from park and recreation agencies, wide disparities exist in the quality of recreation services provided:

Few municipal park and park agencies provide adequate, accessible, professionally-staffed therapeutic recreation programs for the handicapped . . . Park and recreation agencies appear to be insufficiently sensitive to the special needs and recreational desires of the handicapped.[53]

Consequently, an increasing number of cities have been making vigorous efforts to expand their services to handicapped residents. In a special report on this function, the International City Management Association points out that while the delivery of special programs and services is not an easy task,

. . . the problem can be circumvented by a strong commitment to handicapped services. Managers can meet the challenge of providing for, and meeting the needs of, handicapped citizens by working with handicapped individuals, parent groups, and service organizations. The local government's role does not necessarily have to be that of initiator of programs but, rather, that of an active supporter of programs by coordinating, advocating and leading the delivery of services for the handicapped.[54]

The trend toward municipal government's taking a fuller responsibility in handicapped services has been reinforced by the transfer of recreation and park

---

[53]*National Urban Recreation Study: Executive Report.* Washington, D.C., Heritage, Conservation and Recreation Service and National Park Service, February 1978, pp. 59–61.
[54]Betty Cheatham: *Cities and the Handicapped.* Washington, D.C., International City Management Association, Spring 1980, pp. 1–4.

functions from separate departments to comprehensive departments of human services. For instance, in Gardena, California, the newly established Human Services Department provides a full range of services for senior citizens, families and youth, as well as manpower and vocational training programs, counseling, well-baby clinics and numerous other health-related functions.[55]

THE MISSION AHEAD

As this chapter has demonstrated, there has been great progress recently in providing recreation programs to meet the needs of special populations in the United States and Canada.

But more progress is needed. Although there are now many outstanding programs, approximately 90 per cent of the disabled who now live in the community do not have access to programs designed to meet their special needs. Those unmet needs pose a critical challenge to those in this field. The challenge is especially great now because of the sharp cutbacks in funding for all social programs that have been imposed during the early 1980's in the United States and, to a lesser degree, in Canada.

Clearly, therapeutic recreation service must have a fuller level of support from the public and from each level of government—local, state or provincial and federal. To gain this support, therapeutic recreation will need a clearer identity. The field must win wider acceptance as an essential form of human experience as well as a useful rehabilitative tool. Such changes will be tied to the development of a stronger system of higher education in therapeutic recreation service, as well as standardized certification and licensing procedures to ensure that those who enter this profession are qualified.

The major professional organization, the National Therapeutic Recreation Society (NTRS), was not established until 1966. In the brief period since then, the Society has made major strides in helping therapeutic recreation to gain recognition as a profession. NTRS has sponsored research and publications, developed models for professional training and established standards and a highly successful voluntary registration plan. As one example of its contribution, NTRS has

---

. . . been active in establishing and . . . promoting standards for recreation programs in various settings. Working with the Joint Commission on Accreditation of Hospitals, the Society hammered out standards for activity services related to children's, adolescent, and adult psychiatric services, mental retardation services, and alcohol and drug abuse services. These serve to further legitimize and control recreation in community and institutional programs.[56]

---

[55]*Program Brochure of Human Services Department.* City of Gardena, California, 1981.
[56]"National Therapeutic Recreation Society: The First 12 Years." *Therapeutic Recreation Journal*, First Quarter, 1978, p. 7.

Despite these gains, therapeutic recreation is still a relatively young and poorly understood field. To establish a sound basis for practice, it is essential to have a body of knowledge that is based on scientific research and solid empirical findings. The field also needs a convincing and logical rationale to justify itself and to serve as the philosophical basis for its existence. Such a rationale is presented in Chapter 2.

Suggested Topics for Class Discussion, Examination Questions or Student Papers

1. Develop a meaningful definition of contemporary therapeutic recreation service, including a discussion of the 1982 philosophical statement of the National Therapeutic Recreation Society.

2. Describe three distinctly different settings for therapeutic recreation service, showing how its objectives and program content vary according to the nature of the setting and the population group being served.

3. Discuss mainstreaming and integration of the disabled as a key concern of therapeutic recreators.

4. Describe the expanding scope of therapeutic recreation service, including what you regard as the most important developments of the past several years.

2

The Rationale for Therapeutic Recreation Service

Exactly what is the rationale for therapeutic recreation service? Why should recreation be considered a form of therapy or an essential aspect of life for the physically or mentally disabled?

This chapter will present the underlying concepts, values and goals of therapeutic recreation service. It will show how therapeutic recreation has gained the support of leading medical practitioners over the past several decades, and clarify the role of recreation within the rehabilitative services. Several models of therapeutic recreation service will be presented, as well as the principles which help to guide the organization and development of therapeutic recreation in residential institutions and community agencies.

HEALTH VALUES OF RECREATION FOR ALL

It should be stressed again that recreation is *not* solely of value to the emotionally or physically disabled. All individuals have important needs for physical release, creative self-expression and social involvement that recreation can satisfy. A widely accepted definition of recreation presents it as

> . . . an emotional condition within an individual human being that flows from a feeling of well-being and self-satisfaction. It is characterized by feelings of mastery, achievement, exhilaration, acceptance, success, personal worth, and pleasure. It reinforces a positive self-image. Recreation is a response to aesthetic experience, achievement of personal goals, or positive feedback from others. It is independent of activity, leisure, or social acceptance.[1]

---

[1]David E. Gray and Seymour Greben: "Future Perspectives." *Parks and Recreation*, July 1974, p. 49.

Seen in this light, recreation is vital as a form of therapeutic experience for the entire population and a preventative of illness, even among "normal" individuals, in that it helps to minimize emotional strains and to keep the individual functioning in a healthy way. The focus of this text, however, *is* on the use of recreation with persons suffering a significant degree of disability who therefore have acute unmet needs and special problems with respect to leisure. In the past, the people of the United States have been so work-oriented that they paid little attention to recreation and leisure needs. Despite our respect for play as an important economic factor in modern society, we tend to be unaware of its serious social purpose and value. Only in recent years have we begun to accept the physical, psychological and social values of recreation for all age groups and socioeconomic classes.

Therefore, as we examine the rationale for therapeutic recreation service, it is important to ask what support there is for this field. Do medical practitioners understand and support recreation as part of the total treatment plan for the disabled? Medical support and empirical studies showing patient outcomes after therapeutic recreation are essential to gaining fuller acceptance for the field.

Views of Medical Practitioners

The strongest support for recreation as a form of rehabilitative service has come from psychiatrists who have seen diversional activities arouse the interest and improve the morale of the mentally ill. Over the past several decades, leading psychiatrists have given eloquent support to this field.

Dr. Menninger, Co-Director of the Menninger Clinic in Topeka, Kansas, Chief of Army Neuropsychiatric Services during World War II and past President of the American Psychiatric Association, has vigorously supported the use of recreation. In a speech before the National Recreation Congress in 1948 he said,

---

It has been the privilege of many of us practicing medicine in psychiatry to have had some very rewarding experiences in the use of recreation as an adjunctive method of treatment. Along with direct psychological help, hydrotherapy, shock and insulin therapy, many of us have, for years, used various forms of education, recreation and occupation in the treatment of our patients. Within the American Psychiatric Association — a national organization of approximately 4,500 psychiatrists — we have a standing committee on leisure time activities (based on) the assumption that professional recreation experience can contribute to psychiatric practice, and psychiatrists can add to the knowledge of professional recreation workers.[2]

Menninger stressed the value of recreation, not only in the treatment program of mental patients but also in helping former patients to remain well. He outlined three key recreational areas in which psychological needs can be met: (a) competi-

---

[2]William C. Menninger: "Recreation and Mental Health." *Recreation,* November 1948, p. 340.

tive games as an outlet for instinctive aggressive drives; (b) creative activities in art, music or literature as a release for erotic drives; and (c) entertainment activities as a means of providing relaxation and vicarious involvement.

He also pointed out that a conspicuous symptom of many persons who are mentally ill is their inability to feel comfortable with others or to identify with and belong to a social unit. The process of gradually helping a patient become resocialized is readily carried on within group recreational activities, such as parties, ball games, square dances or dramatic productions. Menninger wrote,

Some very concrete evidence of the relation between avocations and mental health was revealed in a survey made at our clinic some years ago. A group of well-adjusted individuals was surveyed as to the type, number and duration of their hobbies. The findings we compared to those from a similar survey of a group of psychiatric patients. In the well-adjusted group, both the number and the intensity of the pursuit of hobbies was far in excess of those of the patients. This cannot be interpreted to mean that, because the individual has a hobby, it necessarily keeps him well. It does mean, however, that a well-adjusted individual learns how to play and does include play as an important feature of his life, much more frequently than does the average maladjusted person.[3]

Another well-known psychiatrist and former President of the American Psychiatric Association, Alexander Reid Martin, took a deep interest in the relationship between leisure behavior and mental health. He pointed out that many otherwise highly successful individuals are unable to deal effectively with leisure in their private lives. Often, they are compulsively driven by work. Martin wrote,

Psychiatry has an extensive and intensive interest in leisure because, in most instances of psychoses and neuroses, the earliest and most unamenable signs and symptoms are disturbances in natural recreative functioning. They include sleeplessness, inability to relax, so-called nervous and mental tension, fear of leisure, and the compulsive need to keep going. Furthermore, the *first signs of recovery are shown in a return to natural recreative functioning.* Improvement is never revealed as clearly in the patient's attitude toward work as it is in his attitude toward leisure and relaxation and in the free play of his body, mind, and feelings, that is, in the free play of his whole personality.[4]

Probably the most eloquent spokesman of the need for recreation in promoting mental health generally, as well as in the treatment of psychiatric patients, has been Paul Haun. His view of play was that it represented an essential aspect of healthy life and constituted a natural rhythmic alternative to work. In making a "medical case" for recreation, Haun wrote,

---

[3]*Ibid.,* p. 343.
[4]Alexander Reid Martin: "Professional Attitudes and Practices." In *Recreation for the Mentally Ill.* Washington, D.C., Conference Report, American Association for Health, Physical Education and Recreation, 1958, p. 15.

It provides patients and appropriate staff members with many familiar social roles through which pleasant and accustomed expressive interaction can occur. It affords the patient a physiological escape from somatic pain and disruptive emotional experiences. It capitalizes upon and supports the non-pathological elements of his personality. It constitutes a path by which he may return from the malignant equilibrium of defensive withdrawal, first to the make-believe universe of the play world and then, after finding this tolerable, to the yet tighter existence of prosaic day-to-day existence. It offers a gratifyingly wide opportunity for instinctual discharge in socially acceptable channels without the need for complicated sublimations.[5]

A similar statement of support was made by Robert H. Felix, a leading psychiatrist for over 30 years and Director of the National Institute of Mental Health. He commented that the problem of filling leisure with satisfying activity is particularly acute in many mental hospitals simply because many patients have so much free time. Beyond this, however, Felix believed that recreation serves as a "great healing force" in providing a means by which leisure can be molded to promote physical and psychological well-being:

The greatest value of recreation is that it can be prescribed as a definitive therapeutic treatment. Particularly in the field of psychiatry . . . recreation plays a positive role in the care and treatment of the mentally ill. Because the activities included in recreation programs usually require some degree of skill and concentration, recreation allows the patient to lose himself in the activity at hand, giving his mind a rest from the mental and physical problems that beset him. It provides a controlled outlet for the release of tensions that otherwise might be directed inward or toward others. It offers a means whereby the patient can acquire and put into practice new knowledge about himself. And recreation helps morale by giving the individual a feeling of satisfaction and accomplishment at having mastered some small skill or compensated for a handicap.[6]

Felix concluded that recreation contributes significantly to the "more rapid physical, mental and social rehabilitation of the patient," and thus has come to be recognized as a clinically oriented discipline, acknowledged by other branches of the medical and health professions.

Support by Other Medical Practitioners

It seems likely that psychiatrists have been particularly supportive of recreation as a valuable form of therapeutic experience because they were fully aware of the character of many mental hospitals. For almost a century, mental health care had

---

[5]Paul Haun: *Recreation: A Medical Viewpoint.* New York, Teachers College, Columbia University, Bureau of Publications, 1964, p. 52.
[6]Robert H. Felix: Preface to *Recreation in Treatment Centers,* September 1962, p. 3.

been carried on in huge, impersonal, custodial institutions. Although treatment approaches varied from time to time, mental hospitals, like other large bureaucratic structures, tended to have an institutionalizing effect on both staff and patients. Patients in particular were robbed of their personal identities, treated in a dehumanized, mechanical way and totally regimented in their behavior. Recreation was recognized as a way of helping them become *people* again, reinforcing their sense of self, their pride in individual accomplishments and their effective relations with others.

However, psychiatrists were not the only physicians to give strong support to recreation. A leading heart research specialist, Dr. Joseph B. Wolffe, formerly President of the American College of Sports Medicine and Medical Director of the Valley Forge Medical Center and Heart Hospital, reported on the specific contribution of recreation in the treatment of patients suffering from acute thrombosis, congestive heart failure and allied illnesses:

A survey of 1,000 patients has shown that carefully selected recreation to suit the patient's problem and personality resulted in reduction both in drug requirements as well as length of hospital stay, when compared to the control group in the institution without the program.[7]

It was found that a special activity program resulted in lessening drug requirements for various types of patients from 30 to 50 per cent and actually shortened their hospital stay by approximately 15 per cent. As an example, Wolffe points out that in the treatment of neurocirculatory asthenia there was a 35 per cent reduction in the need for sedatives and tranquilizers as a consequence of a carefully planned patient recreation program.

The value of therapeutic recreation in the field of physical medicine and rehabilitation has been affirmed by Dr. Howard A. Rusk, formerly Director of the Institute of Physical Medicine and Rehabilitation of the New York University–Bellevue Medical Center in New York City. An internationally known authority in the rehabilitation of the physically disabled, Rusk stressed the need for patients to become involved in their own rehabilitation and in the achievement of greater emotional, vocational and social self-sufficiency. He asked,

What good does it do for a chronically disabled person to learn to walk again if he is so withdrawn and fearful that he will not leave his home? For a handicapped child to realize his highest potential for physical functioning if his emotional and social growth is stunted in the process? For a post-psychiatric patient to be vocationally rehabilitated but unable to make further progress toward healthy social interaction with others?[8]

---

[7]Joseph B. Wolffe: *The Doctors and Recreation in the Medical Setting.* Raleigh, North Carolina Recreation Commission, 1962, p. 19.
[8]Howard Rusk: "Therapeutic Recreation." *Hospital Management*, April 1960, pp. 35–36.

Rusk pointed out that in rehabilitation centers disabled children spend a great deal of time following directions for ambulation and self-care exercises. Often, the recreation session gives them their only opportunity for independent action, with a minimum of adult direction, that will be helpful in achieving social and emotional maturity. Rusk was one of the first authorities to stress the need for providing recreation counseling that would help discharged patients achieve full social independence following their return to community life.

To summarize, it is apparent that a number of leading medical practitioners recognize and strongly support the need for recreation in hospital settings. It should be stressed, however, that therapeutic recreation service cannot rely on such statements exclusively to justify its existence. In addition, a growing number of practitioners and educators have carried out systematic research and evaluations designed to measure the actual outcomes of therapeutic recreation service within specific settings. The findings of several such studies are presented throughout this text.

To develop a fuller understanding of recreation as a form of therapeutic experience, it is helpful to examine its overall relationship to healthful living.

Recreation's Contribution to Healthful Living

Increasingly, we have come to recognize the complex nature of human well-being. The very concept of health implies more than the absence of illness. The preamble to the Constitution of the World Health Organization states, "Health is a state of complete physical, mental and social well-being and not merely an absence of disease or infirmity."

The modern concept of "wellness" implies that an individual is functioning fully and happily in a number of spheres of life, including family and social life, play and work. "Wellness" includes physical, emotional and social well-being. From a holistic point of view, health or "wellness" must be based on a harmonious interrelationship of all personal elements. Instead of seeing work as the primary source of important personal values, as it was commonly regarded in the past, we now see both work and play as vital personal expressions carried on to meet basic needs for self-expression, commitment and a sense of accomplishment.

CHANGING VIEW OF RECREATION

In the past, work was typically thought of as demanding, serious and tiring, while recreation was seen as the opportunity for the rest and refreshment of mind, body and spirit. Martin Meyer, a leading therapeutic recreation specialist in the Veterans' Administration, pointed out that recreation is the time during which we pause, change our pace and recover our energies in order to ease the strains and demands of a fast-paced, competitive society. He wrote,

> The physiological concept of "stroke" and "glide" for the harmonious performance of any body organ applies equally to the total body operating as a synchronized machine in the execution of any task requiring the expenditure of energy. The "stroke" is the thrust, the "glide" the recovery. Our whole life is continuous "stroke" and "glide" and psychologically the "stroke" is our work phase, our vocational pursuit, and the "glide" our recreation, our recovery. The harmonious relationship between work and recreation is essential for . . . good mental health.[9]

Today, we have come to recognize that recreation does not *only* provide rest and relaxation. Particularly for those employees whose work is boring or monotonous, or makes so few physical or mental demands that it provides little challenge or satisfaction, recreation may offer a needed source of personal commitment and creative involvement. Leisure pursuits—including art, music, dance, theater, sports, travel, intellectual or scientific hobbies or community service—may demand much greater commitment, effort or even personal risk than work does.

It is not at all unusual for individuals to become far more involved in their play than in their work. For example, sports fans identify strongly with their favorite teams; rabid partisans may have cardiac seizures at major sports events.

STRESS AS A POSITIVE HEALTH FACTOR

We tend to think of stress as a form of pressure leading to anxiety, inability to function well and even emotional or physical illness. Yet Hans Selye, a physician who has done outstanding research and written extensively on the concept of stress, points out that stress plays a positive role as well. It is a mistake to assume that rest and relaxation are necessarily desirable, particularly in excessive doses:

> . . . simple rest is no cure-all. Activity and rest must be judiciously balanced, and *every person has his own characteristic requirements for rest and activity.* To lie motionless in bed all day is no relaxation for an active man. . . . Many a valuable man, who could still have given numerous years of useful work to society, has been made physically ill and prematurely senile by the enforcement of retirement at an age when his requirements and abilities for activity were still high. This psychosomatic disease is so common that it has been given a name: *retirement disease.*[10]

Selye points out that one of the most fundamental laws regulating the activities of complex living beings is that no one part of the body must be disproportionately overworked for a long period. Stress serves as an equalizer of activities within the body; it helps to avoid one-sided exertion. It is necessary to achieve balance in the

---

[9]Martin W. Meyer: "The Rationale of Recreation as Therapy." *Recreation in Treatment Centers,* September 1962, p. 23.
[10]Hans Selye: *The Stress of Life.* New York, McGraw-Hill, 1956, p. 265.

full range of activities if sound health is to be maintained. Vigorous and challenging recreation can make an important contribution in helping individuals meet their psychological and social needs.

MASLOW'S HIERARCHY OF NEEDS

In a study of personality drives, Abraham Maslow suggested that the primary human needs are those which are concerned with survival. When these needs are satisfied, the individual moves on to progressively higher levels of need. For example, the most basic human drives are to ensure *physiological* well-being through adequate nutrition, freedom from the elements, avoidance of illness and similar threats to health. The second level of human need is based on the need for *safety*, which Maslow characterizes as security, stability, freedom from fear or chaos—the need for structure, order and law. People normally prefer a safe, orderly and predictable world. Maslow points out that when both physical and safety needs are fairly well met, the individual will next require love and *affection:* "He will hunger for (affectionate) relations with people in general . . . and will strive with great intensity to achieve this goal. He will feel sharply the pangs of loneliness, of ostracism, of rejection, of friendlessness, of rootlessness."[11] On the next level, most people in society have a need or desire for a firmly based and high evaluation of themselves, which Maslow refers to as *self-esteem*. This is closely related to the desire for strength, adequacy, a sense of mastery and competence, the capacity for independent action and recognition or appreciation from others. Following the satisfaction of the physical, safety, love and esteem needs, Maslow contends that there are significant needs for individual *self-actualization*, for satisfying the urge to *know and to understand* and, finally, *aesthetic needs*.

It is easy to see how recreation can provide a rich opportunity to meet significant psychological needs. These also may vary according to one's life stage within the overall human life cycle. Godbey points out how at each stage of life, such as later adolescence, early maturity or retirement, different needs may prevail: the need for peer relationships and acceptance, intimacy and connection with others, personal autonomy or accomplishment.[12] Recreation and play may be viewed simply as sources of pleasure or amusement, or may meet other important needs, such as the promotion of family cohesion, physical fitness, or the need for excitement in life.

In addition to the general needs that all human beings have, each of us is likely to have unique needs that stem from our personal make-up, family history and psychosocial development. Although it is all too easy to refer to one group of people as the "disabled" or "handicapped" and to all others as "normal," this tends to be an oversimplification. In an eloquent description of nine disabled adventurers (five blind, two deaf, one epileptic and one with an artificial leg) who successfully climbed 14,410-foot Mount Rainier, Rabbi Sidney Greenberg comments that we are

---

[11]Abraham Maslow: *Motivation and Personality*. New York, Harper & Row, 1970, pp. 35–50.
[12]Geoffrey Godbey: *Leisure in Your Life: An Exploration*. Philadelphia, Saunders College Publishing, 1981, pp. 167–179.

all disabled in one way or another. He points out that not all handicaps are physical or visible, but to be human is to be handicapped, to be flawed. He writes,

---

"There is a crack," wrote Emerson, "in everything God made." Some of us are handicapped by a disturbing sense of inferiority and inadequacy. Some of us carry childhood scars inflicted by constant criticism and bitter rejection.

Some of us feel unworthy of being loved, others cannot give love. Some of us are burdened by guilt, others are filled with rage. Some of us are consumed by envy, others are driven by greed. Some of us have forfeited our self-respect, others never acquired it. Some of us are battered by fear, others are buffeted by frustration and failure. Some of us are imprisoned by selfishness, others are enslaved by alcohol or pills. Some of us suffer heartaches from children, others are tormented by parents . . .[13]

Even for those who do not have such severe adjustment problems, there are likely to be major areas of our lives in which recreation can help to meet pressing needs or fill significant voids.

IMPACT OF HUMAN LONELINESS

Even in a crowded society, many individuals lead lives of great loneliness. An Ohio State University professor of psychiatry, John Whieldon, has found that loneliness is not so much an active phenomenon as a void—the incapacity to develop meaningful relations with others. He writes, "One of the basic processes of childhood is to resolve one's loneliness. To do this, everyone must learn to make meaningful emotional contact with others."[14] The lonely person, Whieldon believes, has never learned to do this or has lost the capacity for it. As a consequence, he or she falls back on a variety of defenses, such as sexual promiscuity, daydreaming, tantrums, narcissism, hyperactivity or the "last defense"—schizophrenia. Numerous studies have indicated the damaging effects of social isolation. The value of recreation in overcoming the problem of loneliness and isolation is clear. Most leisure activities are carried on in groups, and it is possible from earliest childhood to encourage participation in play groups, clubs, teams or musical or theater organizations that help youngsters develop the ability to relate to others.

Recently, medical researchers have begun to gather evidence linking social isolation with heart disease. They have found that many individuals develop coronary heart disease without being subject to such risk factors as cigarette smoking, high blood pressure, high cholesterol levels, obesity, or lack of exercise. The researchers have sought other types of risk factors; one clear risk, based on a number of statistical studies of the incidence of heart disease, appears to be whether individuals are

---

[13]Rabbi Sidney Greenberg: "We Are Each of Us a Flawed Creation." *The Philadelphia Inquirer,* July 25, 1981, p. 7-A.
[14]John Whieldon: "A Study of Those 'Blues' That Start in Loneliness." *New York Post,* June 5, 1964, p. 77.

socially isolated or belong to a close social network. S. Leonard Syme, professor of epidemiology at the University of California at Berkeley, states,

> Social isolation . . . makes sense of (a) statistic we've known for a long time — that divorced, widowed and single people have higher disease rates than married people. It also makes sense of the Type A pattern (the striving, diligent, ambitious behavior linked to coronary heart disease). Type A people don't have time to devote to intimate social relationships.[15]

OTHER CAUSES OF BREAKDOWN IN MODERN LIFE

Tension, strain and boredom are also important characteristics of modern life. Recent research has indicated that about one person out of every four in the United States is using sedatives or tranquilizers. In some occupational groups or social classes today, strain and tension lead to high rates of serious social and familial breakdowns.

What this suggests is that many of our health-related problems in modern society stem from a lack of involvement and physical release, from boredom and from the unfulfilled need for meaningful social contact. To illustrate, one might point to the extremely high incidence of such social diseases as addictive gambling, drug abuse and alcoholism. In a study of motivations for drinking, Riley, Marden and Lifshitz found that Americans drank "to be sociable," "because all of our friends drink" or "to be a good sport." They concluded that drinking, at least to the point where it becomes a compulsive and destructive act, is carried on "for relaxation or for euphoric effect . . . as an escape from worries, responsibilities and frustration. . . ."[16]

PLAY AS PATHOLOGICAL RISK-TAKING

There is growing awareness today that many forms of recreation are carried on to meet the need for challenge and excitement. The arousal-seeking theory of play has been widely accepted,[17] and we have come to recognize that many individuals have a strong need for sensation that leads them into a host of high-risk leisure experiences.

While some activities, such as active sports or outdoor recreation, may be relatively harmless, other forms of activity may represent the self-destructive release of

---

[15]S. Leonard Syme, quoted in David Zinman: "Isolation Is Linked to Heart Disease," *The Philadelphia Inquirer*, March 12, 1982, p. 7-C.
[16]John W. Riley, Jr., Charles F. Marden and Marcia Lifshitz: *In* Eric Larrabee and Rold Meyersohn: *Mass Leisure.* Glencoe, Illinois, The Free Press, 1958, pp. 327–330.
[17]Marvin Zuckerman: "The Search for High Sensation." *Psychology Today*, February 1978, pp. 38–46, 96–99.

neurotic drives. Paul Haun has written extensively on so-called pathological play. In one form, an individual whose hate is self-directed may strive desperately *not* to win and may seek defeat or even physical injury as a punishment for guilt feelings. Beyond this, Haun saw distorted play as a means of blotting out reality.

He described a number of forms of play that are extremely violent or dangerous and afford almost completely unsublimated release for primitive drives, lending themselves "with exceptional ease to sadistic, masochistic, and compulsive distortion by the participant." Some of these types of play, such as speedboat and automobile racing, reckless mountain climbing, bullfighting and fencing with unprotected weapons, occupy a kind of twilight zone, slipping back and forth between pathology and wild adventure. Others are completely pathological in their self-destructive potential:

. . . the most notorious example being that of ''Russian Roulette,'' which is played by spinning the cylinder of a revolver containing a single round of live ammunition, placing the muzzle of the gun at one's temple and pulling the trigger. Another example is the game of ''Chicken,'' in which two contestants drive their automobiles toward each other at the highest possible speed on the same highway lane. The first to weaken and swerve out of the path of certain destruction is said to lose in this singular display of immaturity — and is accordingly labeled ''chicken'' . . .[18]

Such examples reveal the ways in which play may serve as a release for harmful drives. In contrast, there are many forms of play that serve as a constructive means of maintaining emotional balance and preventing neurosis, such as backpacking in the wilderness. This has become an enthusiastic interest of great numbers of Americans of all ages and walks of life; it has been estimated that in recent years no fewer than 20 million Americans have taken up this hobby. In part, the interest in wilderness hiking stems from a desire to get away from the pressure and tension of city life. In part, it comes from the need to meet direct physical challenge and to find out what one is capable of doing and not doing.

Being able to play in constructive and self-enhancing ways is often an indicator of one's mental health and level of social adjustment. Typically, disturbed children and youth often show an inability to engage in normal forms of play; those committed to correctional institutions often lack useful leisure skills. Play serves as a form of release for many kinds of drives that, if bottled up, might be seriously destructive to the individual.

As Martin has shown, many individuals are so committed to work they are unable to free themselves to enjoy leisure; they become addicted to "eating, sleeping and drinking their jobs." In a convincing description of what it is like to be a "workaholic," Professor Wayne Oates describes his own daily performance: At his office, he is "merciless in his demands upon himself for peak performance" and without qualms about "telling off both high and low" when their work is sloppy. Arriving home late, he heads for his study "to make the best of the remaining hours of the day."

---

[18]Paul Haun, *op. cit.*, p. 26.

How does a workaholic know that he is one? Sometimes he finds out only when he suffers a heart attack — or when, as in Oates' case, his five-year-old son asks for an appointment to see him.[19]

It is apparent that for many persons who are not ill or disabled in any serious or permanent way, recreation serves to meet important psychosocial and physical needs. It may be used constructively or, when not understood and dealt with intelligently, may provide an outlet for dangerous drives that can damage the individual. It is essential that *all* individuals be aware of their leisure needs and behavior and that full opportunity be provided in the community for varied, creative and constructive recreational participation.

The ill or disabled person has more difficulty finding an appropriate means of recreation than those who do not have any significant form of physical impairment or mental disability. As a result, disabled persons often encounter great difficulty in learning constructive and rewarding leisure attitudes and skills or in gaining access to a variety of community recreational opportunities.

THE DISABLED IN SOCIETY TODAY

As indicated earlier, the term "disability" today is regarded as preferable to "handicap" because it stresses the concept of disability, which may be overcome, rather than that of handicap, which has a negative connotation in our society. In this text, the term "disability" is used throughout, except in quotations from the past or titles of organizations or projects that continue to make use of the term "handicap."

A statement formulated by the 1960 White House Conference on Children and Youth defines the "handicapped" child as one who

. . . cannot play, learn, work or do the things other children his age can do; or is hindered in achieving his full physical, mental or social potentialities; whether by a disability which is initially small but potentially handicapping, or by a serious impairment involving several areas of function with the probability of life-long impairment.[20]

Disabilities may be mild or severe, single or multiple, and may affect persons of every age, socioeconomic condition, race, religion and region. They may stem from birth defects, environmental factors, illness, accident or a variety of other

[19]"Behavior: Hooked on Work." *Time*, July 5, 1971, p. 42.
[20]*Conference Proceedings.* White House Conference on Children and Youth. Washington, D.C., 1960, p. 381.

causes. Although the impairment may initially be of purely physical nature, it may have secondary effects that limit the individual's social involvement, affect him or her emotionally and create serious behavioral problems. The disabled person's potential for mobility, physical activity, education, holding a job and maintaining satisfying social relationships may all be seriously affected.

As indicated in Chapter 1, it has been estimated that as many as 68 million persons in American society suffer from some significant degree of disability. When one recognizes that for each such person there is also a family unit involved in the problem, it is apparent that meeting the total needs of disabled persons and helping them fit as successfully as possible into the total society are crucial concerns in the United States and Canada.

Attitudes Toward the Disabled

During the past several decades, there has been a radical shift in public concern about the disabled. Social work agencies today provide a variety of welfare services in communities, youth houses, hospitals and residential centers for the disabled. In past centuries, the physically or mentally disabled were often seen as persons who had been cursed by the gods. Often they were cruelly rejected, hidden, ridiculed or even, in some cases, disposed of. We have not *totally* overcome these attitudes, either in the United States or elsewhere in the world.

In a three-year study of attitudes toward the disabled, two German psychologists, Jansen and Esser, questioned several thousand adults and school-age children regarding their feelings toward disabled persons. They found a high incidence of continuing prejudice and aversion. Ignorance appeared to be a major obstacle to social contact with the disabled; those questioned did not seem to know how to approach or deal with the disabled realistically. Jansen and Esser summarized their findings:

Although many of those questioned spoke sympathetically of their attitudes toward the handicapped . . . often they felt revulsion . . . few wished to be friends with them, or to marry one . . . most (63 percent) thought that severely disabled persons should be kept out of sight in institutions; while none recommended that they deserved to die, openly, actually some spoke carefully of the merits of euthanasia. . . .[21]

Attitudes may be defined as positive or negative emotional reactions to an object or individual, accompanied by specific beliefs that tend to induce specific behavior toward the object or individual. Attitudes have three components: a *belief*

---

[21]"Hostility to the Handicapped." *Time,* December 20, 1971, p. 67.

component, an *emotional* component, and an *action* component. While attitudes toward the disabled vary greatly, the May 1977 White House Conference on Handicapped Individuals summarized the research on this subject as follows:

1. Although people make distinctions among types of disabilities, they also are willing to express attitudes toward disabled people in general . . . (and) their attitudes toward people with different handicaps tend to be quite similar.
2. More than 50 per cent of the people in the United States express slightly positive attitudes toward disabled people and indicate that they have sympathetic feelings for them. Other people, however, freely express negative, rejecting attitudes.
3. Many non-disabled persons perceived handicapped people as "different" and in some ways inferior to "normal" people. They are uncomfortable and don't know "how to behave" in their presence.
4. Despite the positive attitudes that may be expressed in public, handicapped persons are often discriminated against. Many people favor segregation rather than integration of handicapped individuals.
5. Individual attitudes vary greatly, as a result of differences in people's knowledge and past experiences. Often they are part of one's generalized approach toward other people; those who reject members of minority groups also tend to reject the disabled.[22]

It is apparent that prejudices toward the disabled have not disappeared. Many people still have feelings that range from excessive pity (which overprotects disabled people and makes them less likely to make independent efforts in their own behalf) to outright rejection and even fear. For example, a recent study by the New York State Department of Mental Hygiene revealed that the public feared former mental patients more than ex-convicts. Believing that they were dangerous and unpredictable, at least one fourth of those surveyed said they would not want to live, work or socialize with former mental patients.

By and large, however, the disabled are increasingly seen as persons who are in many ways like everybody else, with important physical, social and emotional needs that must be met if they are to reach their fullest potential as human beings. In many ways, federal, state and provincial governments have moved vigorously to promote total rehabilitation of the disabled. Increasingly, it has been recognized that disability tends also to be linked with poverty. To eradicate this inequity, strenuous efforts were made in the 1960's to expand programs of vocational rehabilitation for the disabled. Federal support was given to research and training and the development of special facilities. Demonstration projects were initiated first for the physically disabled and later for the mentally retarded, mentally ill, alcoholics, drug addicts, public offenders and disabled persons who were socially and culturally disadvantaged. Under the Rehabilitation Services Administration of the Department of Health, Education and Welfare, hundreds of thousands of disabled persons were served each year. Within this context, recreation has become an increasingly recognized area of service for the disabled.

---

[22]*Awareness Papers*. Washington, D.C., White House Conference on Handicapped Individuals Report, Volume One, May 1977, pp. 93–104.

Justification for Special Therapeutic Recreation Programs

What is the justification for providing special therapeutic recreation programs to serve the disabled in community life? The answer is twofold.

1. Like all people, the disabled have a right to self-expression, social involvement, creative experience and the other important values that can be provided by recreation. They are human beings, and they and their families are taxpayers; they should be served fully by public agencies.

2. Many disabled individuals find most aspects of "normal" life closed to them, such as the opportunity to complete their education, marry and have a family, enter a profession and earn a livelihood or travel freely. For this reason, recreation represents a particularly crucial need. If it is not provided, their lives are cruelly barren and empty. The author has pointed out elsewhere,

---

Those who suffer from disability . . . frequently find difficulty in meeting their recreative needs in constructive and varied ways, in part because serious physical handicaps obviously limit the extent of participation. . . . Much recreative deprivation to the disabled is, however, caused by the reluctance of society to permit them to engage in activity to the extent of their real potential. Sometimes communities or recreation agencies do not make the kinds of adaptations in the design of facilities needed for disabled persons to use them fully. Sometimes recreational and park agencies actively bar disabled persons from their programs because they feel that to serve them would require specialized leadership to a degree they could not afford.[23]

Frequently, park and recreation administrators fear that the presence of blind, retarded or orthopedically handicapped individuals might be distasteful to the general public. Sometimes parents or relatives shelter disabled people excessively, and sometimes they are barred from recreational participation by their own lack of skill or fear of rejection by others. Whatever the reason, many disabled persons are unable to make use of available community recreation resources.

The problem of acceptance in community life is particularly difficult for those who are visibly disabled. Those who have a severe physical disability or crippling deformity are acutely aware of the reactions of others, the threat of social isolation and the direct limitations imposed on their capabilities for full and varied social involvement. Wright points out that while physical limitations themselves may cause frustration or suffering, the more serious deprivation comes from the attitudes of others:

One of man's basic strivings is for acceptance by the group, for being important in the lives of others, and for having others count positively in his life. As long as physical disability is linked with shame and inferiority, realistic acceptance of one's position and one's self is precluded.[24]

---

[23]Richard Kraus: *Recreation and Leisure in Modern Society*. Santa Monica, California, Goodyear, 1971, pp. 364–365.
[24]Beatrice Wright: *Physical Disability: A Psychological Approach*. New York, Harper & Row, 1960, p. 14.

Recreation Potential of the Disabled

Often, disabled people themselves may have a tremendous sense of inferiority, due to their upbringing and the severe limitations that have been placed on them throughout their lives. It is therefore all the more striking to recognize the remarkable achievements of many severely impaired individuals in a wide range of recreational activities. In recent years hundreds of individuals with spinal cord injuries—both paraplegic and quadriplegic—have married, raised families, entered a host of professions and trades and have mastered swimming, wheelchair basketball, track and field, sailing, windsurfing, kayaking, canoeing, archery, hunting, fishing, flying and the use of off-road vehicles. Far from permitting themselves to be defeated by their impairments, such individuals have courageously met the challenge of forging new lifestyles for themselves and opening the eyes of the public to the true potential of severely disabled individuals.[25]

Another category of disabled persons—alcoholics—recently formed an "Alcoholic Olympics" on the West Coast to overcome their limitations through recreation. With dedicated practice, conditioning and enthusiastic competition, these individuals have gained a heightened sense of morale, discipline and power over their lives—as well as increased physical fitness.[26] More and more, disabled individuals within a wide variety of special groups have become convinced of their own potential and have made remarkable strides by participating in numerous activities.

Yet the task of gaining public acceptance for the disabled in community settings remains. This can be accomplished in a variety of ways: through public meetings, demonstration projects, conferences and seminars, and publication of articles and special reports. One ingenious approach used by first-year therapeutic recreation students at Mount Royal College, Calgary, Alberta, was to declare a community-wide Awareness Day to help focus public concern on the needs and capabilities of the disabled. College students and faculty as well as government officials and the public were invited to experience simulated forms of disability, such as maneuvering about the college blindfolded or taking part in wheelchair sports. All local agencies were asked to set up information booths and to distribute literature. Killingsworth comments,

---

. . . the primary purpose of the day was to try to make people aware . . . of the disabled and to let them experience a disability in the hope that this would help make them more empathetic of the disabled. Further, the assignment allowed the students the opportunity to find and utilize valuable community resources. . . .[27]

It is always important that the disabled be seen realistically. Wright points out that people with disabilities are frequently considered to be compensating (that is,

---

[25]Barry Corbet: *Options: Spinal Cord Injury and the Future.* Denver, A. B. Hirschfeld Press, 1980.
[26]Kurt Freeman and Ronald R. Koegler: *From Skid Row to the Olympics.* Castaic, California, Institute of Creative Leisure, 1978.
[27]C. Killingsworth: "Awareness." *Therapeutic Recreation Journal,* Fourth Quarter, 1975, p. 141.

developing strength in one area to make up for weakness in another) when they are merely interested in an activity; they may be regarded as showing a sense of inferiority when they are merely hesitating before committing themselves to an activity because of a realistic awareness of their own limitations. Thus, it becomes extremely important that our attitudes about the disabled be based on an intelligent comprehension of their needs and capabilities rather than on stereotyped and distorted attitudes.

Changing Family Attitudes

The attitudes of family members toward those with disabilities are changing. As pointed out earlier, relatives frequently tend to be overprotective and unconsciously limit the extent to which disabled individuals may strike out independently. A study carried out at the University of Pennsylvania under a grant from the Social and Rehabilitation Service of the Department of Health, Education and Welfare suggested that society sometimes has a vested interest in having its members remain disabled:

> The disabled handicaps the family unit in many ways, most obviously economically and socially. Within the unit, the members attempt, with varying degrees of success, to "negotiate" a satisfying relationship. . . . Despite the sympathy that such a setup might draw from society . . . the interplay of dependent and helper often satisfies the deeper psychological needs of each individual, often retarding the handicapped person's rehabilitation.[28]

In this study it was found that the disabled person typically was not an independent entity but rather the hub of a complex set of family relationships that in effect creates a "disabled family." It was found that both the family and the larger society "use" the disabled, symbolically, to meet psychological needs and are often reluctant to have them move toward true independence.

Nesbitt outlines a number of attitudes through which community educators, recreation and park professionals, and other public and voluntary agency officials justify their failure to provide more effective programming for the disabled. These range from the "futility syndrome" ("What can I do to help? The situation is impossible.") to the "lack-of-training syndrome" ("I can't take handicapped people into my program. I don't have the trained staff to handle epileptic fits, convulsions, slobbering, etc.").[29]

All such "do-nothing" attitudes today are simply rationalizations that stem from a lack of conviction about disabled persons' need for comprehensive recreation programming or their real ability to enter into such programs fully and effec-

---

[28]Nancy Hicks: "Life of Disabled Is Tied to Family." *The New York Times*, September 14, 1969, p. 73.
[29]John Nesbitt: "Special Community Education for the Handicapped." *In* Effie Fairchild and Larry Neal, eds.: *Common-Unity in the Community.* University of Oregon, Eugene, Center of Leisure Studies, 1975, p. 69.

tively. For the sake of the disabled themselves and in the interest of their families and the larger society, those rationalizations must be overcome.

Mainstreaming as a Primary Goal

In recent years, the effort to help disabled persons become integrated members of society on every level has been known as "mainstreaming." Mainstreaming has become a major aspect of therapeutic recreation services and is closely linked to the "continuum" concept of programming. Increasingly, we have sought to close down large, custodial facilities and serve disabled persons within the community. More and more they are becoming part of regular school classes and community programs, including integrated recreation activities.

Salzberg and Langford point out that for most of the past century, mentally retarded and mentally ill individuals were segregated from society in large institutions. Hundreds of thousands of people were institutionalized on the grounds that it was in their own best interests as well as in the interest of society—although often the net effect was that the disabled deteriorated in crowded and poorly operated facilities.

The deinstitutionalization movement, and the resulting transfer of thousands of mentally retarded and mentally ill people from large state institutions into community-based residences, is in part a result of public shock at the living conditions in those facilities. However, in equal measure, it is based upon the principle of normalization which has become a primary guiding influence in directing the care and habilitation of mentally retarded people.

Normalization is defined as making available to handicapped persons patterns and conditions of everyday life which are as close as possible to the norms and patterns of society.[30]

Breaking down the prejudices and barriers that inhibit mainstreaming represents a twofold task. Obviously, it is necessary to help the public understand and accept the disabled more fully. However, it would be a mistake to assume that disabled persons themselves always *wish* to be integrated into ongoing community recreation programs. In many cases, they are not psychologically ready for this step. Shivers and Fait write,

---

The physically disabled individual may accept his permanent disability, but frequently he also feels fear, isolation, and sensitivity about the handicap. . . . He may view his disability as a shameful stigma, as a mark of inferiority, and something which must be kept from view. . . . Disabled people (may) feel that they are not really accepted as members of social groups. . . .[31]

---

[30]Charles L. Salzberg and Cynthia A. Langford: "Community Integration of Mentally Retarded Adults Through Leisure Activity." *Mental Retardation,* June 1981, pp. 127–131.
[31]Jay S. Shivers and Hollis F. Fait: *Therapeutic and Adapted Recreational Services.* Philadelphia, Lea and Febiger, 1975, pp. 184–185

There are numerous examples of such attitudes. In many retirement communities for aged persons, residents actively resist having younger families—particularly those with children—live in the community. Frequently, when blind or deaf persons are encouraged to enter community recreation groups designed for the general public, they respond with fear and resistance. Often, when discharged mental patients return to the hospital, it is because they feel unable to live independently in the community, whereas the hospital and its recreational and social programs represent a warm, accepting atmosphere to them. Geddes points out that although the disabled person may *wish* to be accepted, previous negative life experiences may have resulted in poor psychosocial adjustment that makes it difficult to be accepted by others.

For example, previous frustration, difficulty and embarrassment due to an obvious physical deformity may develop into an adjustment mechanism such as aggression or withdrawal that interferes with group (acceptance). Sometimes the psychosocial problem ends up being a larger, more incapacitating handicap than the condition itself.[32]

She also suggests that integration itself does not always result in desirable outcomes. For example, mentally retarded youngsters included in regular physical education or recreation activities are not always accepted and may have stronger feelings of rejection at the end of the experience than at the beginning. All this suggests that although mainstreaming is a highly desirable goal, it cannot be achieved easily or automatically by administrative decisions or parental pressure alone. Instead, it requires a process of careful education, preparation and skilled leadership in order to succeed.

Ideally, such education should begin early in the lives of disabled individuals. Kay and Kendrigan describe the work of two agencies, the Northwest Special Recreation Association and the Northwest Suburban Special Education Organization. The agencies coordinate 14 park districts in the suburbs around Chicago, providing classes, field trips and other experiences geared to promoting leisure education for the disabled. They point out that

... children with special needs deserve the chance to learn basic skills, to develop appropriate behavior in community facilities, to develop an understanding of safety rules and regulations, and to be taught the positive use of leisure time. These and other concepts constitute the theory and justification for leisure education activities during school hours and for special recreation and education departments to work together to develop a successful leisure education program.[33]

[32]Dolores Geddes: "Physical Activity for Impaired, Disabled and Handicapped Individuals: What's Going On?" *In* Timothy Craig, ed.: *The Humanistic and Mental Health Aspects of Sports, Exercise and Recreation.* Chicago, American Medical Association, 1975, p. 105.
[33]Darla Kay and Keven Kendrigan: "Education for Leisure—A Critical Step to Normalization." *Parks and Recreation*, April 1980, p. 55.

Many disabled children and youth never receive the benefit of such leisure education programs. In addition, many thousands of individuals in hospitals or other institutions are faced with the challenge of being discharged, returning to the community and attempting to develop constructive and rewarding patterns of leisure involvement. It is at this point that the interests of institution and community-based recreational and social agencies coincide. Both must be dedicated to returning disabled persons to the community with skills and attitudes that will permit them to function as happily and effectively as possible within a broad range of relationships.

This has led to the fundamental concept that therapeutic recreation cannot be viewed as a set of isolated services provided without overall direction, but must be organized along with a continuum in which all elements are effectively coordinated. In order to meet the needs of disabled persons at various levels of illness and recovery, it is necessary to develop a logical and orderly progression of services. In turn, these must be designed to fit within a meaningful model of therapeutic recreation service. Indeed, it would be a mistake to assume that *all* therapeutic recreation programs have a similar conceptual base. Instead, they differ widely according to the sponsoring agency and its philosophy of service.

CONTRASTING MODELS OF THERAPEUTIC RECREATION SERVICE

Authorities in this field have identified a number of sharply contrasting approaches to the provision of therapeutic recreation service. For example, Martin describes four such approaches: (1) *fun and games,* in which recreation is seen essentially as a casual experience to be carried on outside of the significant therapeutic program of the treatment center; (2) *personal adjustment,* in which recreation is used to help the patient adjust to changed life circumstances, understand and accept his illness or disability and improve his morale and reduce anxiety; (3) *medical approach,* in which recreation is seen as an integral part of the therapeutic process, with careful prescription of areas of participation intended to contribute to recovery; and (4) *educative,* in which strong emphasis is given to helping the patient develop broader recreative horizons through teaching skills and counseling that will help to prevent residual disability and ensure a successful return to community life.[34]

Similarly, O'Morrow has outlined five basic models of therapeutic recreation: (1) custodial; (2) medical-clinical; (3) therapeutic milieu; (4) education and training; and (5) community models.[35]

---

[34]Fred W. Martin: "Therapeutic Recreation Practice: A Philosophic Overview." *Leisurability,* Ottawa, Canada, January 1974, p. 22.
[35]Gerald S. O'Morrow: *Therapeutic Recreation: A Helping Profession.* Reston, Virginia, Reston, 1976, Chapter 7.

Custodial Model

The custodial model refers to maintaining or acting as guardian for special populations in nursing homes, homes for the aged, mental hospitals, special schools for the mentally retarded and correctional centers. In such situations there tends to be a strong effort to maintain order, to subordinate individual needs to institutional routines and to use various forms of pressure, even punishment, to enforce administrative policies. In general, this model is no longer in vogue, although it persists to a degree in some large state institutions and prisons.

Recreation is not usually seen as a significant form of service in such settings; indeed, custodial programs tend to offer only limited forms of other rehabilitative services. Often, qualified leaders are not employed. Activities consist primarily of movies, dances, mass entertainment and, as in penal institutions, team sports that tend to work off hostility and aggression. Goffman, in his analysis of mental hospitals, prisons and similar custodial structures, comments,

---

Every total institution can be seen as a kind of dead sea in which little islands of vivid, encapturing activity appear. Such activity can help the individual withstand the psychological stress usually engendered by assaults upon the self. Yet it is precisely in the insufficiency of these activities that an important deprivational effect of total institutions can be found.[36]

In custodial institutions, recreation may be used to "kill time," as well as provide some sense of release from the formality and task orientation that normally govern inmate-staff contacts. With voluntary participation, patients or prisoners are permitted to make choices and, to some degree, have a sense of being individuals within the overall institutional framework. Annual parties or Christmas celebrations also help to break down barriers and provide a favorable public image—particularly when the institution is being visited by relatives of inmates or government officials. But that image may have little to do with the normal, on-going life of the institution. Finally, recreation may serve to provide rewards or, when withdrawn, punishments, and reinforce the societal structure and behavioral expectations of the institution through ceremonies, patient or prisoner councils, newspapers and similar activities.

Medical-Clinical Model

Over the past several decades the medical-clinical model has been the most familiar one for institutionally based recreation service. It is characterized, in

---

[36]Erving Goffman: *Asylums.* Garden City, New York, Doubleday-Anchor, 1961, pp. 69–70.

O'Morrow's words, by a "doctor-centered, illness-oriented approach to patient care and treatment." Emphasis is placed on illness or disease, rather than on the whole person, and recreation depends heavily on the diagnosis made by the physician and his prescriptions for needed activity. It is best illustrated within traditional psychiatric hospital settings, in which a doctor works with the recreation therapist to design patient treatment plans that utilize recreation as a specific modality addressed to specific patient needs.

Rosen writes knowledgeably of the needs of psychiatric patients and the ways in which recreation may be used as a specific tool in their treatment. She makes clear that the characteristics of psychiatric patients are such that it is not possible to present activities to them as "normal" people might visualize recreation:

Certainly anyone who has worked with paranoid patients or with guilt-ridden, self-destructive personalities knows that even the most common events of everyday life, eating and sleeping, are frequently connected with fearful and anxiety-provoking fantasies. . . . The peculiar defensive systems erected by psychotic patients shut out and distort the environment and the people in it so that ordinary channels for communication and social interaction are obstructed. Psychiatric treatment is first and foremost concerned with breaking down these barriers, with whatever means are available. It attempts to enable the patient to function within the framework of the social community. Recreative experiences can be utilized to serve this purpose only when they are adapted to the particular needs of the individual patient. Finding the areas of accessibility to psychotic and emotionally disturbed patients may involve a great deal of experimentation in a variety of media. Resourcefulness and imagination in the adaptation of techniques are required. . . .[37]

Although it is possible to make such generalized statements as "strenuous physical activities or certain arts and crafts activities are useful for the release of aggression and hostility" or "group social activities are indicated for withdrawn or isolated patients," these *are* just generalizations. Often, the need to develop a convincing statement of the purpose of a field may lead to precise "laundry lists" of needs and recommended activities that are superficial and misleading. Rosen points out that many of the personal elements intrinsic to the recreative experience defy a systematized method of cataloguing. She comments that it is hazardous to ascribe a specific therapeutic effect to a particular activity:

The practice of listing categories of activities into which patients with specific types of psychopathology can be neatly fitted is little more than a convenience devised by efficient management. In the hands of untrained personnel, the fallacies of such "systems" of selection are obvious.[38]

The treatment of the patient must be directed by the psychiatrist who makes the diagnosis, charts the various techniques that are to be used and evaluates the

[37]Elizabeth R. Rosen: "The Selection of Activities for Therapeutic Use." *Recreation in Treatment Centers,* September 1962, p. 30.
[38]*Ibid.*

patient's progress. The recreation specialist functions as part of the treatment team, planning a sequence of recreational experiences, appraising the patient's reactions and behavior and modifying the treatment plan to eliminate nonproductive activities and focus on those which are most successful in achieving treatment objectives (see Chapters 4 and 5).

When selecting activities for patients, it is important not to rely on classic diagnostic categories as much as on specific observable symptoms, such as disturbances in communication, social control, reality testing and interpersonal relationships.

Therapeutic Milieu Model

Although the therapeutic milieu approach also seeks to use recreation as a significant therapeutic tool in treatment programs, it stems from a markedly different philosophy. Instead of viewing mental illness as a distinct form of disease that can be cured by the physician, those who use the therapeutic milieu model tend to see it more as a problem stemming from the patient's inability to deal realistically and effectively with his or her environment.

In the therapeutic milieu, the patient is taught new attitudes and behaviors that will equip him or her to return to the community, family, job and other environments. Every aspect of the hospital or mental health center environment is an important element in treatment, and all staff members play an important therapeutic role. Within this framework, patients are responsible for their own healthy behavior. Instead of being prescribed *for*, they are encouraged to make choices and decisions for themselves. In contrast to the medical-clinical model of care, where the physician is the major source of decision-making, in the therapeutic milieu model all staff members share meaningfully in discussing patient needs and planning programs with them.

Sometimes this approach is referred to as "milieu therapy." Pattison describes its application in many psychiatric treatment settings today:

The thrust of milieu therapy is not to unlock specific psychodynamic conflicts but rather to provide integrating, guiding, rehabilitating social experiences. This begins with those socializing activities that the most regressed patients can participate in, then on to social activities requiring more ego control and personal-relatedness, and finally to reality-oriented social functions that are part and parcel of everyday living. Seen in this perspective, the adjunctive therapies are experiences in socialization and social interaction. The task of the adjunctive therapist is not that of individual therapist or extension thereof, but that of a social systems specialist.[39]

Similarly, in many community-based treatment centers or halfway houses that serve discharged mental patients, recreation is a means of helping individuals regain social competence and confidence. For example, in one halfway house

[39]E. Mansell Pattison: "The Relationship of the Adjunctive and Therapeutic Recreation Services to Community Mental Health Programs." *Therapeutic Recreation Journal*, First Quarter, 1969, pp. 19–20.

... the club provides opportunities for mental patients, discharged patients, and persons under psychiatric care to participate in social rehabilitation programs, recreation, and other activities. Through this means, they can make social contacts, reestablish social adequacy, reorient social status, regain lost skills, and restore lost self-confidence ... to make the gradual readjustment back into the mainstream of community life. . . .[40]

Education and Training Model

In institutions following the education and training model, various forms of activity therapy are used to overcome physical, psychological or social disability and to equip the client for independent community living. This approach is followed in a wide range of rehabilitation settings, including special schools for the mentally retarded, sheltered workshops, homes for the disturbed and penal centers.

Strong emphasis is placed on occupational therapy, remedial education, vocational training and similar modalities in order to improve the patient's skills, self-concept and social values. Individuals must learn a range of useful skills and interests and must develop favorable attitudes about taking part in them. Bizarre behavior or appearance that tends to repel others (as in the case of many mentally retarded individuals) must be overcome and healthy forms of self-management substituted. Patients and clients learn to seek out appropriate activities and facilities, often with the help of recreation therapists. Particularly in the case of the physically disabled, an important component of therapeutic recreation services lies in helping them learn to travel around the community to available recreational programs, events and facilities. In the case of such groups as the cerebral palsied, recreation may represent the area of service in which problems of human sexuality, courtship or family living are dealt with meaningfully, again as a means of helping the disabled enter as fully as possible into community life and realize their full potential as human beings (see Chapter 8).

Community Model

A flaw in several of the models just discussed is that they describe the role of recreation within the institution as one of preparing individuals to return to community life and fail to deal with the issue of the community's readiness to accept the disabled person. Realistically, patients are discharged from many institutions only to live in neighborhoods where there are *no* clubs, centers or special interest groups they can join on either a segregated or an integrated basis.

The community model, then, implies that a critical aspect of recreation service for the disabled lies in the provision of a wide range of leisure opportunities geared to meeting their needs. Essentially, these are provided by three types of sponsors:

---

[40]Jerry S. Hong and Ralston S. Bauer: "Have You a Halfway House Program?" *Parks and Recreation,* November 1966, p. 914.

(a) public recreation and park departments, (b) voluntary agencies with a specific concern for the disabled; and (c) therapeutic agencies or institutions that develop their own "out-reach" or "satellite" programs to serve outpatients or other disabled persons living in the community.

Multi-Focus Model

In general, none of the models just described exists completely independently of the others. Even most custodial institutions today provide some degree of education and training, and certainly the clinical-medical model has been markedly influenced in most settings by the therapeutic milieu approach. Probably the most accurate way of characterizing the present approach to therapeutic recreation service is in the National Therapeutic Recreation Society's 1982 philosophy statement, which identifies the three major elements of the field: *therapy, leisure education* and *recreational participation* (see p. 5).

This multi-focus model of therapeutic recreation service may be illustrated by (a) the varying roles of therapeutic recreation specialists and (b) the continuum approach to service, which encompasses several different types of experience in sequence.

MULTI-SERVICE ROLES OF SPECIALISTS

As Chapter 1 points out, therapeutic recreation specialists may play a wide variety of roles. Gunn and Peterson write,

---

Many professional therapeutic recreators work in acute treatment settings and function primarily as therapists. Other professionals work in residential, institutional, and community settings where their primary function is to teach leisure skills. Still other professionals work predominantly in community agencies where their primary function is to provide leisure opportunities for special populations. Quite often, a therapeutic recreator is required to perform all three functions in a given setting.[41]

In many situations, all three elements of service may be provided simultaneously within a given program. For example, in some institutions that do not deliberately emphasize recreation as therapy, activities nonetheless may be used to promote specific goals of group or individual treatment. Such programs also obviously have a leisure education value because they help to teach useful leisure skills and promote desirable values.

---

[41]Scout Lee Gunn and Carol Ann Peterson: *Therapeutic Recreation Program Design: Principles and Procedures.* Englewood Cliffs, New Jersey, Prentice-Hall, 1979, p. 14.

THERAPEUTIC RECREATION AS A CONTINUUM

This concept may be illustrated in three ways: (a) a description of the *sequence of settings* in which therapeutic recreation may be carried on; (b) an analysis of the principles of *progressive patient or client care*; and (c) an examination of the patients' *levels of involvement*.

Sequential Settings for Therapeutic Recreation. Today, every effort is made to prevent psychiatric hospitalization in the first place, through the dispersal of community mental health centers that can lead to early diagnosis of illness and the provision of special clinic services that can assist in keeping the patient functioning in the community. However, if this approach does not work and if the patient must be hospitalized because of an acute condition, the following sequence of settings for therapeutic recreation may be developed:

1. *Full Hospitalization.* While the patient is undergoing treatment on an inpatient basis, every effort is made to maintain contact with family and community groups through recreation programs. Outside organizations may provide parties, entertainments and similar programs. Patients themselves may move into the community on special trips and visits. At the same time, a process of recreation counseling is developed that helps the patient become aware of the role of recreation and leisure in his or her own life and develop a positive attitude—as well as knowledge and recreative skills—which the patient may use in the future.

2. *Partial Hospitalization.* Increasingly, instead of discharging patients directly from a custodial setting to complete freedom, the practice is developing of having them visit their homes for weekends or work during the day and return to the hospital at night. An important ingredient in this process is to have patients who are undergoing this process of gradual resocialization take part in community-based recreation activities and social programs. Hospital personnel working closely with community leaders may refer patients directly, assist them with transportation, brief the receiving agency about them and continue to assist them in a variety of ways.

3. *Post-discharge Arrangements.* In a number of communities, "halfway houses" or special social clubs have been provided for discharged mental patients or for those who are undergoing day-clinic treatment. In addition to other services, such as educational counseling or vocational training, such programs may offer a variety of recreational activities to ease the transition of the former patient to community life.

Similar sequences may be found in other types of disability groupings. Mentally retarded adolescents or young adults move from a special school or home, to a sheltered workshop or residence in the community, to full social independence. At each stage along the way, therapeutic recreation may be designed to meet the need for constructive leisure activity and to contribute to the individual's growing capability for community living.

Principles of Progressive Patient or Client Care. This concept is fundamental to medical treatment and the overall rehabilitation process. It implies that at each stage of a patient's illness and recovery (or a client's involvement in a community service agency), all aspects of the program are geared to providing maximum benefit appropriate to that stage and moving the individual along constructively to the next stage.

For example, in an early description of therapeutic recreation service in a military hospital for physically injured or orthopedic patients, service was provided in the following way:

1. *Post-operative and Post-traumatic Phase.* Here, the emphasis is placed on medical care, and on helping the patient make a healthy initial adjustment to the fact of his injury and the period of hospitalization that he must face. At this stage, the recreation specialist makes an early contact with the patient, and identifies interests that may be developed in the following stages.

2. *Traction Phase.* Here, the patient is confined to bed, and obviously limited in mobility, although not under intensive medical care. The emphasis is on providing individual attention to the patient, and helping him occupy his time creatively, by use of such activities as games, arts and crafts and other pursuits that may be carried on individually with limited mobility.

3. *Ambulatory Phase.* In this stage, the patient is able to move around the hospital and take part in varied activities of an individual interest, small-group, or mass nature. The effort here should be on reinforcing old interests and developing new ones that may be appropriate to the residual handicap left by the injury suffered — building on the strengths of the patient, and opening up new areas of recreational involvement for him.

4. *Disposition Phase.* Here, the emphasis is placed on providing experiences that will strengthen the patient's ability to meet his own recreation needs independently and to develop associations and community involvements that will carry over effectively following discharge from the hospital. It is at this stage that the recreation counseling process described earlier is most important.[42]

Mentally retarded clients in a community agency also need to go through a number of stages in order to become increasingly capable of functioning independently, making wise choices and playing meaningful roles in social groups.

Levels of Patient or Client Involvement. Closely related to this concept is the way in which patients and clients become involved in appropriate levels of activity or other forms of therapeutic recreation service. Within a continuum of service, how are such choices made?

It is often difficult for patients and clients to enter activities directly, partly because they may lack skills and confidence, and partly because they may have deeply ingrained negative attitudes about participation in leisure activities. The most obvious answer in most settings would be to *assign* an individual to a given activity or to a group which engages in specific activities. This is an obvious recourse in a hospital or other rehabilitation setting, where patients are regularly scheduled for occupational therapy, physical therapy and other required treatment services.

Prescribed Versus Voluntary Participation. When a patient is *required* to do something, the desirable elements of free choice, self-discovery and pleasure that true recreation should provide are missing. It is the subjective experience of the patient that is most important. As Haun points out, a ball game is not necessarily recreation,

[42]Staff of Oliver General Hospital: "We Prescribe Recreation." *Journal of Health, Physical Education and Recreation*, November 1951, pp. 12–13.

but the absorbed involvement of the patient is. Prescribing calisthenics, softball or dancing may simply result in patients undergoing exercise without receiving the values that should be derived from real recreational experience.

Often, however, it is not feasible to rely on a patient's self-motivation to bring him or her into participation. Streeter writes of the physically disabled individual,

It is terribly hard for seriously damaged people to reconcile themselves to their disabilities. Some of them spend months or years evading the issue by trying vainly to live as they did before their accident or illness. Families, struggling with their own feelings about a disabled patient, may drift away while he is in hospital. Permanent disability and long-term hospitalization often make for apathy and despair.... The complex pathology of the severely disabled, deeply troubled patient makes it specially urgent for him to take initiative and decide for himself what he wants to do.[43]

What solution is there for this dilemma? Obviously, in many cases it will be necessary for the recreation leader to play a strong role in encouraging such patients or clients to participate:

What is important is that, even when it is ''prescribed'' for a given patient, the activity should not be approached in a compulsory fashion. A patient may be introduced to the activity, encouraged to participate, and given help — but cannot be forced to take part — or it is no longer recreation. Thus, the recreation worker will need to be ingenious in his effort to motivate patients and (particularly with psychiatric patients, who often are extremely withdrawn and reluctant to take part in recreation) fairly strong in his efforts to persuade. In the final analysis, however, unless the patient comes to the point of selecting activities for participation voluntarily . . . the approach will not have been successful.[44]

This varied approach to "prescribed" versus "voluntary" participation is illustrated in the breakdown of recreation program activities found in Veterans' Administration hospitals. There, three major phases of recreation have traditionally been provided:

1. *General:* both active and passive services throughout the hospital, in the auditorium, recreation lounge, outdoor areas, dayrooms and on wards. Only a general clearance for these activities is required, usually obtained from the Chief of Staff and the chiefs of clinical services.
2. *Specialized:* activities designed to meet needs based on specific disabilities, particularly of long-

---

[43]George Streeter: "Art Studio: Therapy in an Institutional Setting." *Information Center, Recreation for the Handicapped Newsletter.* July-August 1971, p. 1.
[44]Richard Kraus: *Recreation Today: Program Planning and Leadership.* Santa Monica, California, Goodyear, 1977, p. 184.

term patients in groups. This phase of the program is developed by the cooperative efforts of the medical and recreation staff, usually with recreation workers being assigned to specific services and developing programs for them.

3. *Prescribed:* individualized services which may be provided for individual patients at the specific request of the patient's physician, based on his needs, progress, and past participation in recreation.[45]

To cite a specific example, in a large home for disturbed and dependent boys, recreational opportunities are provided on four levels: (1) *leisure education,* consisting of classes in recreational skills provided during the school day as part of the actual curriculum; (2) *after-school group activities,* in which cottages or units of boys take part as a group in activities scheduled for them on a rotating basis by the recreation staff and cottage parents or unit directors; (3) *individual selection of workshops,* in which each youngster takes part in activities such as music, arts and crafts or nature activities based on his own wishes and conferences with his counselors as well as unit team recommendations; and (4) *voluntary campus-wide participation,* consisting of voluntary involvement in school programs, teams, trips or special events. The principle underlying this structure is that each child needs all four elements: required instruction in skills, participation as part of his living-unit group, activities specially suited to his needs and interests and totally voluntary involvement (or noninvolvement, if he wishes) in community-wide programs.

In general, patients or clients should be helped to move along a continuum from outer-directed, involuntary participation to self-motivated, voluntary activity. In some situations, such as nursing homes, with many severely regressed residents who have suffered brain deterioration, it may not be possible for participants to exercise meaningful choices. Instead, it may be necessary for the therapeutic recreator to select and direct all activities for such patients.

RECREATION AS THERAPY

This question is related to the broader issue, described earlier, of whether recreation *should* be regarded as a form of therapy. It has two sub-elements: (a) whether recreation is *comparable* to other therapies and can justifiably be called a form of therapy; and (b) whether placing emphasis on recreation as therapy may not actually *diminish its value* for patients.

Obviously, regarding recreation as a form of therapy tends to give it a higher status, particularly in a medical setting. For this reason, many therapeutic recreation practitioners have sought vigorously to be accepted as therapists, comparable to occupational and physical therapists. On the other hand, some have argued that recreation, by definition, cannot be presented in a prescribed, required fashion.

---

[45]*Orientation Manual, Physical Medicine and Rehabilitation.* Washington, D.C., Veterans' Administration Department of Medicine and Surgery, March 1966.

Instead, it simply represents the use of an activity for therapy that is customarily performed purely as recreation.

Paul Haun has taken the position that when recreation is conceived of and presented as a therapy, it may lose some of its key benefits and, further, that it is *not* comparable to other medical techniques. He writes,

The hospital recreation worker performs many services essential, in my opinion, to the welfare of the patient. I cannot, however, regard any of them as therapeutic, first because I have never been convinced that recreation in any of its forms is a specific instrument for the modification of a disease process comparable say to penicillin in the treatment of syphilis; second, because I am so fully persuaded of the psychiatric patient's need for recreation *as recreation* that I grudge any dilution of its potency through adulteration with alternative purposes. . . . It is because I believe that recreation is an essential human need that I want it for my patients.[46]

On the other hand, an equally distinguished physician, Howard Rusk, has stated: "I firmly believe that both individual and group recreation for patients have a direct relationship upon recovery—these, in my opinion, are definitely adjunctive therapy."[47]

The distinction between recreation as therapy and recreation which is simply regarded as a morale booster or diversional service has been made by Parker and Downie:

. . . Recreation Therapy is considered a specific clinical service . . . It is an integral part of the treatment process, not just a means for entertaining or providing activities for patients following other treatment . . . It should be noted that the object of the activities used is not to teach skills, but rather to use the cognitive, affective, and sensory motor qualities inherent in each activity. This share of the treatment program is best characterized by the word ''therapy,'' not the word ''recreation.''[48]

When it is used in this way, recreation typically follows a sequence of several steps:

1. Assessment or diagnosis of patient or client's overall status, the nature and extent of disability, along with residual strengths and capabilities.
2. Identification of specific goals for therapeutic recreation as part of the total treatment plan, in combination with other therapies or rehabilitative experiences.

[46]Paul Haun: "Hospital Recreation—A Medical Viewpoint." In *Recreation for the Mentally Ill.* Washington, D.C., American Association for Health, Physical Education and Recreation, 1958, pp. 57–58.
[47]Howard Rusk: *Basic Concepts of Hospital Recreation.* Washington, D.C., American Recreation Society, 1953, p. 7.
[48]Robert Parker and Robert Downie: "Recreation Therapy: A Model for Consideration." *Therapeutic Recreation Journal,* Second Quarter, 1981, pp. 23–24.

3. Selection of appropriate activities or experiences designed to achieve these goals and to accomplish specific behavioral objectives. Adaptation or modification of activities where necessary.
4. Planning and implementation of programs involving these activities or experiences. This may involve several different levels of service simultaneously (see pp. 69–71) or planning of an appropriate sequence of different experiences, each building on those which have gone before.
5. On-going monitoring of the patient or client's participation and evaluation of the program's effectiveness.

Within this model, which is described more fully in Chapter 4, the actual selection of activities and experiences depends heavily on the goals and objectives that have been identified for the specific patient or client or for a specific category of participants. For example, a day camping program provided for mentally retarded children by Camp Spindrift, a project of the Recreation Center for the Handicapped in San Francisco, has the following objectives:

1. To provide fun in the out-of-doors.
2. To offer satisfying contacts with nature, so that the camper may acquire a sense of being at home in the out-of-doors.
3. To provide opportunities for group and individual experiences in a natural environment; to join and contribute to a plan of living for a day, a week, or more.
4. To foster the growth of independence and self-direction in each camper.
5. To acquire new skills, hobbies, and interests that have long-time values.
6. To arouse a sense of curiosity, stimulate spontaneous expression, provide enjoyment, and accelerate the learning process.
7. To provide opportunities for new experiences, for emotional satisfaction, and for spiritual growth.
8. To foster better mental and physical health, courage, and confidence and to exercise mind and body in healthful activity.
9. To offer a range of experiences that will help to prepare the campers for resident camping.
10. To provide opportunities for the development of initiative, leadership, and a sense of responsibility.[49]

It is apparent that these goals are identical to those that might be cited for *any* day camp program. However, in order to achieve them and to make the program meaningful to retarded children, it is necessary to provide a higher degree of skilled leadership, a better ratio of leaders to children, modification of program activities and a much more individualized approach to supervision than in normal programs. For retarded children, these program goals are vital and may contribute to the socialization, growing maturity and improving self-concept of the campers.

---

[49]*Report on Camp Spindrift*. San Francisco, Recreation Center for the Handicapped, Summer 1968, p. 22.

CONCLUDING STATEMENT OF GOALS
AND OBJECTIVES

In summing up the rationale presented in this chapter, the following general goals and specific objectives of therapeutic recreation service may be listed. It is obvious that they vary widely, depending upon the group being served, the nature and degree of disability and the setting in which the service is provided.

General Goals of Therapeutic Recreation

1. To provide constructive, enjoyable and creative leisure activities—a general need for persons of all ages and backgrounds.
2. To improve morale and a sense of well-being and interest in life, as opposed to depression, disinterest, or withdrawal.
3. To help individuals come to grips with their disabilities and build positively on their existing strengths and capabilities.
4. To help individuals gain security in being with others and develop healthy, outgoing social relationships and a feeling of group acceptance.
5. To emphasize positive self-concepts and feelings of individual worth, through successful participation in activity.
6. To help individuals gain both skills and attitudes that will assist them in using their leisure positively and constructively as opposed to negatively and pathologically.
7. To help hospitalized patients build bridges for the successful return to community life, or to help those clients who may be living in the community to function more independently.
8. To contribute to a sense of community and cooperation in institutions or other community residential settings and to promote an atmosphere which encourages progress toward recovery.

Specific Objectives of Therapeutic Recreation

The following list suggests a number of the high-priority objectives of recreation service for specific populations; they are explored in more detail in Chapters 5 through 9.

1. For disabled individuals living in the community, to provide activities and experiences that they can share with their families or that they can carry on independently, thus minimizing their dependence on their families.
2. For psychiatric patients, to provide a positive means of relating to others constructively, coming to grips with reality, expressing aggression or hostility harmlessly and gaining leisure interests that will contribute to their mental health.
3. For the mentally retarded, to promote physical, social and intellectual functioning, to assist in developing social independence, and to promote confidence and the ability to function in the community or at work.
4. For the physically disabled, to provide new skills and interests that compensate for lost

functions or abilities, to provide practice in self-care skills and to assist in reintegration in community recreation programs.

5. For the socially maladjusted, to assist in developing effective social relations with others, to use leisure constructively, to learn to accept the rules and values of society, and to encourage values of good sportsmanship and fair play.

6. For aged persons, to provide creative satisfactions, meaningful social involvement and the opportunity to be of community service.

For other special populations, similar sets of objectives geared to the needs of the particular group may easily be identified. In turn, each of these behavioral objectives may then be transformed into even more specific statements of desired outcomes. It is recognized that such statements tend to use terms which are somewhat diffuse in their meaning. For example, what *are* "healthy social relationships" or "constructive leisure attitudes"? These are value-laden terms which individuals may interpret differently according to age, social status or philosophy. Nonetheless, they are useful in defining the broad areas in which recreation may make an important contribution to the lives of the physically, mentally or socially disabled.

Suggested Topics for Class Discussion, Examination Questions or Student Papers

1. Outline the ways in which recreation is an important aspect of healthy living for all persons, emphasizing its relationship to work and to the modern concept of "wellness."

2. Present the arguments for and against considering recreation as a specific form of medically directed therapy, and take a position on this issue.

3. Briefly summarize the characteristics of three of the different models of therapeutic recreation service presented in this chapter, and show how they might apply to programming for a specific type of disability.

4. Discuss some of the problems affecting disabled individuals in society today, and show how recreation may contribute to their solution.

3

Professional Development in Therapeutic Recreation Service

Because of its rapid growth over the past three decades, therapeutic recreation has become an increasingly prominent specialization within the field of leisure services. Its practitioners have sought to increase its professional status, to improve the body of specialized knowledge on which it rests and to upgrade standards for educating and certifying therapeutic recreation specialists.

This chapter reviews the development of therapeutic recreation and describes the settings in which therapeutic recreation personnel are employed, as well as their job functions. It describes the past and present roles of professional organizations in therapeutic recreation, with special emphasis on current efforts to improve the selection process through registration, certification and licensing and on trends in higher education in the field. It explains the nature of other activity therapies whose personnel have close working relationships with recreation specialists and concludes with an appraisal of therapeutic recreation's present status as a profession.

EMPLOYMENT IN THERAPEUTIC RECREATION

Professional specialization in therapeutic recreation did not suddenly spring into being as an independent area of service. Instead, it developed gradually in a variety of settings. There have been four major stages in the development of therapeutic recreation service:

1. *General Responsibility*. During the early decades of this century, responsibility for supervising or providing recreation tended to be shared by corrective physical educators, occupational therapists, physical therapists, nurses, attendants and other ward personnel.

2. *Beginning Specialization*. Beginning in the 1930's but especially after World War II, some employees were assigned a *special* responsibility for recreation, and

were known as "hospital recreation workers," "medical recreation workers," or similar titles. They tended to be employed chiefly in large federal and state hospitals, particularly those concerned with mental illness or other long-term diseases. In some places they were called "recreation therapists."

3. *Recognition of the Field.* By the 1950's and 1960's there began to be a much wider use of recreation specialists in institutions serving special populations. These institutions included hospitals, homes and training schools for retarded or emotionally disturbed children and adolescents, centers for physical rehabilitation, nursing homes and, to a lesser degree, prisons. At the same time, the term "therapeutic recreation" became widely accepted. College and university training in this field was established.

4. *Extension to the Community.* In the middle and late 1960's therapeutic recreation service was extended to various community settings. This trend was based on three factors: (a) the recognition that hospitals and other residential institutions could do their job properly only if they were able to help discharged patients or clients make successful transitions into community life; (b) the fact that an increasing number of city and county recreation and park departments began to establish special programs for the disabled populations within their jurisdictions; and (c) the expanded role of voluntary agencies providing the blind, deaf or cerebral palsied with recreation, social activities and camping.

During the 1970's and early 1980's the emphasis was on developing a sound base of knowledge and more scientifically formulated professional practices. At the same time opportunities for higher education in therapeutic recreation expanded, research increased, national and state systems of credentialing practitioners were established and more rigorous approaches to evaluating programs and outcomes were developed.

GROWING NUMBERS OF PROFESSIONALS IN THE FIELD

As a consequence of these developments, the image of the professional therapeutic recreation specialists became more sharply defined and increasing numbers of them were employed in treatment centers and community agencies. Although there has been no definitive survey of the number of specialists in recreation service for the ill and disabled, several studies have examined a particular region or type of service.

For example, Phillips reported in 1958 on a study conducted by the National Recreation Association in psychiatric hospitals throughout the United States.[1] Organized recreation programs were found in 456 hospitals providing psychiatric services; approximately 2780 full-time personnel were employed to conduct recreation in these institutions.

A more extensive study of recreation personnel in hospitals was carried out by

---

[1]B. E. Phillips: *Recreation for the Mentally Ill.* Washington, D.C., Conference Report, American Association for Health, Physical Education and Recreation, 1958, p. 1.

Silson, Cohen and Hill in 1959.[2] It was found that in the 1486 hospitals of all types that had organized recreation programs throughout the nation, there were 5236 full-time recreation workers. There were sharply contrasting patterns of employment among different types of hospitals, however, and a considerable number that had no full-time recreation specialists. For example, while almost all Veterans' Administration and state hospitals had full-time employees with recreation titles, only a small percentage of municipal, county and voluntary hospitals had such employees.

A number of studies carried out in the 1960's and 1970's examined the scope of employment and need for qualified practitioners in specific states and provinces. As evidence of the growing numbers of therapeutic recreation workers in the United States, Kelley reported that in the early 1970's, over 800 full-time professionals were identified in the state of Illinois alone.[3] Illinois had about one twentieth of the population of the United States at that time. Assuming similar levels of service elsewhere, there were close to 16,000 therapeutic recreation workers in the entire country. Clearly, the number has grown dramatically in recent years. At the same time, the function and roles of therapeutic recreation specialists have become much more sharply defined.

EMERGING FUNCTIONS OF THERAPEUTIC RECREATION SPECIALISTS

In the late 1950's, Fred Chapman, professor of recreation at the University of Minnesota, analyzed the responsibilities of recreation workers in state, military, Veterans' Administration and private hospitals. The functions were grouped in three categories: *essential* duties, *highly desirable* duties and *desirable* duties.[4] Chapman found that administrative responsibilities (and even such duties as preparing reports, addressing student nurses, ordering supplies or attending professional meetings) were seen as *more* important than providing direct leadership for patient activity programs. This attitude may have reflected a desire by professionals working in medical settings to be seen primarily as therapists and directors of program service rather than as activity leaders, a somewhat less prestigious role. It may also indicate that full-time professional workers essentially *are* supervisors in many situations, with direct leadership carried out by part-time workers, aides or volunteers from the community.

In 1961 an influential statement on the changing functions of therapeutic recreation specialists was developed by the National Curriculum Conference on Ther-

---

[2]John E. Silson, Elliott M. Cohen and Beatrice H. Hill: *Recreation in Hospitals: Report of a Study of Organized Recreation Programs in Hospitals and the Personnel Conducting Them.* New York, National Recreation Association, 1959, pp. 35–39.

[3]Jerry D. Kelley: "A Status Report on Therapeutic Recreation in the State of Illinois." *Expanding Horizons in Therapeutic Recreation II.* Champaign-Urbana, University of Illinois Office of Recreation and Park Resources, 1974, pp. 55–56.

[4]Fred Chapman, survey findings summarized in B. E. Phillips: "Recreational Therapy: Duties of Hospital Recreation Personnel." *Journal of Health, Physical Education and Recreation,* April 1957, p. 60.

apeutic Recreation.[5] Important roles included the following: (a) supervising and administering recreation services; (b) counseling the ill and disabled; (c) providing consultation service for community groups and institutions; (d) interpreting therapeutic recreation to the community and to other professional disciplines; and (e) promoting understanding of the need for expanded community services for the disabled and helping such programs become established.

During the 1960's, in many treatment settings, less emphasis was given to the therapeutic recreation specialist's supervisory functions and more emphasis to his or her serving as a therapeutic agent.

Simon described the concept of "therapeutic use of self":

. . . The hospital must offer a controlled milieu in which the transferences of the patient may be expressed. Psychodynamics teaches us that these transferences are repetitions of relationships which existed in the early life of the individual. It would seem, therefore, that the hospital should present a model of the outside world in which the transference could take place and corrective emotional experiences come about — that the essential difference between the mental hospital and the community should be the presence of personnel trained to understand the patient's reactions and to use themselves therapeutically. In this atmosphere there should exist replicas of all the activities normally experienced by the patient in his community. Whatever the size or structure of the hospital, it should offer the equivalent, in as nearly a similar form as possible, of home and community. This . . . involves basic functions of living, eating and sleeping. . . . Everything is oriented, ultimately, toward re-establishment in the external world.[6]

This approach had considerable influence on the way many recreation personnel functioned, particularly in psychiatric institutions. It also influenced other treatment centers that were concerned with behavioral change, such as special schools for the emotionally disturbed, alcohol or drug rehabilitation centers and correctional institutions. In general, however, formal statements of the functions of therapeutic recreation specialists have not attempted to encompass this "therapeutic use of self" approach. Instead, they tend to describe the more clearly identifiable functions. This is particularly true of job descriptions, as illustrated in the following statement used by the San Francisco Recreation Center for the Handicapped.

Example of Job Description

General Responsibilities

1. Plans, initiates, organizes and supervises an extensive program of recreation activities for an assigned group of mentally retarded and handicapped children, teens or adults.
2. Supervises, trains and evaluates recreation leaders and volunteers in the use of activities for the mentally retarded and handicapped.

---

[5]*Report of Therapeutic Recreation Development Conference.* Sponsored by National Recreation Association's Consulting Service on Recreation for the Ill and Disabled. New York, Comeback, Inc., 1961.
[6]Benjamin Simon: "The New Trends in Rehabilitation." *Recreation's Contribution to the Patient.* North Carolina Recreation Commission, September 1963, p. 11.

3. Incorporates recreation for the retarded and handicapped into an acceptable total philosophy of recreation, and interprets this philosophy to participants, leaders and the public.
4. Consults with the Center Director and with other professional staff members on the place of recreation for the retarded and handicapped in relation to the total recreation program, the program in various segments of the community, and other specialized activity programs.
5. Seeks new programming ideas and adapts them for use in the recreation program for the mentally retarded and handicapped, and sees that they are carried out with appropriate groups.
6. Investigates, recommends, demonstrates, and explains techniques, procedures, adaptations, materials, equipment and supplies for use in the program.
7. Participates in inter-agency planning, research and training, as consultant, leader, or center representative.
8. Serves as community recreation consultant, and interprets recreation and the program for the handicapped and mentally retarded to the general public as well as to interested groups and organizations.
9. Cooperates in promoting, organizing, and directing community-wide programs and events.
10. Prepares instructional materials, budget estimates, and work programs, for assigned groups.[7]

Competency-Based Analysis of Therapeutic Recreation Functions

Still another approach to identifying specific professional functions in therapeutic recreation service has relied on the competency-based approach. With this method, roles and specific tasks performed by professionals are identified, as well as the knowledge and skills required to carry them out. A Temple University study of competencies needed by professionals holding a master's degree in therapeutic recreation identified 30 essential competencies within five major domains of responsibility[8]:

I. Management
1. Ability to formulate a department philosophy of therapeutic recreation which is consistent with the philosophies of agencies providing a therapeutic recreation program.
2. Ability to develop departmental policies and procedures which incorporate the department's philosophy, and which detail how the department will function in providing its recreation service within the structure of an agency.
3. Ability to hire staff through proper utilization of personnel practices and procedures.
4. Ability to prepare, present, and defend an adequate budget for a therapeutic recreation program.
5. Ability to organize and prepare routine reports required by agencies.
6. Ability to participate appropriately and effectively in administrative meetings.
7. Ability to identify funding sources and to develop, write, and submit proposals for grants.

[7] *Staff Manual.* San Francisco Recreation Center for the Handicapped, 1974.
[8] See *Bureau of Education for the Handicapped Project Update.* Report of Department of Recreation and Leisure Studies, Temple University, Philadelphia, February 1980.

8. Ability to utilize public relations to enhance therapeutic recreation programs.
9. Ability to facilitate and promote inter-agency coordination.
10. Ability to provide consultation services.

II. Supervision
11. Ability to effectively supervise staff.
12. Ability to effectively supervise practicum fieldwork students.
13. Ability to effectively utilize and supervise volunteers.

III. Staff Training
14. Ability to identify individual and group training needs of staff and volunteers.
15. Ability to develop learning objectives from identified training needs.
16. Ability to identify and develop training activities to meet specified learning objectives.
17. Ability to evaluate the cost and effectiveness of training programs.

IV. Programming
18. Ability to develop and implement a basic recreation program that incorporates currently accepted recreation principles and goals.
19. Ability to retrieve, interpret, and apply current research to recreation program development.
20. Ability to plan and conduct program evaluation.
21. Ability to organize, service, and maintain equipment and supplies.
22. Ability to function effectively as a member of a treatment team.
23. Ability to assess a client's functional level as a basis for his/her involvement in therapeutic recreation services.
24. Ability to develop treatment plans for clients.
25. Ability to analyze activities to determine their functional elements and potential therapeutic value for clients.
26. Ability to plan and conduct therapeutic recreation activities to meet individual client needs and treatment objectives.
27. Ability to write clinical reports and records concerning clients and their involvement in therapeutic recreation services.
28. Ability to provide leisure counseling services for clients.
29. Ability to implement and maximize integration of clients into the community.

V. Research
30. Ability to plan, conduct, and report research.

In addition to those summarized here, several other studies of job functions of therapeutic recreation personnel are presented in Chapter 12.

PROFESSIONAL AND SERVICE ORGANIZATIONS IN THERAPEUTIC RECREATION

An integral part of the growing professionalization of therapeutic recreation has been the contribution made by professional and service organizations in promoting public awareness of this field, strengthening practices, improving curricula in higher education and developing standards for the selection of personnel. Brief descriptions of several of the most influential organizations follow.

Hospital Section, American Recreation Society

This organization was formed in 1948 in Omaha, Nebraska. It promoted hospital recreation programs in a variety of ways, by (a) sponsoring meetings on therapeutic recreation at the annual National Recreation Congress; (b) pressing for improved standards of training and selection through its Standards and Training Committee; (c) advocating or sponsoring national or regional conferences on hospital recreation, either independently or in cooperation with other organizations; and (d) developing effective relationships with other organizations in the fields of rehabilitation or recreation.

Recreational Therapy Section, American Association for Health, Physical Education and Recreation

This section of the overall organization in the United States serving health, physical education and recreation was formed in 1952 in Los Angeles, California. The Recreation Division of the American Association for Health, Physical Education and Recreation (a department of the National Education Association) had included three sections: *public recreation, voluntary and youth-serving agencies* and *industrial recreation.*

The third one was divided in April 1952 into two autonomous sections: *industrial recreation* and *recreational therapy.* Members of the latter section tended to be more interested in special schools or in adapted physical education programs than in hospital-based recreational therapy. However, the section cooperated closely with other professional groups and, because of its association with colleges and universities that prepared recreation majors, made an important contribution to the field. It also was active in developing conferences, stimulating research and attempting to improve professional standards.

National Association of Recreation Therapists

This organization was founded in 1953. Its initial membership consisted primarily of recreation therapists employed in state hospitals and schools, particularly in the southern and midwestern states. Although many were members of the American Recreation Society, they wished to develop a stronger professional focus on the role of the recreation therapist than was possible in that organization. This group worked closely with other organizations in promoting conferences, research and other action related to therapeutic recreation service. It published a quarterly journal, *Recreation for the Ill and Handicapped.*

Consulting Service on Recreation for the Ill and Handicapped, National Recreation Association

The National Recreation Association did not have a separate branch concerned with therapeutic recreation, but beginning in 1953 it employed consultants who worked with hospitals and other agencies. The National Recreation Association's monthly magazine, *Recreation*, regularly contained a column, "Hospital Capsules," and the organization itself was represented in many professional meetings and conferences.

Council for the Advancement of Hospital Recreation

The membership of these four organizations realized there was a strong need for more effective evaluation of hospital recreation programs and an upgrading of personnel standards as well as a system of certification that might enforce such standards. To meet this need, in November 1953 they formed the group that became known as the Council for the Advancement of Hospital Recreation. The Council was to register qualified practitioners, develop standards for training and clinical practice and promote communication among the other organizations in this field. In 1956, the Council officially adopted personnel standards for hospital recreation director, leader and aide positions and set out to promote a registration system for identifying those in the field who met these requirements. It also attempted to upgrade and improve the overall field of therapeutic recreation and to develop a merger of the existing organizations in this field.

National Therapeutic Recreation Society

Beatrice Hill, formerly a consultant with the National Recreation Association, formed an organization called Comeback, Inc., that was designed to promote professional therapeutic recreation service. However, this was not to be accomplished until the separate organizations representing the field agreed to merge late in 1965, forming the National Recreation and Park Association (NRPA). This organization established a number of separate branches to represent the varied interests of its members. One of these, the National Therapeutic Recreation Society, absorbed the existing organizations concerned with recreation for the ill and disabled and has functioned effectively in this area since that time.

The National Therapeutic Recreation Society has been influential in welding together the separate factions that provide recreation for the ill and disabled. It has also helped define their roles within the spectrum of social and rehabilitative services.

Many of the professions that have become most respected in modern society originally came into being as a result of "social movements." These movements are a response to social problems which can best be dealt with in an organized way. Groups concerned with their solution join together to form a "profession."

Generally, it is assumed that a profession has a hierarchy of identified leadership, a shared body of knowledge, a regular group applying that knowledge to an identified clientele, a system to suport and share knowledge and research, an ongoing training mechanism for the apprentice (usually in universities), recognition and acceptance by other groups (such as other established professions), accepted standards for practitioners and recognition in law through legal certification of the novice (for example, bar exams), and finally, regulative methods and standards with the force of law (disbarment in the case of lawyers).[9]

Usually, the process of combining the separate groups in a given field into a single strong organization is complex and extends over a long period. However, in most cases, a consistent ideology and a vigorous national organization determine whether or not a social movement becomes a profession.

During the first 12 years of the National Therapeutic Recreation Society (NTRS) the organization's primary task was to organize a heterogeneous group of recreators who shared a common ideology: that recreation can be a therapeutic force in the lives of special populations. Specifically, NTRS has made important progress in the following areas:

It has identifed leadership on the national level and provided a forum for potential leaders in the field to make their views known.

It has promoted research in order to produce a systematic body of knowledge and has worked closely with other health-related professions to improve attitudes toward the disabled and to gain support for programs serving them.

It has promoted growth in the field through federal support, university curricula and an enlarged group of practitioners.

It has identified new issues and concerns consistent with the evolving body of theory on therapeutic recreation service and has acted as mediator in the resolution of confusion or disagreement when these have arisen.[10]

One of the key functions of NTRS has been to promote professional development by sponsoring or co-sponsoring conferences and by developing programs and special institutes for the annual National Recreation Congress. For example, it cooperated in the early 1970's in the co-sponsorship of professional conferences on activity therapy with the Joint Commission on Accreditation of Hospitals, the Accreditation Council for Psychiatric Facilities and other organizations representing occupational, music, dance and art therapy and mental centers and psychiatric services for children. At various National Congresses, it has provided pre-Congress Institutes devoted to such themes as the following:

---

[9]"National Therapeutic Recreation Society: The First 12 Years." *Therapeutic Recreation Journal*, Third Quarter, 1978, p. 4.
[10]*Ibid.*, pp. 5–11.

"Programs and Standards for Nursing Homes"
"Psychodrama in Activities Programs"
"Comprehensive Programming for Emotionally Disturbed Children"
"Federal Supports for Therapeutic Recreation"
"Recreation Counseling for the Ill and Disabled"
"Therapeutic Recreation in Correctional Institutions"
"Planning Community Facilities for the Ill and Disabled"
"Recreation Services for Drug Abusers"

The National Therapeutic Recreation Society has appointed official delegates to represent members' views at important national meetings. It has conducted district workshops to develop guidelines for the recruitment, training and employment of disabled individuals in the recreation and park field and has sponsored research efforts with the financial assistance of federal agencies. In addition, it has published the quarterly *Therapeutic Recreation Journal,* which today acts as the spokesman for this united field.

An important function of the National Therapeutic Recreation Society has been to influence government policy and promote improved public awareness of the field. It has done this by vigorously presenting its views before government officials and committees and by pressing for support of special projects serving the ill and disabled. For example, an NTRS special task force on recreation in corrections, chaired by Carroll Hormachea of Virginia Commonwealth University, has fought energetically, through publications, conferences, position statements and similar efforts, to promote a fuller use of recreation as a vital aspect of rehabilitation in penal institutions in the United States.

A recent NTRS president, Carol Peterson, reviewed the society's accomplishments: (a) lobbying to block federal cutbacks in funding programs for special populations; (b) publishing new standards for the practice of therapeutic recreation service; (c) publicizing the International Year of Disabled Persons and cooperating with other organizations on the project; (d) developing a stronger liaison with the Joint Commission on Accreditation of Hospitals; (d) forming a Joint Committee on Community Recreation for Disabled Persons with the American Park and Recreation Society and holding a national forum on this subject; and (e) promoting efforts to gain support for "third-party payments" (reimbursement for therapeutic recreation in treatment settings comparable to that for other therapies and services).[11] Perhaps the strongest efforts of NTRS throughout its existence have been in upgrading standards of selection and hiring.

REGISTRATION, CERTIFICATION AND LICENSING

These three processes represent methods of screening qualified personnel for employment in a given professional field. *Registration* usually refers to the process

---

[11]Carol Ann Peterson: *Report of the President to the Membership and Board of the National Therapeutic Recreation Society,* Annual Meeting, Minneapolis, October 1981.

through which a professional society establishes a series of qualifications for job titles and screens individuals to determine if they have the stipulated qualifications. Those approved are then placed on a list, in this case of registered therapists (see p. 87). In contrast to registration, which involves voluntary compliance by hiring agencies, *licensing* is a legal process through which a government agency screens qualifications and grants approval to persons to engage in certain occupations or professions. Just as one must have a license to drive a car, so one must have a license to practice in such fields. The term *certification* tends to be used ambiguously. In some cases, it is used synonymously with registration. In other health-related or educational fields, certification is established by state law, and all public hiring agencies must comply with its regulations, just as in licensing.

The National Therapeutic Recreation Society maintains a voluntary registration plan that defines standards for various professional levels based chiefly on education and professional experience. A review board assesses qualifications for registration at each level and issues certificates to qualified individuals.

Over the past ten years, support for registration has continued to grow. Approximately 3,000 practitioners were registered by the end of the 1970's. The standards themselves, and the specific job categories they cover, have been revised several times. For a number of years, they included six categories: (a) Therapeutic Recreation Assistant; (b) Therapeutic Recreation Technician I; (c) Therapeutic Recreation Technician II; (d) Therapeutic Recreation Leader; (e) Therapeutic Recreation Specialist; and (f) Master Therapeutic Recreation Specialist.

In October 1981, the Registration Board of NTRS, which has been responsible for issuing credentials since 1967, was formally disbanded. Its functions were transferred to the National Council for Therapeutic Recreation Certification, an independently administered body of the National Recreation and Park Association.

The purposes of the National Council are as follows:

1. To establish national standards for the certification and recertification of individuals who attest to the competencies of the therapeutic recreation profession.
2. To grant recognition to individuals who voluntarily apply and meet the established standards.
3. To monitor adherence to the standards by personnel who have been certified.

It was agreed that individuals who had been registered under the NTRS Voluntary Registration Program would be transferred automatically to certification under the National Council's program. Also, it was agreed that the six existing levels of service would be grouped under a new two-level system: professional (Therapeutic Recreation Specialist) and para-professional (Therapeutic Recreation Assistant).[12]

---

[12]Marcia Jean Carter: "Registration of Therapeutic Recreators: Standards from 1956 to Present." *Therapeutic Recreation Journal,* Second Quarter, 1981, pp. 17–22.

**Certification Standards for Therapeutic
Recreation Personnel**

The 1981 standards for therapeutic recreation personnel are as follows:

Professional Level

I. Therapeutic Recreation Specialist

A. Baccalaureate degree or higher from an accredited college or university with a major in therapeutic recreation or a major in recreation and an *option** in therapeutic recreation. Degree must be verified by an official transcript; student copy not acceptable.

OR

B. Baccalaureate degree or higher from an accredited college or university with a major in recreation *and* two years full-time paid experience in a clinical, residential, or community-based therapeutic recreation program. Degree must be verified by an official transcript; student copy not acceptable.

OR

Provisional Nonrenewable

C. Baccalaureate degree or higher from an accredited college or university with a major in recreation. Degree must be verified by an official transcript; student copy not acceptable. (This alternative permits temporary registration while one acquires the two years of full-time paid experience in a clinical, residential or community-based therapeutic recreation program necessary for renewal of registration as a professional.)

OR

Equivalency Process

D. Baccalaureate degree or higher from an accredited college/university in one of the recreation related or allied health fields *plus* five years of full-time paid experience in a clinical, residential or community-based therapeutic recreation program plus 18 semester or 27 quarter hours of upper division credits in the competencies, identified in the NRPA-AALR Council on Accreditation standards for a professional specialization in therapeutic recreation. Degree must be verified by an official transcript; student copy not acceptable.

Para-professional Level

II. Therapeutic Recreation Assistant

A. Associate of Arts degree from an accredited educational institution with a major in therapeutic recreation or a major in recreation and an *option*** in therapeutic recreation. Degree must be verified by an official transcript; student copy not acceptable.

OR

B. Associate of Arts degree from an accredited educational institution with a major in recreation *plus* one year full-time paid experience in a clinical, residential, or community-based therapeutic recreation program. Degree must be verified by an official transcript; student copy not acceptable.

OR

C. Associate of Arts degree or higher from an accredited educational institution with a major in one of the skill areas (arts, crafts, dance, drama, music, physical education) and one year full-time paid experience in a clinical, residential or community-based therapeutic recreation program. Degree must be verified by an official transcript; student copy not acceptable.

OR

D. Completion of the NTRS 750-Hour Training Program for therapeutic recreation personnel verified by an official certificate of completion.

OR

E. Four years of full-time paid experience in a clinical, residential, or community-based therapeutic recreation program.

*Professional Option

Professional Option is defined to include:

a. a minimum of three courses exclusively dealing with therapeutic recreation content.
b. completion of a field placement experience in a clinical, residential, or community-based therapeutic recreation program which complies with the NTRS Field Placement Guidelines.
c. completion of supportive coursework to include a minimum of 18 semester or 27 quarter units from four of the sixteen areas listed below:

psychology
sociology
physical/biological sciences
special education
human services
adapted physical education

**Para-professional Option

Para-Professional option is defined to include:

a. a minimum of two courses exclusively dealing with therapeutic recreation content.
b. completion of a field placement experience in a clinical, residential, or community-based therapeutic recreation program which complies with the NTRS Field Placement Guidelines.
c. completion of supportive coursework to include a minimum of 12 semester or 18 quarter units selected from psychology, sociology, physical/biological sciences, human services, physical education activity classes.

Note: A major in recreation is identified by the competencies for general education, professional education and professional emphasis of the NPRA-AALR Council on Accreditation.

Despite these efforts, uniform hiring standards have not yet been applied to most practitioners. In part, this is because there is such a diversity of employing agencies that it would be almost impossible to devise any system of certification or licensing that would apply to all positions and be readily enforceable. It also reflects the situation of the overall recreation and park field; certification has been approved in only a few states and Civil Service hiring requirements are generally quite flexible. But there have been increasing efforts, particularly on state levels, to put teeth into the credentialing process.

State Society Standards

In addition to the registration program of the National Therapeutic Recreation Society, a number of state recreation and park societies have developed their own registration plans. For example, the California Board of Parks and Recreation Personnel established a general program of registration for recreation and park professionals in 1955; in 1970, special registration requirements were established for recreation therapists. With guidance from the Therapeutic Section of the California Park and Recreation Society, these requirements have been modified and strengthened. By 1975 they included

---

A baccalaureate or graduate degree with specialization in Therapeutic Recreation, including 18 semester hours in upper-division courses in areas such as psychology, sociology, or the physical and biological sciences. Specific course requirements in aspects of disability, and a survey of recreation for the ill and handicapped, as well as 400 hours of supervised field work, were instituted, accompanied by a special examination administered by the California Board of Parks and Recreation Personnel.[13]

In addition, the Therapeutic Section of the California Park and Recreation Society voted to endorse legislation calling for licensing of therapeutic recreation specialists. The Society succeeded in having therapeutic recreation made part of a bill to certify occupational therapists, but it was vetoed by the state governor. Now, members of the state society are striving to achieve a separate status for their own discipline. Lawrence describes this growing effort in California as "a new maturity in the profession, a political coming of age," pointing out that

---

It represented a realization that existing federal and state laws appear to favor licensed health professionals and that medical insurance and reimbursement through use of public funds tends more and more to cover those services offered to consumers by state certified or licensed professionals. . . . (according to the) HEW Report on Licensure and Related Health Personnel Credentialing: "Under present statutes and regulations when a health profession is licensed by a state, federal health insurance programs typically link qualification for reimbursement to state licensure requirements."[14]

The only state to have approved formal licensing in therapeutic recreation is Utah; it passed a "Recreational Therapy Practice Act" (H.B. No. 361, 1975) outlining requirements for several levels of therapeutic recreation service, with statements of purpose, definitions, exemptions, basis for license suspension or revocation and examples of unauthorized or unlawful practice. This pioneer licensing law has been extremely effective. According to Clark Thorstenson of Brigham Young University, it has had a positive effect on employment opportunities for professionals in Utah:

---

[13]Patricia J. Lawrence: *Position Statement of AB4428 to Include Recreation Therapists.* Legislative Recommendations to Certify Recreation Therapists, to Therapeutic Recreation Section and Board of Directors, California Park and Recreation Society, 1976, p. 1.
[14]Patricia J. Lawrence: *Certification: The Time Is Now.* Report of Therapeutic Section to California Park and Recreation Society, 1976, p. 1.

We have had excellent cooperation from all agencies who have been involved with therapeutic recreation and we have successfully encouraged them to hire only those who are trained in the field . . . we have many more positions in therapeutic recreation than we are able to fill because of lack of (qualified) students. An additional benefit is that those who are licensed have often had an increase in salary. . . . We feel, in general, our image as a profession is increasing and we are much more unified as a group than we previously were.[15]

Obviously, all such efforts to upgrade the profession are heavily dependent on the training provided by college and university programs in therapeutic recreation service. Before describing these in detail, however, it should be noted that, in addition to the National Therapeutic Recreation Society, a number of other national organizations have promoted the overall rehabilitation movement and, through joint projects, have cooperated with therapeutic recreation specialists: the American National Red Cross, American Occupational Therapy Association, American Physical Therapy Association, Association for Physical and Mental Rehabilitation, National Association for Music Therapy, American Association of Rehabilitation Therapists, American Art Therapy Association, American Dance Therapy Association and the National Association of State Activity Therapy and Rehabilitation Program Directors.

Role of AAHPERD and AALR

In particular, the American Association for Health, Physical Education and Recreation (now known as the American Alliance for Health, Physical Education, Recreation and Dance or AAHPERD) has been active in promoting recreation services in general, leisure education and adapted physical education and recreation for the disabled. The Alliance has sponsored conferences and curriculum development task forces, published literature and encouraged research and demonstration projects. One of its most important contributions has been the Information and Research Utilization Center on Physical Education and Recreation for the Handicapped, a comprehensive center providing information, referral service and other forms of assistance. This project was supported for three years in the mid-1970's by the U.S. Department of Health, Education and Welfare's Bureau of Education for the Handicapped as a special demonstration project under the direction of Julian U. Stein, with follow-up grants extending into the late 1970's and early 1980's.

The branch of AAHPERD most concerned with recreation is the American Association for Leisure and Recreation, which has done much to promote professional development in camping and outdoor education, education for leisure, leisure research and various forms of professional recreation service.

---

[15]Clark T. Thorstenson, personal communication, March 11, 1977.

PROFESSIONAL EDUCATION IN
THERAPEUTIC RECREATION SERVICE

The development of special courses in therapeutic recreation did not get fully under way until after World War II. In August 1953, the Standards and Training Committee of the Hospital Recreation Section of the American Recreation Society reported that of the 44 colleges and universities that offered degrees in recreation, only six had graduate or undergraduate degrees in "hospital" recreation. These were Teachers College of Columbia University, New York University, Springfield College, the University of Minnesota, Purdue University and Sacramento State College.

An important step in developing educational opportunities was the 1961 conference on graduate curricula in therapeutic recreation sponsored by the National Recreation Association's Consulting Service on Recreation for the Ill and Handicapped. At this meeting, leading recreation educators and practitioners sought to identify the changing competencies required of specialists in therapeutic recreation and to suggest curriculum models based on these competencies. A number of recommendations were made, chiefly that professional practitioners required graduate education emphasizing mastery of medical and psychiatric terms and the ability to adapt activities for the ill and disabled. It was agreed that graduate students should be trained to meet new demands that went beyond the traditional function of providing activities, such as training personnel, providing consultation services, interpreting the field to the community and to other disciplines and developing strong links to community agencies.

During the 1960's, as the rapid growth in therapeutic recreation programs created a shortage of qualified personnel and as interest grew in this field, the number of colleges and universities offering programs in therapeutic recreation rose steadily. In 1969, the Society of Park and Recreation Educators carried out a study of recreation curricula in the United States that revealed that of 114 institutions with a recreation program, 35 offered a major in therapeutic recreation service. The largest number of programs were in the Great Lakes and Southwest Pacific regions.

By 1975, as a result of increasing interest in professional recreation service in general, the number of colleges and universities in the United States and Canada offering undergraduate and graduate degree programs in this overall field had increased to 345. The third largest area of specialization was therapeutic recreation, with 95 institutions offering degrees. This rapid growth reflected, in part, increasing interest on the part of Canadian colleges and universities. Until comparatively recently, there were few Canadian college or university programs in recreation. Many Canadian therapeutic recreation specialists were receiving their training at such institutions as the University of Illinois or the University of Indiana. Within the past several years, however, a substantial number of Canadian colleges and universities have initiated programs in therapeutic recreation, particularly on the two-year and baccalaureate levels.

A unique development in Canadian recreation education has been the program developed by Aiden Spiller at Fanshawe College, London, Ontario, and documented in his doctoral thesis at the University of Toronto. It is a competency-based in-service program for employed practitioners, with emphasis on a self-directed, tutorial learning process in small instructional groups. Another outstanding recreation education program is the cooperative work-study plan developed at the University of Waterloo; after their first two semesters, students alternate four months of a recreation work placement with four months of academic study. Many field placements are made in therapeutic recreation agencies cooperating with the University of Waterloo.

1980 Report on Therapeutic Recreation Curricula

In a 1980 study of 173 higher education curricula in therapeutic recreation, Stephen Anderson and Morris Stewart examined several aspects of the programs: their titles, types, administrative locations, distribution within regions and the special populations they addressed on both undergraduate and graduate levels.[16] In general, they found that such programs had expanded dramatically during the previous decade and had shifted away from the traditional umbrella of health, physical education and recreation. However, they also concluded that the curricula had expanded faster than the number of well-qualified faculty members and that there was a need to examine the quality and effectiveness of degree programs in therapeutic recreation service.

Courses Offered in Therapeutic Recreation Curricula

A number of studies have examined the specific courses offered in therapeutic recreation in the United States and Canada. In 1970, Donald Lindley examined the courses offered by selected institutions and their relative importance as rated by college educators and practitioners in the field.[17] In an initial study of 30 colleges and universities offering therapeutic recreation curricula, he found that courses tended to be grouped in nine major areas: (a) communication arts–public relations; (b) community institutions and organizations; (c) social science and psychology; (d) medical and psychiatric information; (e) recreation philosophy; (f) recreation administration; (g) recreation programs; (h) evaluation and research; and (i) clinical experience.

On the *undergraduate* level, the most valuable courses were rated in order of importance as follows: field work, introduction to therapeutic recreation, philosophy of recreation, social psychology, community organization in recreation, small group dynamics, foundations of recreation, internship, programming in therapeutic recreation and methods of recreation leadership. Courses dealing with other rehabilitation services, psychiatric and medical information or program elements for specific disabilities fell far below the first ten.

---

[16]Stephen C. Anderson and Morris W. Stewart: "Therapeutic Recreation Education, 1979 Survey." *Therapeutic Recreation Journal*, Third Quarter, 1980, pp. 4–10.
[17]Donald Lindley: "Relative Import of College Courses in Therapeutic Recreation." *Therapeutic Recreation Journal*, Second Quarter, 1970, pp. 8–12.

On the *graduate* level, the most valuable courses, in rank order of importance, were research methods, readings in therapeutic recreation, psychological aspects of disability, readings in recreation, research seminars, professional seminars, psychiatric and medical information and administration in therapeutic recreation.

The actual development of therapeutic recreation curricula has been influenced by the recommendations of task forces established by professional organizations, by federally funded projects intended to develop superior models of professional preparation and by the guidelines for accreditation prepared by the National Recreation and Park Association and the National Therapeutic Recreation Society.

For example, in 1973 the Information and Research Utilization Center (IRUC) in Physical Education and Recreation for the Handicapped, a special service unit of the American Association for Health, Physical Education and Recreation, published a set of guidelines for college and university curricula in physical education and recreation serving special populations. Funded by the Bureau of Education for the Handicapped of the U.S. Department of Health, Education and Welfare, this publication provided a rationale for therapeutic recreation service, identified roles of practitioners and outlined needed competencies for professionals.

Similarly, beginning in the early 1970's the Bureau of Education for the Handicapped gave substantial support to a number of colleges and universities providing professional education in physical education and recreation for the disabled under Public Law 91–230, Title VI, Education of the Handicapped. Eight grants were solely or predominantly recreation oriented and supported master's level or doctoral programs at the University of Illinois, University of Oregon, University of Kentucky, New York University, San Jose State College, North Carolina Central University, Pennsylvania State University and the University of North Carolina. In general, these grants were intended to improve the quality of professional preparation and to help create a pool of high-quality personnel for upper-level positions as administrators, consultants, researchers or educators in therapeutic recreation.

Emphasis on Accountability and Documentation

Within recent years, strong emphasis has been given to the preparation of therapeutic recreation specialists as fully functioning members of the treatment team. Particularly for practitioners functioning in clinical settings, Jewell points out that it is essential that they have skills in clinical writing, activity analysis, patient assessment, prescriptive programming and treatment plan review. In order to document program outcomes, he writes,

---

The therapeutic recreator must have the necessary writing skills to effectively communicate to his fellow treatment staff and to any eventual consumer of the clinical record, the objectives, procedures and results of patient involvement. Specifically, he must be capable of communicating the who, how, when, where, and why for each individual patient involved in his program.[18]

---

[18]David L. Jewell: "Documentation: Shibboleth for Professionals." *Therapeutic Recreation Journal*, First Quarter, 1980, pp. 23–24.

Increasingly, such areas of expertise have been given high priority in therapeutic recreation curricula and in workshops and in-service education programs sponsored by national, regional and state or provincial societies in the United States and Canada.

Community College Curricula

The steady growth in two-year, community college programs stemmed from two basic sources: an awareness of the shortage of trained personnel in the field during the late 1960's and early 1970's, and the general expansion of community college programs in the United States and Canada, many of which sought to prepare young people for positions in the health services or other technically oriented fields. At an early point, Hutchinson described the rationale for such programs:

Those students entering junior (community) colleges who seek a terminal education at the end of two years should be given the opportunity to prepare themselves as assistants in therapeutic recreation settings. A two-year course could develop some to become valuable technicians who, under professional supervision, could contribute much to the recreation program. The functional roles which seem appropriate for them are: movie projector operators and visual aids experts; radio operators, and/or television repairmen; games rooms operators; designers of posters, notices, and other visual materials; organizers of outings, picnics and camp trips; storeroom and equipment attendants; and program assistants.[19]

Despite the original conception of community college programs as terminal, two trends have developed among many community college graduates:

1. Those who found employment tended to move into leadership or supervisory roles rather than be restricted to the kinds of limited tasks described by Hutchinson. Thus, they represented a threat to those already in the profession, who felt that opening up to community college graduates jobs that had formerly required a bachelor's degree represented a lowering of professional standards.

2. The great number of positions expected to materialize for two-year graduates did not appear, and promotional opportunities were sharply limited. Thus, most community college students sought to transfer after graduation to four-year colleges, where they might complete their bachelor's degrees and become fully eligible for Civil Service and other professional positions.

This in turn created a problem of articulation between two-year and four-year colleges. In many cases, the community college curriculum had an extensive range of recreation courses, with comparatively few liberal arts or general academic courses. When students sought to transfer to baccalaureate programs, they found that they were required to take a substantial number of liberal arts credits and, in

---

[19]John L. Hutchinson: "Therapeutic Recreation Education: Programs and Proposals for Sub-Professionals." *Recreation in Treatment Centers*, September 1964, p. 29.

some cases, repeat certain recreation courses on the senior college level. In a number of states, articulation agreements have been worked out between two-year and four-year colleges with the assistance of state recreation and park societies.

In 1978, the Society of Park and Recreation Educators (SPRE), the NRPA branch concerned primarily with higher education in the field of recreation and leisure studies, issued a set of guidelines dealing with four major concerns of community college recreation curricula: (a) quality of faculty and excellence in teaching; (b) trends and priorities in program and curriculum development; (c) two-year/four-year relationships and articulation; and (d) identification and expansion of the job market for two-year degree-holders.[20] In the late 1970's, it was apparent that the number of two-year curricula in recreation and parks had declined.

A document submitted to the Board of Directors of SPRE in October 1981 outlined recommended Standards and Evaluative Criteria for Associate Degree Programs in Recreation, Park Resources and Leisure Services.[21] In addition to standards covering philosophy and purpose, administration, faculty, students, public service, instructional resources and general and professional education course recommendations for both transfer and career-based (terminal) students, the guidelines suggested learning objectives for three categories which represented special-interest areas for many two-year curricula: *Recreation Program Services, Park/Natural Resource Services* and *Therapeutic Recreation Services.*

For example, learning objectives for students enrolled in the National Therapeutic Recreation Society's 750-hour training program for technicians included the following:

Understanding of basic concepts of therapeutic recreation service to special populations.

Understanding of the roles and responsibilities of personnel who provide therapeutic recreation service.

Knowledge about the kinds of facilities and types of personnel involved in delivering services to special populations.

Knowledge about normal growth and development of human beings from before birth to death.

Understanding of ways in which therapeutic recreation can help to serve developmental needs of special populations.

Knowledge about acute and chronic conditions which affect people's ability to engage in recreative activities.

Ability to apply effective communication techniques in working with others.

Knowledge of leadership styles, techniques and processes.

Knowledge about the kinds and levels of activities appropriate for a variety of ages and disability groups.

Ability to apply the knowledge, understanding and skills acquired from the modules of leadership and disabling conditions to leading teaching activities.

Understanding and ability to apply the activity analysis process to therapeutic recreation programs.

---

[20]Don Weiskopf, Larry Williams, H. Douglas Sessoms and Larry Smith: *Guideline Documents for Two-Year College Recreation and Park Education.* Arlington, Virginia, Society for Park and Recreation Educators, September 1978.

[21]*Recreation Standards and Evaluative Criteria for Recreation, Park Resources and Leisure Services Associate Degree Programs.* Report of Two-Year/Four-Year Issues Committee of Society of Park and Recreation Educators, Minneapolis, October 1981.

Knowledge and ability to plan, develop and evaluate a therapeutic recreation program for individuals and special groups.

Ability to demonstrate understanding of leadership procedures and tasks involved in effective administration of activity programs.

Application of the knowledge and skills through actual supervised work experiences in programs serving the ill and disabled.[22]

Accreditation of College and University Programs

Traditionally, recreation education has been closely associated with departments of health and physical education, with the exception of a small number of departments found in schools of forestry, landscape architecture and agriculture. In the past, such curricula have been accredited through the National Council on Accreditation of Teacher Education. Since the mid-1960's, an effort has been made to develop a more exacting accreditation procedure to scrutinize recreation and park curricula thoroughly instead of permitting them to "slide by" almost unnoticed as part of stronger health and physical education programs or schools of education. Several sets of guidelines for accreditation were developed, and in 1975 the National Recreation and Park Association, in cooperation with the American Association for Leisure and Recreation, developed a final draft of evaluative criteria on two levels (baccalaureate and master's degrees) and a set of procedural guidelines. In the following years, a number of pilot accreditation procedures were carried out, and by the late 1970's, the accreditation process was well under way.

By the early 1980's, approximately 30 of the leading college and university curricula throughout the United States had been accredited. While the accreditation standards did not include separate requirements for each program emphasis or degree option, they did involve guidelines through which each of these areas would be examined. In October 1981, the National Accreditation Council adopted a new set of standards based on information from many professional groups. The new standards contain two important areas of improvement. Peterson writes,

First, the specialization (option) of Therapeutic Recreation at the undergraduate level has a much more refined and expanded set of standards by which to judge a Therapeutic Recreation program. In addition to these specialization standards, many standards are incorporated into the professional core standards which reflect a concern for special populations, accessibility, adaptation and modification of activities, as well as facilitation techniques for use with special populations. These are felt to be areas of knowledge, skill and ability that all recreation and leisure curricula should address. In addition, some standards are added related to the accessibility of classrooms, faculty offices and other instructional resources of university and college campuses.[23]

---

[22]*The NTRS 750-Hour Training Program for Therapeutic Recreation Technicians.* National Therapeutic Recreation Society, Alexandria, Virginia, December 1981.
[23]Peterson, *Report of the President, op. cit.,* p. 2.

The new standards are expected to strengthen professional education in all recreation, park and leisure studies programs at preservice levels and lead to a more standardized body of knowledge.

Another major policy decision made at the 1981 Council meetings was to review two-year curricula for accreditation rather than focus on master's degree programs as had been done in the past. This decision met strong resistance from a number of universities with extensive graduate programs which, in many cases, had served as the first level of specialized professional education for many individuals who were already working in the field of therapeutic recreation. The Council's decision meant that individuals who had taken undergraduate degrees in related fields and who had then entered the field of therapeutic recreation service would find a graduate degree in therapeutic recreation less valuable because the master's degree would no longer be accredited.

ROLE OF CONTINUING EDUCATION

Both to offer advanced exposure to theory and practice in therapeutic recreation service for such individuals, and to provide new stimulus, inspiration and awareness of contemporary approaches for all practitioners who have been in the field for a period of years, several different forms of continuing education have become increasingly available. Continuing education refers to special workshops, short courses, clinics or other educational experiences which may be provided by either a college or university or another community agency or professional organization and which are *not* part of a formal degree program.

Carter and James point out that the need for lifelong learning has been reinforced by mandatory continuing education for licensed professionals, including dental hygienists, medical records administrators, medical technologists and occupational and physical therapists:

. . . the professional's desire to remain current, receive peer approval, maintain a level of acceptable educational standards, and maintain active involvement of fellow professionals is rapidly being overcome by the thrusts of state laws and voluntary professional associations' re-licensing requirements.[24]

For example, as summarized in one report, state statutes requiring continuing education for relicensing of professionals includes 45 states for optometrists, 37 states for administrators of nursing homes, 15 states for pharmacists, nine states for nurses, eight states for dentists and six states for social workers.

In the early 1980's it was proposed that practitioners registered under the NTRS Voluntary Registration Plan maintain professional development by participating in

---

[24]Marcia Jean Carter and Ann James: "Continuing Professional Development Programs for Therapeutic Recreation." *Therapeutic Recreation Journal*, Third Quarter, 1979, p. 13.

workshops, symposia, conferences and other continuing education programs endorsed by NTRS. In addition, the NTRS Continuing Professional Development Committee established the following criteria for continuing professional development: ten contact hours of participation per single unit in an organized professional development program endorsed by NTRS and under capable direction.

Specific examples of approved continuing education experiences include the 750-hour training programs for technicians provided by many institutions and agencies under guidelines established by NTRS, and the Therapeutic Recreation Management School sponsored annually by the Recreation Department of the University of Maryland, at Oglebay Park, Wheeling, West Virginia.

It appears likely that in the future such continued professional development will represent a vital part of the retooling process for many therapeutic recreation specialists.

USE AND TRAINING OF VOLUNTEERS

Volunteers also need adequate training in therapeutic recreation programs. In both institutions and communities, the limited numbers of qualified professionals mean that volunteers have an important role.

Clark sums up the values to be gained by the use of volunteers in a Veterans' Administration hospital:

> We believe that volunteers under medical staff leadership and guidance can make a valuable contribution to the care and treatment of patients. We believe the volunteer's contribution is made in two basic types of supplemental service to the patients: first, direct service in which the volunteers participate in hospital-approved programs with and for the patients; secondly, direct service in which the volunteers provide equally valuable assistance as public relations ambassadors to the community, informing friends and neighbors about the care and treatment programs and the role of the community in assisting in these programs.[25]

In addition to these contributions, volunteers are able to relieve professional staff members of many time-consuming tasks that do not require a high level of training. They may provide specialized leadership skills lacking in the regular staff, thus extending the program and offering more highly individualized activities. The fact that they are offering their time without payment, because they *care*, is undoubtedly an important morale "booster" for patients. However, volunteers may constitute a serious administrative problem if they are not properly guided and supervised. Clark suggests a set of guidelines for this process:

---

[25]Thomas J. Clark: "The Administration of Voluntary Services in a Recreation Program." *Recreation in Treatment Centers*, September 1962, pp. 13–17.

1. *Organization.* It is necessary to have one individual who will coordinate and direct the volunteer program, acting as a liaison with community organizations which are the source of volunteers, and assuming this entire responsibility.

2. *Climate.* It is necessary, as a first step, to establish a climate for the constructive use of volunteers within the total scope and philosophy of the agency. Staff members — who may feel threatened by the use of volunteers who work for nothing and may have highly developed skills — should be helped to accept volunteers, and assured that they do not represent a danger to professional, paid personnel.

3. *Establish Need.* Before any volunteers are recruited or accepted, the agency should carry out a survey of its need for volunteers. After these have been established, "job" descriptions might be written for each possible volunteer assignment.

4. *Recruitment.* Generally this is carried on most effectively if there is an advisory council for voluntary services in the community. If not, contact must be made with service organizations that provide volunteers, and all forms of communication (radio, television, announcements, newspapers, and personal contact) should be used to reach potential volunteers.

5. *Screening and Selection.* The potential volunteer should fill out appropriate background forms and be interviewed by the member of the staff responsible for coordinating volunteer services. Such qualities as sincere interest, the ability to work with people and to accept the policies of the agency, dependability, and personal stability should be assessed in this meeting. Then the volunteer should be interviewed by the member of the staff responsible for the program to which he would be assigned.

6. *Orientation and Training.* All volunteers who are accepted should be given a thorough introduction to the agency, in which they are helped to understand its objectives and philosophy, and learn about its structure and operation. Such a process helps to develop an effective rapport between staff members and volunteers. There should also be a preliminary period of instruction of specific skills or methods of carrying out the assignment.

7. *Supervision.* This is a key element in the use of volunteers. A properly qualified, capable supervisor should observe the work of the volunteer, meet with him regularly, offer assistance when needed, help him recognize and solve his problems — and, if necessary, make recommendations for re-assigning or terminating the employment of the volunteer.

8. *Recognition.* Most volunteers do contribute an important service, which should be recognized. This may be done regularly through the year, by praise and recognition of achievements at staff meetings. Providing identification cards or other formal symbols of volunteer roles may be helpful. In addition, it is desirable to give volunteers scrolls or other concrete statements of appreciation, or to hold volunteer dinners or other formal ceremonies in which they are publicly recognized.

THERAPEUTIC RECREATION WITHIN THE TREATMENT TEAM

Another important consideration in this chapter is the place of therapeutic recreation within the treatment team and its relationship with other treatment modalities generally described under the broad heading of *activity therapies.* In many hospitals and treatment centers, recreation has been made a part of larger rehabilitation departments in which recreation specialists must work in close cooperation with occupational therapists, physical therapists and similar personnel. The following section provides concise descriptions of the different disciplines found in hospitals that may be provided as part of the rehabilitation process. It is important that students in the field of therapeutic recreation service become thoroughly familiar with these other specializations.

Activity and Adjunctive Therapies

Before it is possible to consider in a meaningful way the role of the activity therapies, or adjunctive therapies as they are sometimes called, it is essential to examine how they relate to the physician and his or her role. This may be done with respect to two major types of medical settings: *physical medicine and rehabilitation* and *psychiatric care*. Both are part of the broad process of rehabilitation that involves the "cooperative efforts of various medical specialists and their associates in other health fields to improve the physical, mental, social and vocational aptitudes of persons who are handicapped, with the objective of preserving their ability to live happily and productively on the same level and with the same opportunities as their neighbors."[26]

The physician's responsibility today goes far beyond diagnosing, providing necessary surgical or drug treatment and then dismissing the patient. Instead, the physician must be concerned not only with the physical disability but also with the psychological, social and vocational problems of the patient.

How is the whole person to be treated in the field of physical medicine? Krusen writes that rehabilitation, as practiced in modern treatment centers, is a multi-disciplinary service directed by the specialist in physical medicine and rehabilitation, assisted by other specialists in internal medicine, pediatrics, orthopedic surgery, neurology, neurosurgery and plastic surgery. These physicians in turn are assisted by a team of associates in the allied health professions, which might include various types of therapists, as well as social workers, clinical psychologists and vocational counselors.

Within the field of psychiatric treatment, occupational and recreational therapy have, since the 1930's, been operating under a model of prescribing individualized activities designed to meet patients' specific psychodynamic needs during the treatment process. Although there had been examples of the use of various types of patient activities in psychiatric treatment facilities more than a century before, it was not until the beginning of the twentieth century that such programs were widely accepted. The rationale for them, quite simply, was that activity was necessary to combat the demoralizing condition of being "invalided" and institutionalized. Activity was viewed as a valuable antidote to "idleness," which in turn was seen as worsening the condition of the ill and retarding treatment progress. Positive forms of activity—at that time, largely consisting of beginning forms of occupational therapy and recreation—were seen as helping to channel the patient's "attitude toward life" in healthy directions.

A leading psychiatrist of this early period, Adolf Meyer of the Phipps Clinic in

---

[26]Frank H. Krusen, Frederick J. Kottke and Paul M. Ellwood, eds.: *Handbook of Physical Medicine and Rehabilitation.* Philadelphia, W. B. Saunders Co., 1971, p. 1.

Baltimore, stressed the need to appeal to what was "sane and wholesome and natural in patients" and to lead "that healthy core along the road of simple activity." Erikson writes, "Meyer's emphasis was on the intact areas of strength and normal functioning in every patient and on the hospital's responsibility, not only to preserve but to nourish and maximize these aspects in treatment."[27] Furthermore, he stressed the importance of activity in the hospital regimen as a way of encouraging patients to work within the defined limits of reality, balancing self-absorption and fantasy and acting as a remedial normative influence against other distorting factors in their lives.

As the use of occupational and recreational therapy spread in many hospitals, two contrasting approaches were developed: the *clinical-medical approach* and the *milieu therapy approach.*

CLINICAL-MEDICAL APPROACH

The clinical-medical approach to the use of recreation in psychiatric settings was popularized at the Menninger Clinic in particular. Each of the treatment team assumed specific therapeutic roles with specific patients. Activities themselves were used to make psychodynamic diagnoses, and the adjunctive therapist developed elaborate schemes for prescribing specific activities for patients. Pattison comments that this model persists as a dominant model for the adjunctive therapies in psychiatric institutions for two reasons:

For one, it adheres closely to the traditional model of psychodynamic psychotherapy which focuses solely on the one-to-one therapeutic relationship. The adjunctive therapist in his occupational or recreational therapy represents an extension of the one-to-one model of therapy. The activities of the adjunctive therapist are intended to indeed be "therapy"; and the adjunctive therapist becomes a junior psychiatrist of sorts. Thus the work of the adjunctive therapist is determined and controlled by the psychiatrist who is the ultimate authority on the diagnosis and psychodynamic treatment of the patient. . . . [28]

The second reason, in Pattison's view, for this model's continued use is that it supports the professionalization of the various adjunctive therapies. Typically, adjunctive therapists look to the psychiatrist to achieve identity and gain social and professional status. Thus, adjunctive therapists are urged to become educated in psychiatric diagnosis and in psychotherapeutic techniques. However, it is no longer taken for granted that the major value of the adjunctive therapies lies in their specific psychodynamic meanings. Instead, in many institutions, their contribution is seen chiefly in creating a therapeutic environment.

---

[27]Joan M. Erikson: *Activity, Recovery and Growth: The Communal Role of Planned Activities.* New York, W. W. Norton, 1976, p. 27.
[28]E. Mansell Pattison: "The Relationship of the Adjunctive and Therapeutic Recreation Services to Community Mental Health Programs." *Therapeutic Recreation Journal,* First Quarter, 1969, p. 17.

MILIEU THERAPY APPROACH

The concept of "milieu therapy" implies that treatment consists chiefly of providing, guiding and maintaining activities that are therapeutic and thus promoting healthy patterns of social interaction (see p. 65). Adjunctive therapies should *not* be regarded as therapy in a literal sense, but rather as elements of the total treatment process that contribute to varied aspects of the patient's growth and recovery.

In some adjunctive therapy departments, the roles of specialists within the various disciplines have become somewhat blurred. However, today there tends to be a sharper definition of each staff member's area of expertise and responsibility. To some degree, professionals working within such departments tend to see themselves primarily as *activity therapists* and secondarily as practitioners within a separate discipline. Many directors of such departments have become affiliated in recent years with the National Association of Activity Therapy and Rehabilitation Program Directors.[29]

The following section describes a number of activity and adjunctive therapies prominent in the field of rehabilitation today.

OCCUPATIONAL THERAPY

Occupational therapy has been broadly defined by the American Occupational Therapy Association as

---

any activity, mental or physical, prescribed by a physician as a valuable adjunct in contributing to and hastening recovery. Physically, its function is to increase muscle strength and joint motion as well as to improve the general bodily health; mentally, its function is to supply as nearly as possible normal activity through avocational projects and prevocational studies and training.

The U.S. Public Health Service has described occupational therapy in these terms:

Occupational therapy (is) the use of purposeful activity in the rehabilitation of persons with physical or emotional disability. The occupational therapist, as a vital member of the rehabilitation team, determines the objectives of the treatment program according to the individual needs of each patient. This may include decreasing disability during the patient's initial phases of recovery following injury or illness, increasing the individual's capability for independence and improving his physical, emotional, and social well-being and developing his total function to a maximum level through early evaluation and experimentation for future job training and employment.[30]

---

[29]Unlike the National Therapeutic Recreation Society, this organization is composed solely of individuals responsible for activity therapy programs in hospital or other rehabilitation settings. Their backgrounds may be occupational, recreational or in other activity therapies. See Appendix B for address.
[30]*Health Resource Statistics, 1968.* Washington, D.C., Public Health Service, U.S. Department of Health, Education and Welfare, 1968, p. 145.

Occupational therapy may be prescribed to accomplish any of the following objectives:

1. Specific treatment for psychiatric patients—to structure opportunities for the development of more satisfying relationships, to assist in releasing or sublimating emotional drives, to aid as a diagnostic tool.
2. Specific treatment for restoration of physical function—to increase joint motion, muscle strength and coordination.
3. To teach self-help activities—those of daily living such as eating, dressing, writing, the use of adapted equipment and prostheses.
4. To help the disabled homemaker readjust to home routines with advice and instruction as to the adaptation of household equipment and work simplification.
5. To develop work tolerance and maintenance of special skills as required by the patient's job.
6. To provide prevocational exploration—to determine the patient's physical and mental capacities, social adjustment, interests, work habits, skills and potential employability.
7. A supportive measure—help the patient to accept and utilize constructively a prolonged period of hospitalization and convalescence.
8. Redirection of recreational and avocational interests.

Recently, occupational therapy has moved beyond a primary concern with activities of daily living and the development of self-help skills, to a broader focus. Lansing and Carlsen describe it as

---

... a bio-psycho-social approach to health care that concentrates on an individual's abilities to perform, maintain, and balance daily occupational roles.... The premise of the profession is that occupation is a major health determinant: the goal-directed use of a person's potential, capabilities, resources, time, energy, interest, and attention will influence the quality of human development and life adaptation.[31]

Sherrill points out that whereas occupation was once conceptualized as work (vocation or homemaking), it now includes a full range of human endeavors— work, play and self-maintenance. In their concern with improving sensory-motor integration, many occupational therapists are now using equipment previously thought to be within the domain of physical therapy or adapted physical education: scooter boards, cage balls and balancing apparatus.[32]

It is apparent that a number of the goals and concerns of occupational therapy are similar to those of therapeutic recreation service. In fact, occupational therapy includes many clearly recreational activities. However, a clear distinction must be made between therapeutic recreation and occupational therapy in terms of professional preparation. Occupational therapists must graduate from a college or university accredited by the Council on Medical Education of the American Medical Association, in collaboration with the American Occupational Therapy Association. Such

---

[31]Stella Lansing and Pat Carlsen, cited in Claudine Sherrill: *Adapted Physical Education and Recreation: A Multi-Disciplinary Approach.* Dubuque, Iowa, Wm. C. Brown, 1981, p. 49.
[32]*Ibid.*

programs may have as a minimum requirement a four-year bachelor's degree, a one-year certification program following the bachelor's degree or a two-year master's degree program. Normally, the programs include considerable work in the biological sciences, particularly human anatomy and physiology, behavioral sciences and physical and psychosocial dysfunction, as well as courses in occupational therapy principles and skills.

PHYSICAL THERAPY

Physical therapy is concerned with the restoration of function and prevention of disability following disease, injury or loss of a bodily part. It seeks to aid the normal progression of the healing process by serving to relieve symptoms and speed recovery. It is simply defined in Public Law 94–142: "Physical therapy means services provided by a qualified physical therapist."

Latimer suggests that the two major elements in physical therapy are therapeutic exercise and functional training:

Therapeutic exercise includes assisting or teaching the patient body positions and exercises or movement procedures. . . . *Functional training* includes assisting or teaching the patient in ambulation, use of assistive and supportive devices such as crutches, prostheses, and braces, and self-care or activities of daily living.[33]

Among the types of patients served by physical therapy are those with chronic arthritis, rheumatism, forms of paralysis, organic and functional affections of the nervous system, digestive disturbances and various other severe trauma. Generally, physical therapy employs the following types of treatment:

1. Thermotherapy: radiant heat; artificially induced fever.
2. Light therapy: heliotherapy; artificial ultraviolet radiation.
3. Electrotherapy: Galvanic current; low-frequency currents (electrodiagnosis); high-frequency currents (long- and short-wave diathermy); static electricity.
4. Hydrotherapy: hot and cold, medicated, electric baths; douches and showers; whirlpool bath, therapeutic pool; colonic irrigation.
5. Mechanotherapy: massage; general and special exercise; occupational therapy.[34]

In addition, physical therapy includes instruction because it is often necessary to teach patients or their families, or both, about the use of prosthetic and

[33]Ruth Latimer: "Physical Therapy," *In* P. Valletutti and F. Christoplos, eds.: *Interdisciplinary Approaches to Human Services.* Baltimore, University Park Press, 1977, pp. 280, 283.
[34]Richard Kovacs: *A Manual of Physical Therapy,* 4th ed. Philadelphia, Lea and Febiger, 1949, pp. 13–14.

orthopedic appliances and the use of continuing therapeutic exercises and other home treatment procedures. Physical therapy generally is regarded as having three major phases:

1. *Prevention.* To prevent deformity or disability, instruction and practice may be given in corrective posture and movement techniques, muscle reeducation or progressive relaxation as well as preoperative exercise given before surgical procedures.
2. *Diagnosis and Treatment.* Use of physical therapy as a form of testing, to assist the physician in establishing the diagnosis of certain conditions and in determining prognosis and the treatment required; treatment by medically prescribed physical therapy procedures and techniques.
3. *Rehabilitation.* This should begin the day the patient enters a hospital or rehabilitation center and continue until maximum functional or organic recovery is achieved. It includes instruction in functional training, ambulation and self-care activities leading to maximum social and vocational independence.

Among the best known of the exercise systems used in physical therapy today is *proprioceptive neuromuscular facilitation.* Applied particularly to cerebral palsied and other severely handicapped individuals, it entails work with reflexes and voluntary and involuntary muscle action.

Physical therapy is based on medical guidance and precisely stated treatment objectives and is normally applied on a one-to-one basis. The patient is usually in a passive role, although certain tasks may require a vigorous and sustained effort on his or her part. Unlike occupational therapy, physical therapy focuses primarily on the patient's physical recovery and does not directly address itself to social or emotional concerns. Like occupational therapists, physical therapists normally must graduate from an approved program of physical therapy, administered in conjunction with a medical faculty and clinical setting, and they must pass a state board examination.

CORRECTIVE THERAPY

Corrective therapy is the treatment of patients by medically prescribed physical exercises and activities designed to strengthen and coordinate functions and to prevent muscular decline resulting from lengthy convalescence or inactivity due to illness. It places emphasis on functional training and practice in the more advanced stages of rehabilitation and makes use of various types of exercises and modified sports. In addition, it may provide instruction in the use of orthopedic and prosthetic appliances.

The Veterans' Administration employs the largest number of personnel specifically identified as corrective therapists. Generally, corrective therapy in the VA hospitals includes the following types of treatment activities:

1. Conditioning exercises to develop strength, endurance, neuromuscular coordination and agility; reconditioning exercise to prevent both physical and psychological deconditioning.
2. Exercises and resocialization activities for psychiatric patients, specifically oriented toward psychiatric objectives.

3. Teaching of self-care activities, including personal hygiene.
4. Teaching of functional ambulation and elevation techniques, including the use of all types of prosthetic devices.
5. Therapeutic swimming (hydrogymnastic) programs.
6. Corrective and postural exercises prescribed and administered for specific conditions.
7. Conditioning, reconditioning, self-care and motivation activities for aged and infirm patients.
8. Special activities in the reorientation of the blind.
9. Training in the operation of manually controlled motor vehicles, where appropriate.

Corrective therapy may be provided in wards or clinics or in outdoor exercise areas. Normally, prescription for corrective therapy is given on an individual basis, although the program of activity itself may be carried on in a group.

The title "corrective therapist" is normally given to persons who work in this field in hospitals, nursing homes and rehabilitation centers. The minimum educational requirement is a baccalaureate in physical education from an accredited program, which should include courses in anatomy, kinesiology and related subjects, followed by a period of clinical training involving 400 to 600 hours in an affiliated hospital approved by the American Corrective Therapy Association.

ADAPTED PHYSICAL EDUCATION

A field that is closely related to corrective therapy is *adapted physical education*. This term has normally been applied to programs of modified physical activity provided in educational settings to meet the needs of atypical students with physical or psychological disabilities. In some settings the term "corrective physical education" has been used.

In programs of adapted physical education, the activities of students should be highly individualized, with the choice and modification of activity based on medical diagnosis, prescription and supervision. With adapted physical education, all students are able to engage in some form of physical education:

Adapted physical education is for every student who cannot safely or successfully participate in the regular program. Adapted physical education should not be limited to students with postural, orthopedic, and organic conditions. The program should include students with visual handicaps and hearing impairment, as well as those with intellectual limitations, behavior problems, perceptual-motor difficulties, and (other) physical impairments. In addition to students with chronic conditions, adapted programs should provide for those recuperating from injuries and accidents and those convalescing from long or short term illnesses.[35]

The passage of Public Law 94–142, The Education For All Handicapped Children Act, mandated that schools must provide educational opportunities for all

---

[35]See *Journal of Health, Physical Education and Recreation*, May 1969, p. 45.

handicapped children, including physical education, as part of overall special education. Aufsesser points out that school systems throughout the United States have expanded physical education programs for children with a broad range of disabilities. These students are included in the regular physical education program where possible and in special classes where necessary. He writes,

---

The major implication of mainstreaming is that many mildly handicapped children will be placed in regular physical education programs in the future. The moderately and severely handicapped children will remain in the adapted physical education program in a safe environment and with a good chance of success — where they can receive quality instruction from trained specialists.[36]

The range of such programs is broad, including not only physical fitness and movement education activities but also such play-related activities as rhythms, dance, games, sports and swimming for all disabled children in the school population. Auxter points out that a major purpose of adapted physical education is to help students gain the skills they will need to enjoy recreation in the community. To achieve this goal, adapted physical educators must find potential resources and programs for the disabled in the community and assist in planning needed educational experiences.

Sherrill suggests that the emerging role of today's adapted physical educator involves far more than simply teaching modified movement experiences to disabled children and youth. Instead, adapted physical educators must work not only with handicapped students but also with parents, siblings and significant others (peers, teachers and friends). She writes,

---

The only way to teach the whole child is to understand the total environment in which the child lives. Such desired social outcomes of physical education as self-worth, acceptance by others, and rich, full leisure depend more on family and neighborhood interaction than on school training. Thus the teaching-learning process must be a partnership between school and family.[37]

This statement implies that there should be a close working relationship between adapted physical educators and recreation professionals in community life if the needs of disabled children and youth are to be fully met. Adapted physical educators and corrective therapists tend to share similar objectives and employ many of the same types of activities. However, adapted physical educators make greater use of modified games and sports, while corrective therapists rely more heavily on various types of individualized exercises and functional training activities.

---

[36]Peter M. Aufsesser: "Adapted Physical Education: A Look Ahead, A Look Back." *Journal of Physical Education and Recreation*, June 1981, p. 32.
[37]Sherrill, *op. cit.*, p. 32.

Other Activity Therapies

In addition to the therapies just described, a number of other specialized techniques are used in various rehabilitation settings and are frequently included under the general heading of "activity therapies."

EDUCATIONAL THERAPY

Educational therapy is the conscious utilization of instruction in academic areas of education to develop the mental and physical capabilities of hospitalized patients. Instruction given at various levels may be accredited by recognized educational authorities. It may be restricted to classwork in such subjects as English, mathematics and the physical or social sciences, all carefully geared to the capabilities of those taking part and with teaching methods designed to meet individual needs.

In addition, in some programs of educational therapy, discussion groups serve to promote motivation and social involvement. Such sessions may include current events discussions, travelogues and seminars on problems of aging, human relations and similar topics. Educational programs of this type are becoming increasingly important in treatment plans for chronic, long-term geriatric patients and in some cases have been blended with "sensitivity training" or "encounter group" methods to promote interaction, awareness and involvement on the part of aged patients. One approach to using discussion groups in this way has been called "remotivation therapy."

Educational therapists usually hold a college degree with a major in education and have had several months of training in a clinical setting.

MANUAL ARTS THERAPY

Manual arts therapy is the use of industrial arts for actual or simulated work which helps patients prepare to return to jobs and the community.

In part, such therapy is used to appraise patients' reactions, functional ability, emotional status and aptitudes in order to help them plan realistic rehabilitation goals for post-hospitalization employment or involvement in a sheltered workshop. In addition, manual arts therapy may have the same goals as occupational therapy, in terms of direct stimulation and improvement of the patient's physical and mental functioning. Typically, seven broad categories of manual arts therapy are metalworking, woodworking, electrical work, graphic arts, applied arts, agriculture and hospital industries. Within these categories, the demands of many jobs can be duplicated and the patient's level of performance evaluated.

The normal preparation of a manual arts therapist consists of a college degree with a major in industrial arts, agriculture or some other related field, followed by two to seven months of training at an approved hospital or rehabilitation center.

INDUSTRIAL THERAPY

This field consists of the therapeutic use of activities related to the operation of the hospital. Formerly, it was known as "hospital industry"; it involves the patient working as a laborer, carpenter, kitchen worker, electrician, plumber, clerk-typist, laboratory technician, psychiatric aide or nursing aide. In some settings such assignments of patients (e.g., unskilled labor, laundry help, grounds maintenance and the like) have represented little more than a form of cheap labor that helps to keep the hospital going. However, when properly supervised, industrial therapy has real value for patients.

The distinction between industrial and manual arts therapy is that the former generally involves performing real work that is significant to the operation of the hospital, while the latter is basically a form of modified instruction and treatment within a clinic or workshop. Industrial therapy is not normally carried on under the guidance of specially trained therapists but is most valuable when selective placement techniques are used and patients are carefully observed and evaluated.

There is a growing body of opinion that work in itself is an important form of therapeutic experience and makes a significant contribution to the patient's feeling of self-worth and importance, as well as to his growing readiness for discharge to the community and ultimate vocational adjustment. This view is based in part on the high value that modern society places on work as a human endeavor. It also is based on the nature of work that relates patients to reality-based situations, providing a structure to their lives and a sense of concrete accomplishment.

VOCATIONAL ADJUSTMENT

In some situations, manual arts and industrial therapy are combined with vocational or career counseling in a treatment program designed, when possible, to enable patients to return to the community and hold a meaningful job. According to the Pennsylvania State Mental Hospital Manual cited earlier, Vocational Adjustment Services are intended to help patients find productive, satisfying work that allows them to realize their highest vocational potential, either in the outside society or in the institutional community:

Vocational Adjustment is the planned utilization of work activities in a realistic manner to meet the needs of the patient/resident, who for some reason is presently not able to compete in the normal work role expected by society. Its operation is based on planned work activity that combines a variety of learning and counseling techniques to provide the motivation to foster the development of goals (emotional, social, academic, financial, and vocational), appropriate to the individual.

The vocational adjustment program involves finding, developing, and providing the opportunity for realistic and therapeutic work experiences based on the current needs of the individual patient/resident, and utilizing existing work and training areas throughout the institution and community.[38]

---

[38]*Pennsylvania State Mental Hospital Manual for Evaluation of Occupational Therapy Programs.* Pennsylvania Department of Public Welfare, 1974, p. 3.

ACTIVITIES OF DAILY LIVING

Another activity therapy found in many rehabilitation programs today is called A.D.L., or activities of daily living. It involves group and individual experiences in self-care, home management, shopping, cleaning, cooking and similar tasks. In some hospitals, for example, patients may live in an apartment where they are responsible for self-care before being discharged or moved to an off-grounds semi-independent residence. In some cases, A.D.L. is one of the assigned responsibilities of the activity therapist, who might be an occupational therapist or therapeutic recreation worker. In other situations, it might be defined more specifically as "home-making therapy" and assigned to a specialist known as the "homemaking rehabilitation consultant." Such individuals are usually college graduates with a degree in home economics or occupational therapy, followed by in-service or graduate training in work with the physically or mentally disabled. Degrees or work experience in such fields as dietetics, nutrition or home economics or practical experience in homemaking and child care are also valuable attributes.

The homemaking rehabilitation consultant adapts knowledge of home management, family finance, nutrition and similar subjects to meet the needs of disabled persons who have housekeeping responsibilities to which they will return on discharge. The specialist may either provide direct retraining in these areas or, as a resource specialist, counsel other persons on the rehabilitation team. His or her goals should be to strengthen the skills of patients in these areas and to help restore their confidence in handling family problems, at which they may have failed in the past.

MUSIC THERAPY

The use of music for therapeutic purposes is found more widely in psychiatric treatment programs than in physical rehabilitation settings. Emphasis is placed on the use of music to promote group dynamics, nonverbal communication and individual expression. Both improvisation and instruction in technical skills are stressed, with the emphasis usually on instrumental music.

Music is generally viewed as a medium through which disturbed patients may be reached and involved and in which they may find not only emotional expression and release but also a growing sense of self-worth. It is regarded as a supportive therapy that facilitates other treatment methods. A number of colleges offer degree programs in music therapy today. To meet the standards of the National Association for Music Therapy, qualified music therapists must complete a six-month internship in approved psychiatric hospitals affiliated with their institution.

ART THERAPY

Like the field of music therapy, art therapy is generally regarded as a form of treatment that provides the opportunity for healthy self-expression and growth, self-awareness, communication and relating to society. Art has been used widely in the past as a means of understanding the dynamic elements in a patient's illness (it is chiefly used in psychiatric therapy) and helping him express himself and recognize the source of some of his own difficulties through nonverbal expression.

In a special issue of *Prism*, devoted to the "arts and the handicapped," Rubin points out that many people, artists in particular, question whether it is appropriate to "dilute" an art experience by using it for anything other than an aesthetic aim. In part, their concerns are justified, because many individuals calling themselves art, music or dance therapists have a minimum of clinical knowledge, training and sensitivity. They have often made use of mechanical, noncreative art projects, or have misinterpreted the patient's work in clumsy and inaccurate diagnoses.

Essentially, Rubin suggests, there are two kinds of special values in the arts:

One of the most profoundly therapeutic aspects of the arts for the handicapped (as for all people) is the enhancement of good feelings about the self through pride in the development of skill and the creation of worthwhile products. In some approaches to the arts in therapy the primary emphasis is on the deep pleasures and internal integration gained from creative activity. . . . In others the emphasis is on gaining a better understanding of those conflicts and fantasies inhibiting the full flowering of the personality.[39]

In the first approach, the "art" in "art therapy" is emphasized, while in the second, the "therapy" aspect is primary. In both, however, the net effect is an important contribution to the reintegration of the patient. The same principles apply to other creative experiences, such as writing (including poetry and fiction) and the performing arts. In recent years, there has been a growing recognition of the value of creative expression in healthy personality development. Art therapy generally focuses on the freer forms of artistic expression, such as drawing, painting, modeling and sculpture. It is commonly seen as a highly flexible, individualized experience in which patients select their own project and proceed at their own pace, with the encouragement and help of the art therapist. In some settings, an art studio is simply made available for patients' use, unlike other forms of therapy that may be prescribed and carefully structured for them.

Art therapy may also be used for specific hospital projects, such as the design of Christmas cards and the provision of posters or other art work for departments of public information, recreation or volunteers. A number of colleges and special schools have initiated special training programs for art therapists that include course work in psychology, psychopathology, rehabilitation and therapeutic methods, as well as art techniques.

DANCE THERAPY

Like art and music therapy, dance therapy is based on the view that expressed feeling, meaningfully shared, can aid in the integration of the personality and

---

[39]Judy Rubin: "The Arts, Handicapped and Therapy." *Prism No. 4*, Pittsburgh, Pennsylvania, Museum of Art, Carnegie Institute, Spring 1981, p. 5.

growth in the ability to relate to others. It is particularly useful in work with individuals for whom words are difficult or impossible.

Dance therapy utilizes the tools of basic dance movement and rhythmic action as a means of nonverbal communication. In many hospitals, both psychiatric and physically disabled patients may be involved in social forms of dance, such as folk, square and social dancing, as part of the overall recreation program. When dance is applied as therapy, it consists of a simplified and unstructured form of modern or creative dance, permitting highly individualized, free personal movement. The dance therapist aids individuals or groups of patients in discovering their own capabilities for expressive movement, using simple music, drum rhythms or even vocalization and other improvised sounds as accompaniment.

To be most effective, dance therapy is conducted in close consultation with psychiatrists and other hospital personnel, with close atttention given to the psychodynamic needs and recovery process of individual participants. There has been an increasing amount of research and special training in this field, encouraged by the American Dance Therapy Association.

PLAY THERAPY

Play therapy is generally carried on with younger children in hospitals or psychiatric treatment centers. In the hospital, it may be used with both general medical and psychiatric patients. In one general hospital it was described as having the following goals:

1. To offer diversional activity to the child while undergoing medical treatment, thus continuing as much normal play as possible.
2. To help alleviate tension or feeling of homesickness, thus aiding orientation by establishing a better rapport with hospital personnel and other children.
3. To promote normal development, in spite of physical, mental or emotional disability.
4. To promote staff and parental understanding of the purpose, use and selection of play experiences and equipment.[40]

When used as a form of treatment with disturbed children, play therapy is normally monitored by specially trained therapists with a strong background in guidance and psychotherapeutic principles and techniques. Usually, it is unstructured; children are encouraged to use a variety of media—toys, play equipment, clay, finger-paints, construction materials, dolls, clothing and similar materials—in a completely free way. They play either individually or in small groups, with a therapist who encourages them, helps them resolve difficulties and talks with them about what they are doing and why, but does *not* instruct or guide them in any formal way. Play therapy is used as a means of understanding disturbed children and diagnosing the bases of their illness and also of helping them express themselves in

---

[40]Eloise C. Parker: "Play Therapy." *American Journal of Occupatinal Therapy,* September-October 1952.

nonverbal ways. For severely disturbed children, play may be the only way to encourage self-expression and communication and may represent the first step in communicating with a therapist and beginning treatment.

BIBLIOTHERAPY

This field consists of the guided use of reading to promote patient recovery. Ordinarily, it is facilitated by hospital librarians who become specialists in understanding patient needs and who help them select books, magazines or stories that will meet their interests and promote specific aspects of reintegration. Generally, it does not constitute a separate field with its own area of training but represents the work of librarians who become knowledgeable in the area of psychodynamics and who work closely with medical personnel in understanding and guiding patients' reading programs.

HORTICULTURE THERAPY

One of the oldest forms of therapy is horticulture therapy, which is based on the concept that seeing a plant develop from a seed or cutting and learning to understand the life cycle by growing a plant can be therapeutic for many individuals. Patients who need help in overcoming feelings of isolation and withdrawal may benefit from working in a greenhouse with others and sharing materials with them.

At Friends Hospital in Philadelphia, for example, horticulture therapy is an important element in the overall Department of Adjunctive Therapies. Using two modern greenhouses, a potting shed, and ample vegetable and flower gardens, patients meet in regular groups for instruction and supervision in their individual or group projects. Potting, propagation, identification and arrangement of plants, and various horticulture crafts may also be linked to service projects for the hospital or the surrounding community. In terms of carry-over value, horticulture therapy may lead to a long-lasting hobby interest or even a new field of personal study or vocational involvement.

Other Group Therapies

Each of the activity therapies just described may, to some degree, be part of the responsibility of therapeutic recreation specialists or may overlap with therapeutic recreation service. For example, in some hospitals or treatment centers, recreation workers conduct arts and crafts, music or dance programs and activities of daily living. Similarly, recreation specialists may provide adapted sports in some situations, although they would not normally be responsible for the kinds of one-to-one, medically prescribed services provided by physical therapists.

In addition to the services described here, many other forms of activity therapy may be found, such as "poetry therapy" or "photography therapy." Activity therapists also may be expected to conduct special programs such as "remotivation therapy," "reality orientation" and "sensory training," and to apply principles of behavior modification or reality therapy in their ongoing programs (see pp. 136–143). In such cases, they may be given in-service training or encouraged to attend outside institutes to become qualified in the use of these special methods.

WORKING WITHIN THE TREATMENT TEAM

In many institutions or agencies, therapeutic recreation is not a separate department, but is an integral part of a department of rehabilitation or adjunctive therapies. The therapeutic recreation specialist must be prepared to work knowledgeably and cooperatively as part of the treatment team.

Sherrill suggests that such patterns of cooperation should be developed as part of professional preparation. She writes,

It is important that prospective adapted physical educators, special educators, occupational therapists, physical therapists, recreators, and related others become acquainted and work together as early as possible in the undergraduate years. These professions have far more commonalities than differences. . . . each is extending its role and scope in response to new legislation; and each is dedicated to the self-actualization of handicapped persons.[41]

Valletutti and Christoplos urge that all professionals cooperate as fully as possible in serving disabled populations, regardless of traditional disciplinary boundaries and territorial protectiveness. They write,

Interdisciplinary team members should be viewed as *individuals* with insights and skills to contribute to the team rather than as representatives of a discipline. Team membership is thus envisaged as a state of mind and members as unique *contributors* to the whole team process.[42]

In addition to working closely with other activity therapists, the therapeutic recreation specialist must also coordinate his or her efforts with medical practitioners, dietetic and nutritional services, other health aides or health educators, nursing and related care services, psychological and social services, speech pathologists, the clergy and, of course, representatives of the community or concerned voluntary organizations. Within many hospitals, five or six of these disciplines may work closely on the treatment team in diagnosing patient needs, determining their pro-

---

[41]Sherrill, *op. cit.*, p. 51.
[42]Valletutti and Christoplos, *op. cit.*, p. 6.

gram and formulating treatment plans. It is essential that therapeutic recreation specialists be accepted on this team and that they play a significant role if they are to gain respect for their field of service and make a significant contribution to the overall treatment process.

To make the team work effectively, Witt writes, it is necessary for the specialist to provide accurate information to other team members and to collaborate closely with them in order to provide meaningful service and avoid duplication of efforts. It is helpful for each member of the team to become familiar with basic medical terminology and concepts and, when possible, to extend his or her own area of special competence by developing secondary therapeutic skills, as well as generalized skills of team management and administration. Above all, it is necessary to put the overall success of the team before all matters of individual prestige and to avoid personal or professional biases or defensiveness.[43]

STATUS OF THE FIELD

To what degree is therapeutic recreation recognized as a specialized field? As the earlier chapters of this text indicate, there has been a steady growth in the field of therapeutic recreation, first in hospitals and other treatment centers and more recently in community-based programs.

However, community recreators too often tend to see their function with respect to therapeutic recreation as limited to sponsoring senior citizens' clubs or providing an occasional special program for the mentally retarded or physically disabled. Few have fully accepted the view that this area of service represents a major responsibility of municipal recreation and park departments. Fewer still have developed meaningful links with institutions in order to facilitate post-discharge or outpatient programming for disabled persons.

In too many hospitals, the view held by administrators or key medical personnel is that recreation is chiefly a diversional activity and thus deserves lower priority than other services that are more closely related to treatment goals. In part, this attitude stems from the fact that, unlike occupational therapy and physical therapy, both of which are certified fields requiring clinical training under medical supervision, therapeutic recreation does *not* require such training. In many institutions, those working in recreation have come from other disciplines and have little specialized preparation for their work.

This problem is made more complex by the fact that many therapeutic recreation specialists today work in settings in which medically oriented training is *not* essential. The recreation leader who works in a senior center, a home or school for the retarded, a correctional institution or similar setting may require varied kinds of information related to that disability and its treatment goals and procedures, but it is not basically medical information.

Thus, it is essential that fuller attention be given to the nature of professional

---

[43]Jody Witt: "The Team Concept as Interpersonal Ping Pong." *Journal of Leisurability*, Ontario, Canada, April 1974, n.p.

education in therapeutic recreation service today, as well as to the kinds of selection, accreditation, registration or certification procedures that might be used to ensure a higher standard of professionalism among workers in this field.

Reimbursement and Effect on Recognition

Since so many treatment programs today are largely supported by federal funds such as Medicare, it is important to understand the place of recreation within such structures. For example, Park points out that for a number of years, federal Medicare regulations stipulated that such institutions as nursing homes had to have activity programs and activity directors to be eligible for Medicare funds. However, no regulations stipulated minimal standards for programs or professional staff, and it was only through the efforts of the National Therapeutic Recreation Society in cooperation with the Public Health Service that guidelines were developed that recognized therapeutic recreation as a professional discipline and included meaningful personnel classifications. Despite this progress, in many institutions throughout the United States in which occupational therapy and physical therapy represent reimbursable services, to be paid for by Medicare funds, recreation is *not* billed as a significant medical service. As a consequence, in such treatment centers, recreation is seen as an unimportant aspect of the overall rehabilitation program and is poorly supported.

The fact is that recreation therapy in hospitals *is* reimbursable through Medicare, Medicaid and third-party carriers. The Medicare-Medicaid Guide states the following under Regulation Section 6095.75 (Determination of Cost of Services to Beneficiaries):

For reimbursement purposes, the reasonable cost of recreational therapy furnished by a hospital to inpatients where such services are ordinarily furnished by the hospital to its inpatients should be included in computing the cost for routine services.[44]

Therapeutic recreation is also reimbursable in the psychiatric setting as an "active treatment," defined in the Government Programs Reimbursement Manual as a service furnished while the patient is receiving either active treatment or admission and related services necessary for diagnostic study and meeting the following criteria: (a) provided under an individualized treatment or diagnostic plan; (b) reasonably expected to improve the patient's condition or for the purpose of diagnosis; and (c) supervised and evaluated by a physician. Richard Patterson, Director of Activity Therapy at Mercy Hospital and Medical Center in San Diego, California, has done a systematic study of federal reimbursement procedures and points out that therapeutic recreation may be billed, just like occupational therapy,

---

[44]Richard Patterson: *The Development of a Self-Sufficient Therapeutic Recreation Service.* Mercy Hospital and Medical Center, San Diego, California, unpublished report, March 1977, pp. 1–2.

physical therapy or electroconvulsive or drug therapy, provided that it is planned for a particular patient and is prescribed, supervised and evaluated by a physician. In addition, it is necessary to document the treatment in medical records, giving progress notes, program descriptions and treatment plans in the accepted style of the regulatory agency and with such frequency as to give a full picture of the therapy administered.

Patterson concludes that, by following reimbursement guidelines properly, it is possible to lay the foundation for an income-producing, self-sufficient therapeutic recreation program within the general or psychiatric hospital. At the same time, he points out that there are certain pitfalls or dangers in this process, and that although it may upgrade the status of therapeutic recreation as a service and improve the morale of recreation practitioners, it may have a negative effect on the provision of recreation in the treatment setting.[45]

With growing interest in the question of third-party reimbursement—both as a funding source to support programs and as a recognition of professional status—the National Therapeutic Recreation Society has established a committee to promote third-party reimbursement for recreation therapy in hospitals and treatment settings. In 1982, under the leadership of Ray E. West, research was carried out to gauge the extent to which therapeutic recreation service is being reimbursed and to learn about the policies of insurance companies and federal agencies.

Also, there is a strong movement throughout the therapeutic recreation field to develop more rigorous and precise standards of practice to support a higher level of professional recognition. Recently, for example, Navar and Dunn edited a new publication dealing with the standards applied by the Joint Commission on Accreditation of Hospitals for child, adolescent and adult psychiatric, alcoholism and drug abuse treatment centers. This report had significant implications for therapeutic recreation service with respect to such processes as preparing policy and procedure manuals, documenting goals and activities, assessing clients and evaluating programs.[46]

Need to Clarify Roles and Responsibilities

As the first three chapters of this text have explained, the roles and responsibilities of therapeutic recreation specialists are extremely complex and varied. The objectives and methods of practitioners often differ greatly according to the setting in which they are employed and the needs of their patients or clients.

Therefore, it is necessary to define more sharply each of these specialized areas of service as to the needs of those served and the unique responsibilities or functions of the therapeutic recreation specialist in each of them. It is quite apparent that this varies widely from institution to institution—even within a particular area of service, such as psychiatric care. It is clear also that the other fields of professional

[45]*Ibid.*, pp. 3–5. See also *Medicare and Medicaid Guide.* Chicago, Blue Cross Association, June 11, 1974, pp. 6097, 8063, 8066.
[46]Nancy Navar and Julia Dunn, eds.: *Quality Assurance: Concerns for Therapeutic Recreation.* Champaign-Urbana, University of Illinois Department of Leisure Studies, 1981.

service described earlier also impinge on recreation. Occupational therapists frequently assume major responsibility for recreation in their institutions. Corrective therapists frequently conduct modified games and sports. Music, art and dance therapists often provide services that might be regarded as recreational.

Again, it should be the responsibility of college and university educators in this field and of those in professional organizations to carry on systematic research to clarify roles and functions. It would be appropriate for them to make recommendations regarding the assignment of responsibilities that might be helpful to those responsible for organizing services in institutions, communities or in federal or state-wide systems of rehabilitation. There is a related need to conduct more effective research on methodology in therapeutic recreation service and on the legitimate outcomes of such programs.

Strengthen Ties with Professional Preparation Programs

Key to the continued upgrading of therapeutic recreation service is the need to strengthen ties between agencies in the field and programs of professional preparation. This may be done through cooperative arrangements developed directly between recreation practitioners and faculty members in colleges or universities, or it may be part of a more comprehensive linkage, in which several disciplines are involved.

As an example, all ten psychiatric hospitals in the Province of Ontario are directly linked to one or more of Ontario's 15 universities, either as teaching arms of medical faculties or peripherally, using such tools as Telemedicine (a two-way audio-visual hook-up that allows for consultations, patient interviews, patient visits with relatives, counseling and lectures at a distance). In many cases, professional staff members in hospitals also have university affiliations. Several facilities boast significant research departments with funding available from the federal and provincial governments, in addition to private foundations. Similar arrangements have been established on a lesser scale in a number of areas of the United States (see p. 241).

A Challenge to Professionalism

Within the overall field of therapeutic recreation service, there has been widespread acceptance of the view that professionalism is a highly desirable goal. Van Andel, for example, describes the process of developing a set of program and personnel standards designed to help the field of therapeutic recreation service become a more viable, respected profession.[47] In general, strong support has been given to

---

[47]Glen E. Van Andel: "Professional Standards: Improving the Quality of Services." *Therapeutic Recreation Journal*, Second Quarter, 1981, pp. 23–26.

registration, certification, accreditation and similar efforts at upgrading the professionalization of therapeutic recreation service.

Yet, not all educators or practitioners have accepted this position. As an example, the very notion that it would be possible to define a college curriculum that would "produce" qualified practitioners based on a standardized educational model has been challenged. O'Morrow, in a recent discussion of the accreditation process, suggests the need to develop more than one track of professional preparation; he concludes that no uniform standards of accreditation will ever be practicable. Indeed, he suggests the risk that raising the standards of professional qualifications and imposing stricter accreditation requirements may be viewed by the public as "perpetuating the self-interest of the profession," rather than meeting a legitimate social need.[48]

Another leading educator, Peter Witt, suggests that some of the motivations for gaining a higher level of professional status are "potentially dangerous to the very public we so vehemently say we are trying to protect." Witt predicts that the certification-accreditation process

---

. . . will ultimately diminish the number of people entering the field and allow a closed group of "professionals" to control salaries, working conditions, etc. We will finally achieve the power, recognition, and status we have all been missing for so long.[49]

Further, he concludes that many of the attempts in therapeutic recreation service to acquire the "trappings" of professionalism are really efforts at white-collar unionism, which confuse the rhetoric of "quality of service" and "public protection" with job protection, and the search for higher salaries and status. Clearly, this issue needs to be debated within the field so that, in O'Morrow's words, therapeutic recreators place the welfare of society ahead of their own individual, institutional and professional interests.

A Positive Stance for Professionals Today

Beyond these concerns, in the early 1980's many practitioners and educators in the field of therapeutic recreation service recognized that their discipline was increasingly threatened by the sluggish economy and by deep budget cuts in human services. In a letter to the editor of the *NTRS Newsletter*, Joanne Ardolf Decker commented on budget cuts that had resulted in elimination of programs and services and on the "apathy and depression" caused by such assaults. However, she

---

[48]Gerald S. O'Morrow: "Therapeutic Recreation Accreditation: Its Problems and Future." *Therapeutic Recreation Journal*, Second Quarter, 1981, pp. 36–38.

[49]Peter A. Witt: "Professionalism/Certification/Accreditation: What's At Stake?" *Leisure Commentary and Practice*. Denton, Texas, North Texas State University Division of Recreation and Leisure Studies, March 1982, pp. 1–2.

continued, this made it all the more necessary for professionals to unite in support of their national organization, to

---

... take an open stand as guardians of the services we believe to be *essential* to quality of life for our clients. . . .

There is a current need for NTRS and every local and state body of therapeutic recreation specialists to set a plan of action to create high visibility for recreation programs and educate others about the importance of recreation services. We must become a creative, viable force giving each other ideas of how to create a high profile for our services while supporting each other during this time of crisis. It's high time to become a united force . . . and stay alive![50]

Without question, Decker's message is an important one for all therapeutic recreation practitioners. It is not enough for them to upgrade the quality of their work and to gain the recognition of other professionals. It is also critically important that the public—including legislators, civic officials and policy-makers—become fully aware of the role played by recreation in the lives of the ill and disabled, and of the human values and rehabilitative functions recreation serves.

Suggested Topics for Class Discussion, Examination Questions or Student Papers

1. Identify and describe several of the major functions of therapeutic recreation specialists in hospitals or other treatment settings today. In what ways do these extend beyond the direct conduct of recreation programs?

2. How does the National Therapeutic Recreation Society promote professional development in this field today? Be specific with respect to standards for the credentialing of professional personnel and the accreditation of higher education programs.

3. Contrast the work of specialists in other fields of activity therapy (such as occupational or physical therapy) with that of therapeutic recreation specialists. Describe both similarities and differences in goals and methods, and indicate how specialists in various fields can work together cooperatively within the treatment team.

4. Therapeutic recreation is today practiced widely not only in medical and other institutional settings, but also in many community agencies. Recognizing that therapy is often not the primary thrust of such programs, what are other typical emphases for practitioners in community settings?

---

[50]Joanne Ardolf Decker: Letter to the Editor. In *National Therapeutic Recreation Society Newsletter*, Alexandria, Virginia, January 1982, pp. 2–3.

4

Program Planning in Therapeutic Recreation Service

This chapter is concerned with program development in therapeutic recreation service. It examines the basic orientation of the sponsoring agency, its administrative structure and other logistical details of the program setting. Several recent approaches to program planning are presented as well as a number of guidelines for scheduling activities and involving patients or clients in activities. The chapter also describes several special techniques which may be used as part of therapeutic recreation programming, including leisure counseling and leisure education. In conclusion, it covers a number of guidelines for therapeutic recreation program planning in various settings.

FACTORS AFFECTING THERAPEUTIC RECREATION PROGRAM PLANNING

Therapeutic recreation program planning depends on certain key factors, such as (a) the type of sponsoring agency or department; (b) the agency's administrative structure and staffing capability; (c) the overall philosophy of the treatment staff and the services offered by other disciplines or agencies; (d) the service model being followed (medical-clinical, education and training or others); (e) the exact nature of the population being served—its degree of disability, age, diversity, stage of recovery or rehabilitation and so on; (f) the physical resources and setting of the agency or department; and (g) the nature of patient or client involvement in program development.

It should be understood at the outset that in many places, program development is approached on a rather casual basis, without a systematic process of goal-setting or patient/client assessment. Often, when a new program is being introduced in a general hospital or nursing home, the recreation specialist in charge is likely to begin with the tentative introduction of a few obviously needed activities or services, gradually adding to them for a more comprehensive program.

In such situations, it may be desirable to work in close cooperation with other professionals and to solicit their advice and suggestions. For example, Evans writes of the process of developing a diversified recreation program in a 217-bed hospital concerned with short-term patient care in Guelph, Ontario. Here, it was necessary to develop appropriate treatment goals and activities for a wide range of patients, including postoperative, stroke and burn patients, diabetics, cardiac convalescents, pediatric and geriatric populations and those in other categories. The bulk of the case load was referred by doctors and head nurses, and it was necessary to work closely with the director of nursing, the occupational therapist and the physical therapist, as well as volunteers and representatives of community agencies.[1] Obviously, within this framework no single set of goals could easily be developed, and it was necessary to adapt to the needs and expressed interests of patients, as well as the recommendations of staff members.

In large hospitals or treatment centers, programs may follow rather inflexible guidelines set forth in manuals or presented at in-service training programs. Several factors may influence the selection of program formats, including the "expressed desires" of those being served, current practices in similar institutions, tradition and the views of the program director. The contemporary trend in therapeutic recreation service, however, is toward prescriptive programming, and it is this approach that is emphasized in this chapter and the next.

Sponsoring Agency or Department

As Chapter 1 points out, therapeutic recreation service is provided in many different types of agencies or community settings. The nature of each agency or department affects its goals and choice of service models. Numerous examples are given throughout this text of varied types of organizations in which recreation represents an important program focus—although its specific objectives differ sharply from setting to setting. Another key aspect of the agency or institution is its administrative structure, staffing pattern and available facilities.

Administrative Structure

Administrative structure varies considerably from institution to institution. Recreation may be provided as a separate service, with its own departmental title, or may be part of a larger department. In a regional study of recreation in psychiatric institutions, it was found that recreation was most frequently located within a separate department (42.7 per cent) and next as a service within a department of psychiatry (13.3 per cent), occupational therapy (12 per cent), activity therapies (10.7

---

[1]Lorna Evans: "The Guelph General Hospital Story." *Journal of Leisurability*, Ontario, Canada, January 1974, pp. 27–31.

per cent), rehabilitation service (5.3 percent) and within several other less frequently found structures.[2]

Recreation may be provided as an institution-wide service, with a single centralized staff organizing and providing services for the entire patient or client population, *or* it may be decentralized so that each unit of the institution has its own treatment staff (usually including medical, nursing, activity therapy and social service personnel). The effect of such varying patterns of organization may be to encourage the development of rather rigid program schedules and services or more informal and flexible programs involving a high degree of patient choice.

It is apparent that the extent to which therapeutic recreation is administered independently (although staff members obviously may interact closely with others on the treatment team) affects the degree of autonomous decision-making and planning on the part of its director and staff. If recreation is part of another administrative unit, such as "recreation and camping" or "recreation and social service," this too will affect its program emphasis.

Staffing Capability

The standards and hiring expectations of agencies and departments strongly influence the kinds of staff members who are employed and their capabilities for programming and leadership. For example, a department that requires staff members to hold degrees in therapeutic recreation from accredited colleges or universities, or to be registered with the National Therapeutic Recreation Society, is likely to have much higher expectations of them than agencies which hire individuals with more limited backgrounds. Similarly, some departments may seek only generalists, while others may be able to employ individuals with highly developed specialized skills in arts and crafts, music, leisure counseling or other areas.

The nature of the hiring agency will have much to do with staffing patterns. For example, in most governmental institutions, staff members are normally identified by professional titles and Civil Service grades, although on the job they may be assigned different titles within the table of organization. A Civil Service title might be *Recreation Therapist II*, while within a given institution the title might be *Senior Activity Leader*. Program responsibilities are customarily assigned to personnel according to rank, with upper-level staff members, such as directors, supervisors or senior therapists, assuming major responsibility for planning, coordinating and directing services while lower-level personnel provide direct program service and activity leadership. The numbers of recreation staff members may vary greatly, with as many as 30 or 40 activity therapists, including 10 or 12 recreation specialists, in a large state hospital, and as few as one or two leaders in a small nursing home or sheltered workshop program.

Such factors tend to influence both the flexibility with which staff members

---

[2]Richard Kraus: *Recreation and Related Therapies in Psychiatric Rehabilitation.* New York, Herbert Lehman College and Faculty Research Foundation, November 1972, p. 17.

may be assigned to various functions and the extent to which they can be involved in patient assessment, meeting with the treatment team or similar services.

Philosophy of Treatment Staff and Related Services

A less tangible but equally important factor in therapeutic recreation program development is the philosophy of an agency's administrators. If they have a limited view of recreation's potential contribution, the program itself may be restricted to a relatively minor role—used to fill up "idle" hours when patients are not undergoing other, more "serious" therapies or services. Administrators may view recreation as a morale booster and emphasize only large-scale diversional activities. It is essential for the recreation staff to present a strong case for recreation as a type of treatment and to strive to develop a program that proves this case.

The activities offered by other therapeutic disciplines may also influence the development of a therapeutic recreation program. For example, a hospital with a strong corrective therapy unit may have it run all sports, games, fitness and outdoor recreation activities. In some situations, occupational therapists provide extremely rich arts and crafts activities; as a result, recreation specialists may offer limited arts programs. Ideally, even when specialists in other areas offer such activities, recreation specialists should be doing so as well—but with different objectives and techniques.

Choice of Service Models

Probably the most important influence on a program is the service model under which it operates. As Chapter 2 demonstrates, these may encompass a wide range of possibilities, including *clinical* and *nonclinical* approaches, or, more specifically, custodial, medical-clinical, therapeutic milieu, education and training and community models (pp. 62–67).

In an effort to clarify the varied functions or stages of therapeutic recreation service, the 1982 philosophy statement adopted by the membership of the National Therapeutic Recreation Society identified the three key functions of therapeutic recreation service: *therapy, leisure education* and *recreational participation.*

Within a particular department or agency, one of these may be emphasized heavily and the others given less weight. In some settings, all three may receive equal emphasis. It is important to recognize that the distinctions made among these three functions are somewhat arbitrary. For example, it is possible to become educated about leisure *while* engaging in a recreational activity. Therapy itself may be enjoyable (although prescribed, not voluntary) and the very act of taking part in recreational activity may have strong therapeutic benefits. It is the particular goal of a given area of service that determines the way it is presented. For instance, painting, a form of artistic expression, may be presented as therapy, leisure education or recreation, and may have benefits in any of these three roles.

DEVELOPMENTAL GOALS

In some settings, recreation may have a developmental purpose—essentially as education for its own sake—rather than therapy or leisure education. Geddes cites many examples of how physical activities promote physical, intellectual or social-emotional goals among disabled individuals.[3] Later chapters will show in detail how recreation helps the mentally retarded to gain the confidence to function in the community, develop appropriate behavior, gain a sense of independence, learn to care for themselves and live independently. Such goals are not therapy, education for leisure, or recreation in the sense of being purely diversional. Instead, the goals are either educational or habilitative—not rehabilitative, which suggests regaining skills (which such individuals have not had before), but habilitative in the sense of learning to function effectively in a new environment.

Nature of the Population Being Served

The nature of an individual's disability is a key factor in program development. It influences not only the goals of therapeutic recreation service but also its potential limits.

Some individuals may be alert and active, even hyperactive. Others may be autistic or highly regressed, showing little or no response to stimuli. Some may be physically capable but unable to relate to reality. Others may have severe physical impairments but be highly intelligent and positively motivated to participate in leisure activities.

Each population—whether it be the mentally ill, mentally retarded, physically disabled, dependent aging or socially deviant—has a unique set of capabilities and deficits, which imposes a special set of goals for therapeutic recreation service. However, the problem is more complex than simply determining what the characteristics and needs of a given disability group are. Within each category, each patient or client is an *individual*. He or she may be classified as a moderately mentally retarded young adult—but may be very different from every other person in his or her club or sheltered workshop, in terms of temperament, experience and personality.

Similarly, some individuals who suffer spinal cord injuries and become paraplegic or quadriplegic want to curl up and die; life represents a challenge they do not even want to try to meet. Others with the same degree of dysfunction are optimistic and daring, and venture into an incredible range of vocational and recreational challenges, including high-risk outdoor recreation activities that many able-bodied individuals would avoid.

Programs must be designed to meet the needs of patients or clients who may be at different stages of recovery; one person is just getting over the immediate effects of a major trauma or illness while another is ready to get a job and begin a new life.

---

[3]Dolores Geddes: *Physical Activities for Individuals with Handicapping Conditions.* St. Louis, C. V. Mosby, 1978, pp. 20–25.

Program planning to meet such diverse needs obviously requires sensitivity and flexibility—particularly when the therapeutic recreation specialist is working not only with *individuals,* but with *groups* of individuals, all with different needs and interests. Here lies a major challenge for the therapeutic recreator. Numerous examples cited in Chapters 6 through 11 show how that challenge can be met.

Physical Resources and Setting of Program

Still another important factor in program planning has to do with the facilities, equipment and other physical resources of the agency or department.

Obviously, the number and type of available facilities play a major role in helping to determine program services. Many large psychiatric or chronic disease hospitals have auditoriums, lounges, music rooms and even swimming pools, arts and crafts shops, outdoor ballfields, picnic areas and tennis courts. On the other hand, it is not uncommon to find some hospitals in which all activities are carried on within the ward or in a crowded day room.

Although it is clearly much easier to run a rich activity program in a well-endowed complex, this is not the sole criterion in determining a program's effectiveness. In some penal and correctional institutions, for example, there may be facilities that are hardly used because of lack of staff or administrative support or because problems of security and staff coverage militate against diversified programming. Even though it is important to make the fullest possible use of available resources, it is also possible to "make do." In many nursing homes, for example, cafeterias or dining rooms are also used as meeting rooms, and auditoriums also double as gymnasiums in many agencies. In addition, many hospitals or special schools make use of other public, voluntary or commercially owned facilities in the community at large.

What is critical is that facilities be obtained, improvised or borrowed to serve all of the major elements of a diversified program. The use of facilities must be carefully coordinated with other hospital or agency services to avoid overlapping usage and to ensure safety and administrative efficiency. For example, arts and crafts rooms, swimming pools, meeting rooms or other facilities may be used by more than one discipline or by different units of a hospital. These are usually assigned according to schedules worked out by the administrative heads or supervisors of various units or services and cleared by the institution's buildings and grounds staff. When off-grounds facilities are to be used or when patients take a trip to attend some community event, it usually must be cleared through administrative channels, with, in some cases, medical clearance or the permission of parents or guardians.

In addition, there are usually clearly stated hospital or agency guidelines governing the use of all facilities or the scheduling of all trips. These may include (a) permissions and approval from administration and authorization from parents or guardians; (b) regulations regarding staff members taking patients of the opposite sex off grounds; (c) nature of transportation, including use of hospital-owned or private vehicles; (d) role of volunteers in assisting with transportation and supervision; (e) required ratios of accompanying staff; (f) regulations controlling participation of patients in outside activities, as opposed to involvement as spectators; (g) regulations governing emergency situations, accidents or lost or runaway patients or clients; and (h) cooperative parties, picnics or other special events sponsored with parents, community groups or other assisting groups.

It is essential that architectural barriers be eliminated from facilities serving the orthopedically handicapped or those with other serious physical impairments.

A closely related concern is transportation of the disabled to recreation facilities in the community. Since public transportation is frequently not adaptable to the special requirements of the disabled, vans and buses must often be equipped with hydraulic lifts for loading wheelchairs. Some community-based programs have volunteers transport disabled individuals to recreation programs. Obviously, the ability to arrange transportation and to provide accessible facilities for the disabled are important factors in therapeutic recreation planning.

Patient/Client Involvement in Planning

Therapeutic recreation programmers must involve those being served in planning their own programs as fully as possible. In the past, clients were usually treated as if they were not capable of making intelligent decisions, as if they were young children being served by all-wise adults. Today, there is a strong conviction that disabled people themselves must take responsibility for their own lives to a much greater degree and should play a stronger role in speaking out in patient councils or before the boards of voluntary agencies. At hearings before city councils or legislative committees, it is common for disabled participants to join with staff members and other advocates to forcefully make their needs known.

PATTERNS OF INVOLVEMENT BY PATIENTS AND CLIENTS

How are disabled participants to be involved in programming? To what degree are they given free choice in institutional settings, for example, as opposed to being assigned to activities through prescriptive programming?

At the simplest level, therapeutic recreation planners should ask disabled individuals to be members of program development committees, or survey them through the use of "interest-finder" questionnaires.

There is no typical patient program involvement. As an example of the varied patterns of involvement, the regional study of recreation in psychiatric facilities, described earlier, found that there was an almost equal incidence of hospitals reporting that patients were involved in activities through "complete free choice" (40 per cent), "assigned individually" (38.7 per cent) or "assigned by group" (46.7 per cent), with many institutions using a combination of several methods.[4] Although the most desirable situation might appear to be one in which patients

---

[4]Kraus, *op. cit.*, pp. 21–22.

took part in only those activities that they chose for themselves, in many cases the nature of their illness is such that if given free choice they would engage in *no* recreational, social, work or educational activities at all. The rationale for this approach is expressed in the following passage:

> ... disruptive, asocial and socially unacceptable behavior, often called emotional disorder, may perhaps best be seen as chronic social disruption. For these people, perhaps, a living and learning program of activities might best meet their needs.... An answer then seems to be that the disabled would benefit most from a structured learning situation. The activity therapies can be seen as a part of milieu therapy, which definitely implies a structuring of the environment. Structure involves certain regulations, directions and control, and in a sense at least, certain limitations of freedom for the individual. Such limitations ... have the very purpose of giving greater freedoms in certain other directions.... Various kinds of structure and prescribed activities, with the proper kinds of supervision, have a therapeutic effect.[5]

Optimally, over the course of treatment patients move from prescribed to voluntary participation. And, through group action, they may plan and conduct many aspects of the activity program themselves. Certainly in senior centers or clubs for the physically disabled, the most successful ventures are those in which the participants play a major role in program development.

Mainstreaming as a Planning Focus

It must be stressed that integration of the disabled, along with the process of "normalization," represents a key objective of all therapeutic recreation programming. Gunn and Peterson point out that most disabled individuals do not live, work or play exclusively with other disabled people. Instead, they represent an important part of our society; to treat them separately is to deny them the fullest possible self-expression and the right to enjoy the good things of life. The goal of "mainstreaming" and "normalization" is to enable disabled persons to live as much as possible like other people. Gunn and Peterson write,

> The most important mainstreaming principle is *integration* into regular programs — both physically and socially. For handicapped people to achieve and maintain normative behaviors, appearances, and interpretations and for them to be accepted by society, maximum integration into the cultural mainstream is essential. This is achieved in the field of recreation only when *all* programs and facilities are accessible to the handicapped and totally staffed by persons with some basic knowledge about the needs of persons with handicapping conditions.[6]

---

[5]*Activity Therapy Manual.* Longview, Ohio, State Hospital, 1973, p. 21.
[6]Scout Lee Gunn and Carol Ann Peterson: *Therapeutic Recreation Program Design: Principles and Procedures.* Englewood Cliffs, New Jersey, Prentice-Hall, 1979, pp. 42–43.

Ideally, *all* disabled persons should be served in the same settings as the non-disabled population. The reality is that this is not always feasible. Many disabled individuals suffer from such severe physical, mental or social impairments that they would be unable to function successfully in integrated situations. In some cases, integration might result in the disabled suffering repeated failure and rejection—and this would be contrary to their best interests.

For these reasons, later sections on mainstreaming will demonstrate a variety of patterns for integrated and segregated programming. Some moderately disabled individuals may participate fully in integrated programming with the nondisabled—particularly if the activity lends itself to such a process of mainstreaming. Other disabled persons may function partly in integrated programs and partly in special programming for the disabled. For still others, segregated programming is the most realistic solution. For examples of such programming variations for disabled campers, see page 175. Ideally, the program should be a continuum, moving patients or clients from segregated programs toward higher levels of independence and integration.

APPROACHES TO THE PLANNING PROCESS

How are therapeutic recreation programs planned and developed?

First, it is necessary to identify the program's goals and objectives. *Goals* are broad statements of purpose or major outcomes that the program seeks to achieve. Typical goals of therapeutic recreation programs are to (a) provide participants with opportunities for satisfaction in order to enhance the quality of their lives; (b) provide therapeutic experiences which help to minimize dysfunction or contribute to the process of physical or emotional recovery; (c) help the individual to learn more about leisure activities and develop a positive attitude toward participating; and (d) contribute to the participant's ability to function autonomously in community life by providing satisfying group experiences.

Objectives are more concrete statements of purposes and serve as a means of achieving the major goals. Sponsoring agencies may have direct objectives, or the objectives may be expressed in terms of behavioral changes desired in participants. A number of examples of specific sets of objectives for different populations of disabled individuals are cited in the chapters that follow. In some cases, objectives simply state the specific skills to be learned or behaviors to be changed. In others, objectives set goals for participation. Whenever possible, objectives should be designed so that the extent to which they have been achieved is measurable.

To meet objectives, a number of specific techniques may be used: (a) *patient or client assessment*, an evaluation of the behavioral status and needs of individuals being served, which helps to establish objectives; (b) *interest finders, intake forms, interviews* or other techniques to determine what the past experience of clients or patients has been and what types of activities they would like to engage in; (c) *activity analysis*, a study of various program elements in order to determine the kinds of behavioral skills they require, the types of group structures and social interaction they provide, their cognitive, psychomotor and affective components and benefits and similar elements; (d) *activity adaptations or modifications* to make specific activities appropriate for individuals with impairment, in order to ensure success and goal-achievement; and (e) *systematic ways of observing and measuring outcomes,* to help improve a program while it is being carried on and to determine its ultimate success.

Several of these techniques are described in detail in this chapter and the next, and also are illustrated in the other chapters dealing with specific types of disabilities.

Developing Group and Individual Activity Plans

After the goals and objectives are set, a program is established to achieve them, both for the overall patient or client population and for individual participants.

The program may have a variety of elements. Typically, it could include (a) mass activities providing passive entertainment or diversion, such as watching films or television; (b) mass activities involving participation, with some degree of instruction or direct leadership, such as a dance, parties, carnivals, card-playing or bingo; (c) small-group creative activities, perhaps involving direct instruction, such as arts and crafts, chorus, hobbies, sports, dance or horticulture; (d) social clubs for those clients or patients who form a cohesive group; (e) group therapy sessions related to remotivation, sensory training, reality therapy and similar elements; or (f) individual activities in which clients or patients pursue their own interests separately or on a one-to-one basis with staff members.

Within this range of program activities, participants may be involved in several ways. All involvement may be of a purely *voluntary* nature, with individuals making their own choices. Or, all participation may be *prescribed and involuntary,* and carefully monitored by members of the treatment team. In most treatment settings, there is a blend of both types, with participants engaging in some activities of their own choice and in others scheduled by therapists.

Different activities and different levels of participation may be planned to accomplish different goals; i.e., a patient may take part in an arts and crafts program to gain creative satisfactions, participate in a social club program to improve his or her patterns of interpersonal involvement, and take trips to museums or theaters to prepare for the positive use of leisure after discharge from a treatment center.

Ideally, a patient or client should be involved with several levels of group activity, such as *individual, small group* or *mass activity.* Preferably, the patient's overall involvement in therapeutic recreation should also include a balance of activities—both physically strenuous and quiet, intellectually demanding and undemanding, challenging and simple.

Activity Scheduling

Once a variety of activities have been selected, it is necessary to schedule them according to a daily as well as weekly or monthly cycle of activities. In the past, many institutions tended to follow an extremely rigid and segmentalized schedule of activities, with weekly schedules posted in all locations and patients assigned to activities at regular times during the day or evening. Today, scheduling tends to be more flexible, with a much higher degree of patient choice in the selection of activities. Schedules are normally worked out through the cooperative effort of all team members in order to meet their particular needs and avoid overlapping and duplication. In most situations, certain services—particularly those connected with medical treatment or prescribed physical therapy—are given priority when assigning blocks of time. It is important, however, that other services be given significant blocks of time and that these scheduling commitments then be respected, rather than arbitrarily changed or canceled because of the decision of medical or nursing staff members.

TIME BLOCKS

There are usually morning, afternoon and evening sessions in which certain key activities are offered each day. Other, more specialized program elements may be offered less frequently. Each of the major elements in the activity program should be assigned appropriate times, including (a) scheduled time for small-group activity; (b) open hours for informal arts and crafts or sports; (c) time for social programs and group discussions; (d) time for religious activity, either on-site or off-grounds; (e) appropriate time for trips and community involvement; (f) time for major events or institution-wide programs, such as large parties, carnivals or bazaars; (g) assigned hours for special therapies, like *sensory training* or *remotivation;* and (h) opportunities for one-to-one or small-group leisure-counseling sessions.

Time blocks must be tailored to the available facilities as well as to staff schedules. For example, leaders or therapists must have hours assigned to group meetings, filling out reports or records, in-service training and other administrative duties. Some of these duties must be assigned to regular weekly time slots; others may fill gaps between other leadership activities. In developing schedules, it is important not to have major blocks of time, such as evenings and weekends, when *no* activities are offered. In some institutions, Civil Service personnel are employed on a weekday schedule from 9 A.M. to 5 P.M., leaving only part-time workers or aides assigned to evening hours or weekends and these periods extremely barren of activity. This is particularly true because other therapeutic services are not usually scheduled at these times—resulting in a great deal of empty time for patients. To alleviate this problem, some institutions stipulate that activity therapists must work an alternating schedule so that they will have some evening session responsibilities—or duty every third weekend, with days off *during* that week.

Such scheduling should provide both a skeletal framework of regular activities with participation of a prescribed or voluntary nature and enough flexibility to permit the introduction of new activities, events or groups on relatively short notice. As much as possible, patients' needs should be the primary basis for scheduling decisions rather than the convenience of staff members or the goal of administrative efficiency.

In some settings with many patients or clients, several different types of activities may be scheduled simultaneously. In others, with a limited number of participants or staff members, only one or two activities may be provided at any given time.

The preceding section has described a relatively straightforward and familiar approach to selecting and scheduling program activities. Over the past several years, a number of authorities have developed more systematic approaches to planning and carrying out therapeutic recreation programs.

Systems Analysis in Therapeutic Recreation

Peterson has developed a model of program planning in therapeutic recreation with three basic elements: *input* (combination of clients, resources, personnel and materials), *transformation process* (involving in this case some form of service or program involvement) and *output* (referring to changed patient or client behavior).[7] The key to this sequence is the element of *feedback*, in which the programmer seeks ongoing information to determine whether the system is working as anticipated or whether it needs to be modified.

Peterson devised a matrix, or grid, of therapeutic recreation services of three types (preventative, sustaining and remedial) that in turn are provided on administrative, supervisory, leadership and educational levels. She points out that specific therapeutic recreation systems must function within the framework of a larger agency, institution or department that in turn exists within the suprasystem of the overall society. These surrounding or higher systems provide input to the therapeutic recreation system in the form of patients or clients, staffing and other resources at the same time that they impose agency or societal expectations, values and constraints. The heart of Peterson's method is based on the definition of systems analysis as

---

a systematic approach to helping a decision maker choose a course of action by investigating his full problem, searching out his objectives and alternatives, using an appropriate framework — insofar as possible analytic — to bring judgment and intuition to bear on the problem.[8]

On the basis of this understanding, Peterson has designed a program planning procedure founded on fundamental principles of systems analysis and applied it to the actual problems and situations found in therapeutic recreation service. She describes it as a flexible tool rather than a totally fixed procedure. It contains seven stages that might be applied, with some degree of elaboration or modification, to any therapeutic recreation setting:

---

[7]Carol A. Peterson: "Application of Systems Analysis Procedures to Program Planning in Therapeutic Recreation Service." *In* Elliott M. Avedon: *Therapeutic Recreation Service: An Applied Behavioral Science Approach.* Englewood Cliffs, New Jersey, Prentice-Hall, 1974, pp. 80–103.
[8]E. S. Quade, cited in Peterson, *ibid.*, p. 136.

1. *Conceptualization and Formulation.* The planner or analyst identifies the components in the process (agency, clients, resources, current status of program and purposes or objectives).

2. *Investigation.* This stage involves fuller study of the clients, the agency and the environment in relation to program goals and identification of the most promising alternative program elements or strategies to achieve objectives.

3. *Analysis of Alternatives.* The planner analyzes the probable outcomes of each alternative program element or strategy based on known factors in the situation or overall system. In some types of systems, this is done with computer analysis; this approach tends to be used less frequently in therapeutic recreation service.

4. *Determination of Strategy or Course of Action.* The planner selects an appropriate course of action and identifies needed service components, resources, leadership, facilities and so forth.

5. *Design of Program.* In this key stage, the planner formulates specific goals and objectives of the program (usually stated in clearly measurable and quantifiable behavioral terms). He or she designs the actual program sequence, activities, schedules and so on and constructs criteria and evaluation methods for each element of service.

6. *Operations Planning.* As a continuation of the previous stage, detailed schedules, staff assignment and training, preparation of facilities, acquisition of needed supplies or equipment and similar operations are planned and put in motion.

7. *Implementation.* The plan is put into action. As in all systems operations, it is continually reviewed and needed improvements or changes are carried out. If feedback indicates that elements need to be redesigned, or objectives rethought, this is done. Full evaluation would be carried out after a period of time in order to give the operation sufficient time to achieve its stated goals.[9]

Peterson's approach, which she illustrates with the example of a nursing home's therapeutic recreation program, may be applied to many other types of settings. It may be used to design an entire program or to solve a single limited problem in an agency.

Computer-Based Activity Analysis and Prescriptive Programming

A second line of development for providing a more rational and scientific basis for selecting and prescribing appropriate recreation activities for disabled populations has explored the use of the computer. In the past, activities have been selected with a limited concern about their specific elements, applications and outcomes. Similarly, behavioral objectives for patients and clients have been stated in extremely broad terms. A number of studies during the past several years, however, have sought to sharpen both the understanding of the specific elements inherent in recreational activities and the methods for modifying them for varying levels of skill or making them progressively more challenging. Recently, investigators have explored the potential of computer analysis in determining program goals, client

---

[9]Adapted from Peterson, *ibid.*, pp. 137–155.

needs and appropriate forms of activity prescription. Such approaches show considerable promise for providing more precise and sophisticated methods of designing programs in order to meet specific treatment, rehabilitative or educational goals.

BERRYMAN-LEFEBVRE MODEL

Under a three-year grant from the Bureau of Education for the Handicapped of the U.S. Office of Education, Doris Berryman and Claudette Lefebvre of New York University have developed preliminary models intended to assist institutions or community agencies in providing effective and comprehensive therapeutic recreation services for disabled children and youth. In the investigators' words,

---

. . . there is a great need to systematically analyze and organize existing information on utilization of play and recreation activities to achieve specific education, learning and/or treatment goals; develop a conceptual model for comprehensive analysis of play and recreation activities to determine the sensory-motor, cognitive, affective and social dimensions inherent in those activities; and, utilizing the information derived from these analyses, design a therapeutically-oriented recreation program for disabled children and youth which will assist in developing perceptual-motor, cognitive and social skills and abilities.[10]

Following the design of these models and computer programs storing activity analysis data and client demographic and behavioral assessment information, Berryman and Lefebvre moved ahead to carry out pilot demonstrations of the project in Hempstead, New York. Clearly, this approach offers significant promise for helping to make therapeutic recreation a more significant and respected form of service, particularly within institutions or agencies operating under the *medical-clinical* or *education and training* models. Like the Peterson systems analysis method, however, it does raise a serious question as to whether it is possible to reduce an area of human service to a computerized model with precise diagnoses and quantifiable outcomes. Certainly, within such fields as psychotherapy or social work, although the broad directions of treatment may be indicated, it would be unlikely that the exact outcomes of treatment or the effects of different types of therapeutic strategies could be either predicted or measured objectively as a practical form of everyday programming. Beyond this, as earlier chapters have shown, a major thrust in recent years has been *away* from prescriptive programming by therapists and in the direction of milieu therapy, in which all concerned (patients and staff alike) serve as therapeutic agents, chiefly through a process of social interaction and overcoming problems of self-management and group living. Nonetheless, it seems clear that

---

[10]Doris L. Berryman and Claudette B. Lefebvre: "A Computer Based System for Comprehensive Activity Analysis and Prescriptive Recreation Programming for Disabled Children and Youth." *In* Betty van der Smissen, ed.: *Indicators of Change in the Recreation Environment—A National Research Symposium.* State College, Pennsylvania, Penn State HPER Series No. 6, 1975, pp. 99–116.

within the *medical-clinical* model of service there will be continuing efforts to develop new and more effective models of therapeutic recreation service delivery.

COMPTON-PRICE LINEAR MODEL

One medical-clinical model has been developed by David Compton and Donna Price. Entitled the *Linear Model for Individual Treatment in Recreation* (LMIT), it represents a detailed model for planning, implementing, recording and evaluating program service for an individual client.[11] Its seven stages, or phases, are similar to those in other systems approaches—including developing a personal profile of the client, determining objectives and planning activities for the treatment unit, implementing the unit treatment plan and evaluating its results.

The unique element of LMIT is the utilization of a rating system that evaluates performance over time in six developmental areas: cognitive, communicative, motor, self-help, social-emotional and expressive. The important point about the use of this type of performance evaluation is that it specifies exactly the types of tasks to be performed as well as the exact behavioral outcomes of planned or prescribed activity. Use of such instruments is essential if systems analysis or computer-based planning is to contribute to the successful development of therapeutic recreation programs. Compton describes the essential purpose of LMIT or similar models:

. . . to provide the practitioner with a greater degree of accountability for the ''purposive intervention'' in therapeutic recreation; to utilize the most current and relevant techniques from related areas; to develop precision in the delivery of therapeutic recreation services; to provide the therapist with a step-by-step systems analysis of the delivery of therapeutic recreation services to individuals; for application primarily to those individuals who have accentuated needs, especially the more profoundly handicapped; and for application to clients regardless of their age, sex, diagnostic category or severity of dysfunction.[12]

Despite the fact that Compton and Price's model is primarily concerned with young children, a similar approach might be used with any age group or type of disability. Peterson's major example was the development of an activity program for a nursing home. It is important to stress that the initiation of such a program is expensive. Although it is possible to employ computer experts, train observers and mount a substantial budget for program planning in a federally funded project, such as Berryman and Lefebvre's, in most situations this would not be feasible.

Realistically, it is likely that through experimental work by leading researchers and theorists in this field, new program principles and uses of activity with specific disability categories will be developed and will then be applied directly by practitioners in treatment settings. New guidelines or formulations for developing pro-

---

[11]David M. Compton and Donna Price: "Individualizing Your Treatment Program: A Case Study Using LMIT." *Therapeutic Recreation Journal,* Fourth Quarter, 1975, pp. 127–134.
[12]*Ibid.*

grams tend to be disseminated through the professional literature, by professional organizations or, in many cases, through networks of organizations that guide member agencies or institutions in their basic policies.

RELATED TREATMENT MODALITIES

A final element to be considered in this chapter is the use of special therapeutic techniques by therapeutic recreators. In the following section, a number of such methods are described in detail. All of them are concerned with behavior and so are most appropriate for populations with psychiatric disability or forms of social deviance. However, any serious physical disability also may be accompanied by emotional and psychological effects. Therefore, these methods may in some cases be useful with those who have physical impairments.

Sensory Training

Sensory training is a group experience specially designed to assist residents of nursing homes or hospital geriatric units who are classifed as suffering from organic brain syndrome or institutional neurosis. Organic brain syndrome, often called *senile dementia* in the aged, is "commonly due either to vascular degeneration interfering with the blood supply to the brain, or to senile degeneration of the brain substance itself. Its manifestations include memory defect, intellectual deterioration, uninhibited behavior and loss of emotional control."

Institutional neurosis is the term applied by Whitehead to the effects of institutionalization on patients who, on being subjected to regimentation, lose their sense of individuality and independence and suffer an erosion of personality.[13] Geriatric patients, who are particularly vulnerable, tend to refuse to respond to the limited stimuli in their isolated environments. Such individuals, commonly referred to as "disoriented," seem to have little or no awareness of time or space; often, they do not respond to even the simplest occupational or recreational tasks. The rationale for sensory training, according to Leona Richman, who helped develop the method, is to make use of participation in a closely knit group and the impact of selected stimuli, guided exercises and social interaction to prevent further atrophy of the senses and, hopefully, to improve alertness. She describes the method in the following terms:

1. Sensory training is designed for the patient who is regressed, blind, or wheelchair-bound, and does not participate in off-ward activities.
2. Sensory training is a structured, sequential process, which is a shared group/individual experience.

---

[13] Anthony Whitehead: *In the Service of Old Age: The Welfare of Psychogeriatric Patients.* Baltimore, Penguin Books, 1970, p. 33.

3. The program provides the person with differentiated stimuli to improve his/her perception and response to the environment.

4. All sense receptors are stimulated: auditory, olfactory, tactile, vision, taste, proprioception, and kinesthetic.

5. Sensory training is specifically ordered, structured and designed to increase sensitivity to stimuli by the individual's discrimination, and response to stimuli. A "response-feedback" system is inherent in the group interactional setting.[14]

The method, as formulated by Richman, formerly an occupational therapist at Bronx State Hospital in New York City, involves a group situation in which patients are brought to a room available at the same time every day and relatively free from distractions. Patients should be comfortable in the familiar environment. The sessions themselves involve from four to seven patients at a time and last from a half hour to an hour. Patients are greeted by the leader, who introduces herself to them and encourages them patiently to respond; if they do not know their names, they are helped to reply. Patients are encouraged to greet each other by their first names. The leader shakes hands with each patient, since touching is an important form of communication. She also speaks loudly, slowly and clearly, with as much repetition as necessary. When the introductions are over, the leader helps orient group members to the time, place, date and the fact that they are in the hospital or nursing home to be helped; a blackboard may be used for this purpose.

Body image training becomes an important part of the session in order to give patients a fuller sense of self and to lay the groundwork for later perceptual-motor development. Each group member is asked to identify and move various parts of his or her body—naming and bending the joints, for example, or having them move in imitation of the leader. In a sitting position, they go through various flexion and extension movements.

Next, in order to stimulate patients' awareness of the environment, the leader provides a number of *tactile* stimuli. Material or objects of various kinds are passed around one at a time, so patients have an opportunity to handle them and describe the feeling of touching them in their own words. The leader stimulates them with questions: "Is it hard? Soft? Is the surface smooth? Rough? How does it feel? What do you call it?"

In turn, the leader introduces a number of stimuli that are then identified and discussed: *olfactory* stimuli—smells from liquids, foods or other objects (perfume, coffee, garlic, and so forth); *auditory* stimuli—various sounds; *visual* stimuli—various objects or pictures (patients may be asked to look at themselves in mirrors and say what they see, or they may be asked to describe other patients and what they are wearing); and *taste* stimuli—candy, cookies or other foods or seasonings.

Throughout the session, verbal exercises or questions are used to encourage alertness, awareness and communication. During *hearing* exercises, for example, the leader may bounce a ball and ask group members to count and tell how often it was bounced. Throwing a ball gently from patient to patient may encourage them to remember and call out each other's names. Songs and rhythm instruments may be

---

[14]Leona Richman: *Manual of Sensory Training Techniques.* Geriatric Unit, Bronx State Hospital, New York, 1968.

used, always with the goal of stimulating group members to respond, to interact with each other and to become aware of what is happening.

It is generally believed that at least ten or more sensory training sessions are needed before concrete progress begins to show. As patients improve, they may be moved on to a more advanced sensory training group, in which, rather than simply responding by repeating the leader's words, they express their individual ideas, engage in discussion and take part in more complex body movements, songs, dances or group interaction activities.

This method, like others described in this chapter, may be seen both as a therapeutic and as a valuable recreational experience. It makes use of basic recreational activities and often has a playlike and enjoyable atmosphere, particularly when patients begin to be more fully involved, to respond and to laugh.

Remotivation

Remotivation is a somewhat similar technique that promotes interaction. It may be used by recreation leaders, nursing personnel or aides in a nursing home or hospital to help disoriented geriatric or mentally ill patients improve their cognitive and social functioning.

Remotivation, which is closely linked to the "reality orientation" approach, is a method evolved by Dorothy Hoskins Smith at the Philadelphia State Hospital in 1956 and assisted by Smith, Kline and French Laboratories as it spread rapidly to other hospitals and nursing homes throughout the United States and Canada. Before long, it was recognized by the American Psychiatric Association as a valuable technique for use with disoriented aged persons and chronically ill mental patients. Through the 1960's, the American Psychiatric Association provided workshops, seminars and demonstrations to train leaders in remotivation, with assistance from Smith, Kline and French. By the late 1960's over 15,000 leaders had been trained in the method.

Remotivation consists of a series of meetings involving between ten and 15 patients and a leader; the sessions last from 45 minutes to an hour. Meetings are held once or twice a week and are usually designated for patients who have not responded to other hospital therapies. Patients are encouraged to attend but are not forced to do so. The goal of remotivation is to help disoriented or regressed patients begin to be aware of their environment and relate to the hospital staff and other individuals. Remotivation meetings are highly structured and follow a five-step sequence, shown below with the approximate amount of time given to each phase:

---

1. *Climate of Acceptance (5 min.).* The leader addresses the group and expresses appreciation to its members for coming to the meeting. The leader moves around the group greeting each member, calling them by name, or introducing herself to them. She compliments them on their appearance, and attempts to establish contact or arouse response in other ways. The purpose of the first step is to help the patient to realize that he or she is in a new different setting, away from the regular daily routine, and to establish a comfortable, relaxed social atmosphere.

2. *Bridge to Reality (15 min.).* The leader uses a clipping, poem, article, or other piece of printed material, which is intended to gain the interest and attention of the group. She may read from it, slowly and clearly, or may move around the circle asking other participants to read a line or two, if they are able to do so. Patients are asked to comment on, or respond to this statement. In some "bridges," a theme is presented which may reflect the patient's past experience, and they may be asked to discuss it, based on the past. Photographs may be helpful in arousing such interest.

3. *Sharing the World We Live In (15 min.).* Here the leader develops a topic for group discussion and response. The theme may stem from the idea presented in step 2, or may be different. It should have to do with awareness of what things are like today, and should involve information close to patients' experiences or personal interests. Ideally, it should not be a disturbing or highly controversial subject. The leader should be prepared with specific questions and information, and should encourage all group members to contribute to the discussion.

4. *The World of Work (15 min.).* Extending the previous step's emphasis on the reality of present-day life, the intent is to discuss work as a form of human activity. The patient is encouraged to think of work in relation to his or her own life — either in terms of work he or she had done, or is presently doing in the hospital, or might do in the future. This step is particularly useful with psychiatric patients who might return to community life, and less so to disoriented geriatric patients who are not likely to do so.

5. *Climate of Appreciation (5 min.).* The leader thanks each group member in turn for coming to the session, and tells them that she is pleased with them. She announces when the next meeting will be held, and urges them all to attend.[15]

Records of the participation of individual patients in remotivation sessions are kept, with detailed information as to their involvement, understanding and reaction to different aspects of the experience. As patients progress, such records may provide the basis for recommending that they be moved along to a higher functioning group or encouraged to become involved in other hospital programs.

Reality Orientation

Reality orientation is a very similar kind of approach that is used with disoriented or chronic patients in an effort to help them focus on reality and relate meaningfully to their physical and social environment. Gladin points out that it has two separate aspects: (a) a 24-hour-a-day method basing all contacts with the patient on an "attitude therapy" approach that is part of reality orientation and (b) specific therapeutic sessions carried on in a classroom-like situation.

In the first aspect, patients are dealt with in a consistent, interpersonal style that emphasizes the reality of who they are and why they are there and points out what their behavior is like, how they affect others and why the institution operates as it does. Gladin indicates that the following therapeutic attitudes are helpful:

---

[15]M. Alice Robinson: *Remotivation Technique: A Manual for Use in Nursing Homes.* American Psychiatric Association and Smith, Kline and French Laboratories, n.d.

Kind firmness used with depressed or uncooperative patient.

No demand made on the patient who is out of control.

Active friendliness used with the withdrawn and apathetic patient.

Passive friendliness used with the suspicious patient.

Matter-of-fact manner used with patients who are manipulative, seductive, and those approaching more "normal" behavior.[16]

This approach is very similar to reality therapy developed by William Glasser, which emphasizes patients' accepting reality, responsibility and awareness of right and wrong.[17] It deals concretely with the individual's present behavior and seeks to correct and improve it rather than to delve into the past causes of illness or deal with problems through a traditional psychoanalytic approach (see Chapter 6). The second aspect of reality orientation consists of classes for small groups of disoriented or confused patients to help them become aware of the present and the reality of their lives and surroundings. Both basic and advanced classes use a "reality orientation board" as a teaching tool; this contains such information as the following:

Title card (name of agency or institution)
Location card (city or state)
Today is—
The date is—
The year is—
The next meal is—
The weather is—
The next holiday is—
Today's activity is—
Activity director is—

As Gladin describes the method, patients are drilled in learning and reciting accurate information, such as that listed above. In more advanced classes, they would deal with other aspects of the hospital or nursing home—the daily schedule, their living circumstances, their family and home background or other relevant information. As indicated, this method is similar to remotivation but more specific and limited in the areas of information covered.

Behavior Modification

In a sense, all activity therapies are designed to be a form of behavior modification, since it is their purpose to substitute new, more constructive values and forms of behavior for past negative, limited or destructive attitudes and behaviors.

---

[16]Catherine B. Gladin: "Reality Orientation and Remotivation in Health Care Facilities." *In* Jerry D. Kelley, ed.: *Expanding Horizons in Therapeutic Recreation II.* Champaign-Urbana, University of Illinois Office of Recreation and Park Resources, 1974, pp. 111–114.

[17]William Glasser: *Reality Therapy: A New Approach to Psychiatry.* New York, Harper & Row, 1965.

However, the term "behavior modification" has become popular in recent years as a distinct form of treatment. Dunn defines it as " . . . the systematic use of the theories of learning to weaken, maintain, or strengthen behavior through the use of selected reinforcers and under specified conditions."[18]

Behavior modification may be used to describe a wide range of techniques, including brainwashing of prisoners, use of aversive conditioners to work with sex criminals, addicts or alcoholics and many other methods—some of which have a dubious reputation. As it is most commonly used in therapeutic settings with the emotionally disturbed or socially deviant, behavior modification relies heavily on the use of positive reinforcement, which may be defined as "any pleasant event which follows a behavior that strengthens the future frequency of that behavior," or, more simply stated, a reward. Obviously, a reward need not simply be an object, such as money or a piece of candy, but can involve privileges, verbal praise, a hug, a smile or other forms of positive reinforcement. Modeling, or demonstration of appropriate behavior, is also a useful behavior modification technique.

To discourage inappropriate or undesired behavior, negative reinforcement such as withdrawal of privileges, criticism or other penalties may be used. Rawson describes the rationale of behavior modification:

Behavior modification theory places heavy emphasis upon the early extinction of socially maladaptive behaviors and immediate and consistent reinforcement of socially appropriate behavior. Put in its simplest terms, the basic assumption of this theory is that most behavior, good or bad, is in fact learned, and it was originally learned because it was reinforced socially or otherwise. Therefore, deliberate, consistent manipulation of reinforcements as a consequence of specific behaviors leads to unlearning of previous behaviors (which no longer lead to positive reinforcements) and simultaneous learning of new alternate behaviors which now lead to positive reinforcements.[19]

The author describes the program of behavior modification at the Englishtown Park therapeutic camp, a residential short-term camp in Indiana for children with behavioral problems. It demonstrates how behavior modification cannot simply be a casual dispensing of praise and blame, rewards and punishments, but must instead be based on a systematic identification of the behavioral problems of each subject and determination of appropriate therapeutic goals:

Before each child arrived at camp, an intensive "behavior prescription" was drawn up for him, based upon study of family case histories, school and teacher reports, psychometric case findings, and parental reports. Based on this, the teacher-therapists sought to achieve specific behavior modification goals, using a number of positive and negative reinforcements to either reward or inhibit behavior. Positive reinforcements were: (a) verbal praise; (b) physical gestures of affection and approval; (c) award of candy pellets; (d) award of gummed stars on name badges, which could be

---

[18]John M. Dunn: "Behavior Modification with Emotionally Disturbed Children." *Journal of Physical Education and Recreation*, March 1975, p. 67.
[19]Harve E. Rawson: "Residential Short-Term Camping for Children With Behavior Problems: A Behavior-Modification Approach." *Child Welfare*, October 1973, p. 513.

traded for candy bars, soft drinks, or ice cream; (e) fancy certificates of merit given in public cer-
emonials; and (f) the right to participate in highly desired activities, such as evening swimming or
overnight campouts. Negative reinforcements were: (a) complete ignoral (turning one's back on a
child, despite his attention-getting pleas); and (b) withdrawal from a highly desired activity for a
period of several minutes.[20]

A prescription is written for each child, outlining major problems and desired
and undesired behavior and suggesting appropriate forms of reinforcement to modify behavior in desired directions. A typical prescription, after outlining goals and
methods, states, "Be very firm and consistent with this camper at all times and make
sure he understands your expectations, repeating them often; utilize maximum peer
pressure where possible to alter inappropriate behavior, including halt of coveted
activity for entire group."

Behavior modification can obviously be applied in all types of settings, but it
is most effective in situations of sustained contact and interpersonal involvement—
as in a camp or other residential situation, as opposed to a community mental health
center where clients may come for only a few hours a week. In some cases, the
method used is a contract outlining specific desired behaviors as well as behaviors
or deficits to be eliminated. Based on whether the client lives up to the contract,
certain rewards or other positive reinforcers are given. As in reality therapy, behavior modification is not concerned with exploring and understanding the past roots
of the individual's disturbance. Instead, emphasis is on the here and now, and it is
assumed that if the client is helped to behave constructively and rationally, this will
help to reduce his problems significantly.

Token Economy

A somewhat similar approach, used in a number of large psychiatric hospitals,
is the "token economy" system. Maxmen, Tucker and LeBow describe the token
economy method as a treatment that systematically applies certain principles
derived from general experimental psychology, particularly operant learning. It
seeks

. . . to strengthen the patient's desirable behaviors and weaken his socially maladaptive ones by
utilizing tokens as tangible and serviceable intermediaries between the patient's desirable activities
and the positive reinforcers that are available to him. For example, a withdrawn patient may receive
tokens for socializing with other patients, which he can then exchange for privileges or commodi-
ties he desires, such as watching television.[21]

---

[20]*See* Richard G. Kraus, Gay Carpenter and Barbara J. Bates: *Recreation Leadership and Supervision: Guidelines for Professional Development.* Philadelphia, Saunders College Publishing, 1981, pp. 207–209.
[21]Jerrold S. Maxmen, Gary J. Tucker and Michael LeBow: *Rational Hospital Psychiatry: The Reactive Environment.* New York. Brunner, Mazel, 1974, p. 26.

In a hospital residential unit, the patient may receive tokens for carrying out assigned responsibilities, such as bedmaking, washing or other services. He may also display adaptive behavior in other areas of social interaction or activity therapy that is rewarded and reinforced by tokens. Tokens themselves are positive reinforcers and are generally concrete objects that have little or no inherent value, such as paper money or "scrip," colored poker chips and foreign coins of low value. They must be easy to carry and difficult to counterfeit. They gain their power as reinforcers by being essential for acquiring desired privileges—buying tobacco or going on a trip or to a movie, for example. It is desirable to give immediate reinforcement for most patients in psychiatric situations, and since there are limited ways in which this can be done directly, the use of tokens (which can be granted immediately) acts as an intermediary between the desired behavior and the deferred reward.

In hospitals employing this method, tokens are used as a means of structuring an entire network of recreation, as well as other amenities of living. The approach is therefore known as the "token economy" method because it represents an entire economy of exchange within the institution. In addition to serving as a means for channeling reinforcers, tokens are a continuing form of motivation, a stimulus to think in terms of deferred rewards and to plan for the future. Finally, as preparation for returning to community life, they represent working for wages and an experience in saving and spending—all important areas of preconditioning for independent community living.

Leisure Counseling and Leisure Education

A final important therapeutic approach to be discussed in this chapter consists of two closely related functions: leisure counseling and leisure education.

LEISURE COUNSELING

Although not a specific form of recreation in itself, leisure counseling is directly concerned with attitudes, values and habits and can make a major contribution to patients' readiness to function successfully in community life. Pointing out that leisure counseling has become an increasingly important part of the total therapeutic recreation program in psychiatric institutions, McLellan and Pellett state,

> The objective of leisure counseling is to determine the patients' leisure interests and then to assist in locating activities in the home community to meet their interests. The leisure counselor also helps the patients examine the feasibility of their activity choices in terms of cost, accessibility, and personal skills and capabilities.[22]

---

[22]Robert W. McLellan and Lane Pellett: "Leisure Counseling—The First Step." *Therapeutic Recreation Journal*, Fourth Quarter, 1976, pp. 161–165.

Extending this description somewhat, it should be stressed that not only psychiatric patients but also other special populations are normally in need of effective leisure counseling. Although much of the literature refers to leisure counseling as a form of therapy used in institutions, it has also been used widely with the physically disabled, the mentally retarded, the socially deviant and, indeed, with non-disabled populations as well. A precise definition of leisure counseling is provided by Gunn, who characterizes it as

a helping process which uses specific verbal facilitation techniques to promote and increase self-awareness, awareness of leisure attitudes, values, and feelings, as well as the development of decision-making and problem-solving skills related to leisure participation with self, others, and environmental factors.[23]

Leisure counseling may be carried out in a variety of ways: through informal, one-to-one interchange between activity staff members and patients or clients; through regularly scheduled individual counseling sessions; or through group counseling. Each client's recreational interests should be evaluated. Efforts to expand and enrich these interests and skills should be planned as part of the treatment process. One goal of counseling should be to have patients engage in community recreation programs while institutionalized. Finally, counseling should provide not only guidance to help discharged patients find desirable leisure outlets in the community but also follow-up assistance to help them function there effectively.

Six component parts, or phases, may be identified in this process:

1. *Procedures designed to evaluate each patient or client's present and past recreational interests.* This involves such techniques as reading the case record, using a "recreation inventory" during an initial leisure counseling interview and interviewing family, friends and associates. The inventory (see p. 219) might include such categories as games and sports, social activities, cultural events, hobbies and arts and crafts, and might deal not only with established interests but also with other leisure interests the individual would like to engage in.

2. *Planned efforts to expand and enrich interests and skills and to examine values and outcomes during treatment.* Usually, this phase involves regular small-group meetings that focus on leisure use. They may be under the leadership of a multi-disciplinary counseling team but are most often directed by a single staff member. Social workers or activity therapists, including recreation specialists, are frequently given this responsibility. In group discussions, they explore leisure interests and opportunities and examine problems they may have had in the past as well as their present leisure activities and future plans. At the same time, according to Olson and McCormack, patients in recreation counseling groups go to group activities together

[23]Scout Lee Gunn: "A Systems Approach to Leisure Counseling." *Journal of Physical Education and Recreation,* Leisure Today, April 1977, p. 8.

... and thus accumulate a backing of common social experiences. They ordinarily bring these experiences into the group discussions and comment on their reactions to them. This serves as a point of departure for observations about their pre-hospital experiences in the social-recreational area and of expectations about the future.[24]

Hitzhusen also emphasizes the importance of learning by doing and of the interaction between recreation experiences and counseling.[25] Along with group-centered activities, patients should also be guided in their choice of hospital recreation programs in order to enrich skills and build positive attitudes toward participation.

3. *Efforts to have patients engage in community recreation programs while institutionalized.* To the greatest degree possible, patients should become directly involved in community recreation activities while still in the institution or treatment program in order to build a bridge to the future and give them a realistic exposure to available community programs. Olson and McCormack, for example, describe one patient who was referred to and became part of a community orchestra before discharge and remained with it after leaving the hospital.

4. *Involvement of community groups in recreation activities carried on within the hospital.* Mobilizing community resources is important to the success of any leisure counseling service. Many institutions, therefore, encourage community groups to become involved in the hospital or other rehabilitation center program by sponsoring regular programs in which patients may take part. Again, this allows a patient to build a bridge to the community by establishing favorable personal contacts and developing confidence.

5. *Guidance to help discharged patients find desirable leisure outlets in the community.* Throughout this process, the patient's leisure attitudes, values and goals for future leisure participation are being clarified. While still in the treatment program, he or she develops a conscious plan of involvement for the future—identifying programs, groups, clubs and hobby interests. To make this work, it is essential that hospital personnel become thoroughly familiar with potential recreational resources. O'Morrow lists "a directory of community recreation resources" as one of the "usual missing ingredients" in a recreation counseling program.

6. *Follow-up assistance to help patients function effectively in the community.* Referral, initial visits to a community recreation program while still hospitalized and follow-up observation and counseling are the final step to ensure that patients make a satisfactory adjustment to community programs. Despite the fact that some institutions do not feel this is a necessary or appropriate step, it is often critical that disabled persons be given temporary assistance when returning to the community. In some cases, as shown in Chapter 6, they may attend a community-

---

[24]W. E. Olson and J. B. McCormack: "Recreation Counseling in the Psychiatric Service of a General Hospital." *Journal of Nervous and Mental Diseases*, April-June 1957, p. 237.
[25]G. Hitzhusen: "Recreation and Leisure Counseling for Adult Psychiatric and Alcoholic Patients." *Therapeutic Recreation Journal*, First Quarter, 1973, p. 19.

based mental health center or other day-clinic program through which they can continue to receive leisure counseling assistance. However, the effort should be on breaking the dependency and encouraging them to establish their own independent interests and group affiliations.

In another text, the author describes comprehensive leisure counseling programs at the Binghamton, New York, State Hospital and at the Mental Health Centre in Penetanguishene, Ontario, Canada. The latter program in particular places strong stress on the use of a variety of diagnostic and exploratory procedures, including videotaped interviews, the use of printed recreation interest inventories, administration of psychological projective tests and specially designed sessions to measure the patient's actual behavior in a variety of different social and recreational settings.[26]

It should be stressed that although the chief emphasis has been on the need for leisure counseling in psychiatric settings, it is obviously of considerable importance for those with other forms of disability as well. It is being used today, for example, in penal and correctional settings.[27] Within the past several years, realization has grown that many individuals who have no specific psychological or physical impairment at all can benefit greatly from leisure counseling. Cross describes several community-based programs that approach leisure counseling not so much as a therapeutic service but as a developmental learning experience and that serve both the disabled and the nondisabled in Los Angeles, Milwaukee and the Borough of Etobicoke, Ontario, Canada. The Milwaukee program in particular has become known as a leading community-based center for leisure counseling for a general population.[28]

Criticism of Leisure Counseling. As leisure counseling became more and more popular during the late 1970's and early 1980's, various professional groups criticized the fact that individuals with relatively little training in this field were presenting themselves as skilled "counselors." Some authorities encouraged practitioners to go far beyond leisure counseling to deal with lifestyle attitudes, values and behavior patterns; in some cases, leisure counseling took on the aura of psychotherapy.

Chinn and Joswiak point out that leisure counseling has been widely referred to as a panacea and has been described and criticized as a fad. Increasingly there have been calls for standards and ethics in leisure counseling. Chinn and Joswiak suggest that leisure counseling should simply be regarded as part of the repertoire of the trained professional that, with continued refinement of its theory and techniques, can make a valuable contribution to therapeutic recreation service.[29] They also suggest that leisure counseling should properly be regarded as

---

[26]Kraus, Carpenter and Bates, *op. cit.*, pp. 214–215.

[27]Bob Brayshaw: "Leisure Counseling for People in Correctional Institutions." *Journal of Leisurability,* Ontario, Canada, January 1974, pp. 10–14.

[28]Ken Cross: "Leisure Counseling: An Overview with a Community Center Emphasis." *Recreation Review,* July 1976, pp. 22–26.

[29]Karen A. Chinn and Kenneth F. Joswiak: "Leisure Education and Leisure Counseling." *Therapeutic Recreation Journal,* Fourth Quarter, 1981, pp. 4–7.

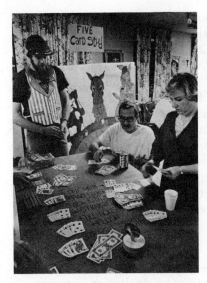

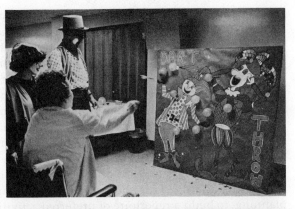

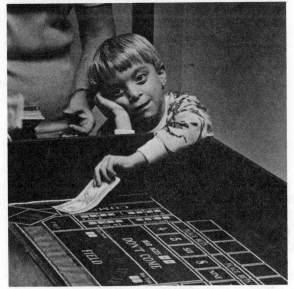

Patients enjoy social recreation activities and carnival stunts as part of special-events programming at Williamsport, Pennsylvania, Hospital.

> . . . a subset of leisure education, (which) facilitates the process of problem-solving, decision-making, and conflict management regarding leisure interests, awareness, values and opportunities . . . (with) one of the keys to the appropriate terminology . . . whether or not counseling techniques are used.[30]

LEISURE EDUCATION

Leisure education was identified as one of three major elements in therapeutic recreation service by the 1982 philosophical statement of the National Therapeutic Recreation Society. Essentially, leisure education helps patients become aware of

---

[30]*Ibid.*, p. 6.

and knowledgeable about leisure resources; obviously, it is somewhat similar to leisure counseling. How are the two to be distinguished from each other?

As Chinn and Joswiak suggest, leisure education provides a full understanding of leisure and its uses and encompasses a wide variety of techniques, such as behavior management, task analysis, a "learning center" approach or individualized prescription. In contrast, leisure counseling tends to be problem-centered and to rely on counseling methods, such as conflict management or values clarification.

In the past, leisure education primarily was aimed at elementary and secondary school students and dealt with constructive leisure knowledge, skills and attitudes. Today, it is being used increasingly with the severely handicapped, providing a framework for individualized program development. Voeltz and Wuersch comment that leisure activity skills should be taught as part of comprehensive longitudinal planning, to build a repertoire of preferred activities for severely handicapped individuals. They write,

---

Recreators will undoubtedly shift their focus away from taxonomies and developmental sequences, and move to refine strategies to teach meaningful leisure behavior, which is functional in integrated community environments, for even the most severely handicapped person.[31]

Disabled individuals must be helped not only to learn skills but also to become able to make meaningful choices, to enjoy activities and express their feelings about them and to use available community resources. Dunn suggests a number of specific goals and program possibilities that might be employed in a community-based residential facility for former psychiatric patients who are in the process of "transition" to fully independent living:

Goal: To provide opportunities for increased awareness of leisure.

Program Possibilities: (a) discussion groups on topics such as "What is leisure?", leisure-oriented current events, or "What do you do for fun?"; (b) identifying leisure-oriented commercials on television and radio; (c) participation in the leisure education program.

Goal: To teach leisure-related experience skills necessary for successful leisure functioning.

Program Possibilities: (a) . . . education on how to use public transportation; (b) appropriate dress for various leisure experiences; (c) appropriate behavior at various leisure experiences.

Goal: To teach the use of a variety of community resources related to leisure and leisure participation.

Program Possibilities: (a) field trips into the community, i.e., recreation centers, libraries, shops, restaurants, ball games; (b) exercises in using information in newspapers, phone books, and on radio and television; (c) discussions on costs of various activities.[32]

---

[31]Luanna Voeltz and Bonnie Biel Wuersch: "A Comprehensive Approach to Leisure Education and Leisure Counseling for the Severely Handicapped Person." *Therapeutic Recreation Journal*, Fourth Quarter, 1981, p. 34.

[32]Julia Kennon Dunn: "Leisure Education: Meeting the Challenge of Increasing Independence of Residents in Psychiatric Transitional Facilities." *Therapeutic Recreation Journal*, Fourth Quarter, 1981, pp. 20–21.

Both leisure counseling and leisure education are important elements in a total program of therapeutic recreation service. Ideally, they should not be separate components of service, isolated from the day-by-day involvement of patients and clients in ongoing programs. Instead, they should be part of an integrated approach to treatment and rehabilitative service, with leisure counseling contributing to and drawing material from the individual's involvement in recreation programming. Similarly, leisure education should not be restricted to something that prepares patients or clients for some distant day, but should be an ongoing service that contributes to their growing competence in the use and enjoyment of leisure as a vital part of living.

Other Related Services

This chapter has outlined a number of basic approaches to planning therapeutic recreation programs and has presented a number of relatively new techniques and treatment.

It should be recognized that many other types of activities—some of which are *not* clearly recreational in nature—may fit into the overall program. For example, in senior centers, daily activities may include a "nutrition" (hot lunch) program; seminars, discussion groups or social action programs dealing with problems of the aging; legal, family or housing counseling; or other special health, dental or vision services—all as a part of the overall program.

Similar examples might readily be given of other related services which are provided for special populations. Obviously, they may be part of the responsibility of a therapeutic recreation specialist who plans and coordinates the total activity program, although he or she may not be an expert within each area of service and would need to bring in skilled resource persons.

GUIDELINES FOR THERAPEUTIC RECREATION PROGRAM PLANNING

In conclusion, a number of important guidelines for program planning in therapeutic recreation are presented. Obviously, these may vary somewhat in their application according to the type of disability being served or the setting or resources of the agency under consideration. As a general picture of *how* programs should be planned and implemented, however, they serve as a practical model.

1. Program planning should be based on a coherent philosophy of the place of leisure and recreation in human life. At the same time that specific therapeutic objectives are identified, program activities should also provide such general values of recreation as pleasure, emotional release, sociability, healthy physical exercise and creative self-expression.

2. Emphasis should be placed on using and serving the healthy, positive aspects

of each patient or client's personality and physical make-up rather than focusing only on disability or pathological aspects of behavior.

3. Although there is an important place for prescribed or assigned participation in activity, patients should also be given the opportunity for free choice within a flexible therapeutic recreation program. Regimentation that contributes to institutionalization and dependency should be avoided.

4. Programs should cover a wide range of active and passive social, physical, creative, intellectual and service activities. Patients or clients should be encouraged to begin at their present level of skill and interest and should be helped to move toward more deeply involving and challenging activities.

5. Through both participation and leisure counseling sessions, the program should help patients and clients become aware of the place of leisure and recreation in their lives and help them develop more constructive plans for their own involvement, either in the community or in a continued residential setting.

6. Programs should be planned with the help of professionals from other disciplines on the treatment team or should, at least, be made thoroughly familiar to them in terms of rationale, schedules and outcomes. This communication can be achieved through regular reports, invitations to events and input from recreation and activity staff members at team meetings.

7. Programs should be scheduled at appropriate times, both to allow for other hospital or treatment services to be provided without conflict and to space needed leisure activities through the day, evenings and weekends.

8. Important health and safety principles should be observed, with medical supervision in all necessary areas, such as use of medication, effects of exercise on physical disability and appropriate ways of dealing with patients in acute phases of illness and treatment.

9. Whenever possible, programs should not be limited to the institution or treatment setting but should involve community resources. This may mean carrying on activities in the community or inviting members of community groups to take part in or to assist programs in the hospital or agency.

10. Program planning should encourage patient or client initiative to the fullest. This may be done by having individuals or small groups of patients take responsibility for planning activities, contributing to policy decisions or leading their own activities. It may also involve, on a broader scale, patient councils that help to set priorities and make policy decisions on activity programs.

11. Just as the therapeutic recreation specialist is more than an activity leader, so the activity program should include the various special treatment methods described in this chapter or other nonrecreation services when appropriate.

12. There should be an ongoing, consistent and systematic effort to assess patient needs and capabilities, define program objectives and measure outcomes of participation regularly. To the extent that therapeutic recreation specialists are made accountable and demonstrate what they have accomplished, their status within the overall rehabilitative structure will be enhanced, and it will be possible to continue to modify and improve the program.

Each of these guidelines is illustrated and reinforced in the chapters dealing with specific disability areas, the modification of activity, community-based programs and services, and research and evaluation.

Suggested Topics for Class Discussion, Examination Questions or Student Papers

1. Outline the key considerations in program planning within any therapeutic recreation agency or department.

2. What are several of the ways in which patients or clients may be involved in programs (i.e., through assigned groups, individual prescription, voluntary participation in mass activity and so on)? Show how these might be combined in a total program schedule in a given institution or community setting.

3. Summarize the goals and methods used in one of the special techniques, such as *sensory training*, described in this chapter.

4. Apply one of the systems analysis approaches to program planning presented in this chapter to a specific hypothetical setting. Philosophically, how does this approach relate to the *milieu therapy* model described in Chapter 2?

5

Patient/Client Assessment and the Selection and Modification of Program Activities

Although therapeutic recreation specialists fill many roles, such as supervisors, educators, community organizers, advocates or consultants, many of them still have as a primary responsibility the presentation of *activity programs* for special populations. Even the head of recreation or activity therapy in a large hospital must direct other leaders, aides or volunteers in planning and presenting leisure activities.

This chapter provides a fuller discussion of the following elements: (a) patient or client assessment, in terms of both individuals and groups; (b) development of goals and objectives as part of treatment plans; (c) activity analysis and selection; and (d) modification of activities to achieve objectives. The chapter also explores several basic areas of activity in depth, describing their values and suggesting modifications.

PATIENT AND CLIENT ASSESSMENT

Assessments may be made in several ways. Typically, in many institutions or community agencies, they are done by means of *interest inventories* or *activity preference checklists*. The patient or client may be asked to fill out a form listing a range of available leisure activities, indicating pursuits that he or she is familiar with or would like to try. The individual may be asked to describe his or her skill level in the activity or the frequency of past participation. Often, an assessment is made routinely when a patient or client first enters the program.

A second approach to assessments would be through *observation* and *functional analysis* of the individual's behavior in social situations or recreation activities. Typically, staff members would observe the patient or client in such situations and would note and document his or her ability to interact with others, to engage successfully in activities, to master the required skills and to grasp the concepts underlying specific activities.

A third approach might come through the *treatment team's analysis* of all that is known about the patient or client's background: emotional, cognitive, psychomotor, medical, educational, vocational or avocational. The data may be obtained through interviews, observation and past treatment records.

Altogether, these sources of information are used to develop an overall picture of the patient and to formulate a treatment plan. This plan might focus on one or another of the patient's primary needs for therapeutic recreation service (*therapy, leisure education* or *recreation*) or a blend of the three. The plan would outline not only the recommended activities but also specific behavioral objectives, appropriate styles of leadership or instruction and desired patterns of group involvement.

THE TREATMENT PLAN: GOALS, OBJECTIVES AND METHODS

Gunn and Peterson suggest that there are five basic steps to individualized program planning: (a) client assessment; (b) goal determination; (c) specification of objectives; (d) preparation of the individual plan; and (e) evaluation. Following the first step, it is necessary to develop individual program goals. They write,

---

Individual program goals are broad statements that reflect needs and are directly determined by analyzing assessment data. Unlike objectives, goals are not directly measurable, but rather provide direction in the actual planning of individualized programs. The first step in determining individual program goals is the formation of a problem list.[1]

The problem list should be drawn from all presenting problems that have appeared in the assessment, including psychomotor, cognitive and emotional problems. The problems should be described as specifically as possible, in terms of observed behavior rather than in general diagnostic terms. Since the problems are to guide the formulation of a therapeutic recreation program, they should be relevant to therapeutic recreation rather than to other disciplines such as medical or nursing care. The problems should then be translated into a statement of needs, and the needs into goals for desired behavior. For example, Gunn and Peterson suggest several goals for a specific patient:

---

1. To increase ability to interact verbally with others in social settings.
2. To increase attention span and awareness of realistic surroundings.
3. To increase ability to make decisions regarding leisure participation.
4. To improve body image.[2]

---

[1]Scout Lee Gunn and Carol Ann Peterson: *Therapeutic Recreation Program Design: Principles and Procedures.* Englewood Cliffs, New Jersey, Prentice-Hall, 1979, p. 79.
[2]*Ibid.*, p. 81.

Goals are designed to help the patient change his or her behavior. Goals are determined in part by the nature of the disability and the limitations it imposes, and in part by the characteristics of the individual.

Specific behavioral objectives are then developed for participation in prescribed elements of the therapeutic recreation program. Behavioral objectives should be stated concisely and contain the following elements: (a) a description of the client's specific behavior or skill that can be directly observed and measured by others; (b) the circumstances in which (when, where and how) the behavior will take place; and (c) standards or conditions of performance under which the behavior will be shown.

In some cases, behavioral objectives may include any of the following:

Initiating conversations with others and responding appropriately to their remarks.

Taking part in a group game, comprehending the needed actions or strategy and showing the desired actions.

Performing a given physical skill correctly, at an assigned level of performance (skating, running, throwing, swimming, dancing, gymnastics or other psychomotor activity).

Carrying out a given activity correctly a required number of times.

Agreeing to a deadline for reducing specific forms of antisocial behavior, such as cursing, losing one's temper, striking others or alcohol or drug abuse.

Each behavioral objective may be broken down into step-by-step behaviors that are to be learned, or into several parts that are to be achieved within a given period of time.

Appropriate goals are often stated in general terms by a doctor or other department head and interpreted specifically by the therapeutic recreator. All goals, objectives and recommendations for the patient or client's involvement in activities should be detailed in the individual's treatment plan, the guide to his or her participation over a period of time.

Importance of an Individualized Treatment Plan

Particularly in a medical setting, where therapeutic recreation service is to be established for third-party reimbursement, the individualized treatment plan must meet certain important criteria. Ingber has defined these as follows:

Standard:

The therapeutic recreation staff (must) develop and implement an individualized treatment plan for each patient referred to the service.

Criteria:

The plan is based on complete and relevant diagnostic data.

The plan is consistent with the treatment goals for the patient and is considered reasonable and necessary medical care expected to improve the client's condition.

The treatment objectives are stated in behavioral terms that permit the progress of the individual to be assessed.

The plan is documented in the medical record of the patient.

The plan is periodically reviewed, evaluated and modified as necessary to meet the changing needs of the patient.

The plan reflects patients' physical, social, mental and emotional functioning as well as leisure functioning and potential for achieving treatment objectives.

Where appropriate, the plan reflects the patient's goals and expectations of benefits to be derived from the Therapeutic Recreation Service.

When applicable, plans indicate precautions, restrictions, or limitations as determined by the physicians or other health care professionals.

When feasible, the patient and/or his/her family assists in developing and implementing the therapeutic recreation treatment plan.

The plan differentiates between short-term, long-term and discharge goals.

The plan indicates the type, duration, and frequency of treatment activities.

Appropriate recreation experiences and activities are used as therapeutic modalities by which the treatment objectives can be achieved.

Provision is made for each client to participate at his/her optimal level of functioning and to progress at his/her own speed in relation to the treatment objectives.

Provision is made to modify activities to assure success experiences and sequential development for each client.

Provision is made for instruction in activity skills and for participation at varying levels of proficiency. Special aids, devices, and adapted recreation equipment are available.[3]

It should be stressed that not all therapeutic recreation programs make use of so systematic a procedure. Some do not, simply because they are operating at a relatively unsophisticated level or because they do not have sufficient numbers of qualified staff members, in proportion to the patient load, to be able to develop and utilize individualized treatment plans. Still others prefer to rely on a more flexible approach; they make no attempt to prescribe specific objectives for each patient. However, the clear trend today is toward precise definition of treatment goals and objectives, particularly in medical facilities.

SELECTION OF ACTIVITIES FOR PARTICIPATION

After the treatment plan is set, the next step is to select specific activities and to develop a schedule. Several factors play an important part in the selection of activities:

Leisure Skills Preference.   What skills does the patient or client already demonstrate, and which activities has he or she indicated a desire to learn?

---

[3]See Fern Kaufman Ingber: *Issues and Guidelines for Establishing Third-Party Reimbursement for Therapeutic Recreation.* Ray E. West, ed. National Therapeutic Recreation Society, July 1978, pp. 21–22.

Physical and Mental Characteristics.   Without assuming that any impairment would necessarily limit participation in a given activity, what *are* the present characteristics of the individual, and what are their implications for successful participation and for possible modification of an activity?

Age-Appropriateness of Activity.   Are the skills and social behaviors involved appropriate for the individual? Would other nondisabled participants of the same age consider them suitable?

Access to Materials and Events.   Would the client have access to needed equipment or supplies in his or her home, and would transportation be available to special events or settings to facilitate involvement in the activity?

Influence of Home Environment.   Would relatives, friends or other helpers be available in the individual's home or neighborhood to reinforce leisure skill development and assist in participation?[4]

Each of these factors will influence the appropriateness of a given activity for a patient or client in terms of both its initial benefits and its carry-over value. In addition, such basic demographic information as the individual's name, age, sex, race or national background, marital and family status, occupation, level of education, referral source and previous records of treatment and past recreational experiences will be helpful in the selection of appropriate activity.

Depending on the individual's functional status and needs, and on the resources of the program, involvement may include the following possibilities: (a) free choice of involvement in small- or large-group activities; (b) prescribed involvement in classes, social activities, hobbies, trips or other programs; (c) required participation during a given period, with the stipulation that a choice of some area of activity must be made; (d) consultation between patient or client and recreation specialist to determine appropriate involvement; or (e) free choice to participate or not.

In some settings, each of the above options is presented to a patient or client as an element within an overall program. To illustrate, at one or more times in a weekly schedule, he or she is assigned to individually prescribed therapy or leisure education. At other times, the individual is expected to participate with his or her unit in other activities. At still other times, the individual may select from among several different choices or may choose not to participate at all (see p. 127).

ACTIVITY ANALYSIS

With the growing sophistication of much therapeutic recreation programming, stronger emphasis is being given today to the systematic analysis of program elements and activities. Such analysis seeks to determine the kinds of capabilities that are necessary to participate successfully in a given task. The analysis also identifies the nature of the social interaction involved in a program activity and the extent to which it involves cognitive, affective and psychomotor skills and learning values.

---

[4]Paul Wehman and Stuart J. Schleien: *Leisure Programs for Handicapped Persons.* Baltimore, University Park Press, 1981, pp. 26–33.

Activity analysis is an important part of program planning in therapeutic recreation service for the following reasons:

1. It facilitates the process of individualizing instruction by identifying the component parts and skills of an activity, a necessary step in determining whether or not it will be suitable for given patients or clients.
2. It helps determine whether specific activities will be useful in achieving desired program outcomes or behavioral objectives.
3. On the basis of the preceding two elements, activity analysis can be used to develop instructional strategies—i.e., how to present or modify the activity, what steps to present first, how to reinforce learning and how to transfer skills involved to other activities.
4. When the dynamics of an activity are better understood it is easier to assess the patient or client's success with the activity and with achieving behavioral objectives.
5. Finally, the activity analysis is useful both in justifying the selection of specific activities as part of the treatment plan and in demonstrating outcomes for other practitioners who need to understand their therapeutic benefit.

Specifically, activity analysis involves identifying and describing the following elements:

Physical Elements

These include the use of specific body parts, including the arms, legs and hands, in various movements, such as throwing, catching, running, jumping, twisting, pulling or crawling. The description of the physical elements should include each fundamental movement pattern, as well as a detailed analysis of smaller coordinations, hand-eye demands or manipulations.

In addition, the physical elements in an activity may include balance, rhythm, endurance, timing, agility and speed, along with the perceptual demands related to seeing, hearing or feeling. The analysis indicates the physical requirements of the activity, provides a measure of their relative importance and suggests the minimal level of ability that an individual must have in order to accomplish the activity.

Because an individual does not possess the usual physical requirements does not necessarily mean that he or she cannot participate. For example, basketball normally requires great agility, including the ability to leap; however, individuals in wheelchairs can play it with great pleasure. Bowling and archery are sports requiring good vision; yet the visually impaired can enjoy both of these sports, and do, in many programs.

Cognitive Elements

Some activities require knowledge and memory as important elements, such as cards, quiz games and other mental activities. Success in other games may depend on an understanding of strategies, rules and basic concepts of play. If these are complex, and if the individual is not able to comprehend them at all or to concentrate on them over a period of time, participation in the activity must be at a very low level or highly modified. Academic skills such as the ability to read, write or do mathematical calculations are found in numerous hobbies, cultural pastimes and other forms of recreation. Again, both the minimum and normal levels of cognitive ability needed to take part should be determined.

Social-Interaction Elements

Activity analysis is also concerned with the nature of social interactions inherent in different activities. Both the demands of socializing and its contribution to a participant's treatment program should be analyzed. The ability to function as a member of a group, to accept the give-and-take of shared decision-making or program planning, to respect others for their human qualities and personal strengths and not to condemn them for their weaknesses or deficiencies—all these are important aspects of recreational programming.

Avedon has developed a classification system of social interaction patterns that is useful in determining whether or not a given activity would be appropriate for an individual or treatment group. It includes eight distinct patterns: (a) *intraindividual*, carried on totally by and within the mind of the individual; (b) *extraindividual*, in which the participant is involved with other environmental elements, but not other people; (c) *aggregate*, carried on as part of a larger group, but not in direct interaction with other members of the group; (d) *interindividual*, in which two individuals play with each other, often in competition; (e) *unilateral*, involving three or more participants, in which one player at a time competes against all the others; (f) *multilateral*, including games for three or more, in which all compete equally; (g) *intragroup*, with two or more persons cooperating to reach a mutual goal; and (h) *intergroup*, in which two or more teams compete against each other.[5]

Understanding the interaction patterns of various activities helps us understand the dynamics of involvement and the therapeutic potential of each activity. Some individuals may be able to participate at only the simplest, most nonthreatening level, while others are ready to engage in activities demanding complex interaction with others or fairly high competitive pressures.

On the basis of the elements described in the preceding section, appropriate activities should be selected as part of a treatment plan. These activities should be grouped as part of an overall sequence of involvements that will meet the individual's therapeutic needs and will achieve the behavioral objectives. A major purpose of such selection and grouping is to ensure that the activities will not only improve the patient or client's initial skill level but will contribute to other needs and have a meaningful carry-over value. Wehman and Schleien write,

---

[5]Elliott M. Avedon: *Therapeutic Recreation Service: An Applied Behavioral Science Approach.* Englewood Cliffs, New Jersey, Prentice-Hall, 1974, pp. 162–170

As behavioral programming replaces diversional activities for disabled persons, the question of generalization or transfer of learning must be seriously addressed by leisure service personnel. Specifically, the skills taught to handicapped learners must transcend specific activities, instructional sessions, and leisure settings if normalization is to be achieved.[6]

They point out that the following guidelines will be helpful in maximizing the benefits of skill development programs:

1. Programs of available activities should be made appealing and relevant to potential participants, and should provide a variety of different skills appropriate to their chronological ages.
2. Even when carried on in segregated or sheltered environments, activities should resemble community-based, integrated settings as fully as possible, in terms of the tasks, group make-up and physical environment of the program, to permit learning that will be useful for carry-over.
3. Emphasis should be placed on developing a variety of competencies with uses in other situations, rather than too narrowly focused a range of skills.
4. Programs should not be limited to instruction, but should include play (actual participation for "fun") to stimulate both motivation and enjoyment, and to help participants improve their leisure attitudes and reinforce their interest in recreation and leisure.
5. Developmental instruction should make use of individualized teaching based on the strengths, weaknesses and observed progress of each participant, and employ appropriate sequential techniques.
6. Self-confidence should be instilled in the patient through repeated success at different levels of involvement.[7]

These guidelines can best be achieved through the intelligent modification of activities, in addition to effective selection.

MODIFICATION OF ACTIVITIES

In general, modifications are called for when the participant is unable to take part successfully in an activity in its original form. Modifications may be aimed at achieving very specific treatment goals—i.e., to promote socialization or verbalization, or to overcome particular blocks the client may have to social involvement or physical activity. It may also be desirable to present simplified versions of certain activities as a preliminary step to taking part in the activity as it is normally carried out. Such modifications are *not* unique to therapeutic recreation service; many simplified, so-called "lead-up games" are played with children in the lower grades to teach them the basic skills for more familiar team sports in the upper grades.

Wehman and Schleien suggest that five types of possible activity adaptations

---

[6]Wehman and Schleien, *op. cit.*, p. 11.
[7]Adapted from M. L. Hutchison, cited in Wehman and Schleien, *op. cit.*, pp. 11–12.

should be considered: (a) adaptation of *materials and equipment;* (b) adaptation of *rules or procedures;* (c) adaptation of *skills sequences;* (d) adaptation of *facilities;* and (e) adaptation of *lead-up activities.*[8]

A wide variety of special equipment has been developed to permit the blind, orthopedically disabled and other special populations to take part in sports like bowling, archery, swimming and baseball. In bowling, wheelchair-users utilize special ramps for releasing the ball. Adams, Daniel and Rullman describe many other examples of special equipment,[9] and a number of additional illustrations are presented in later chapters of this text.

Rules or procedures may be readily modified to permit successful play. Orthopedically handicapped, neurologically impaired or mentally retarded individuals may be permitted to strike at a ball mounted on a tee instead of swinging at a ball thrown to them. They may be permitted an indefinite number of strikes, until they hit a ball. Card games may be simplified for participants who have difficulty distinguishing among pictured cards. Disabled pool players may be allowed to aim at any ball on the table, rather than in a defined sequence.

Skills may be broken down into simpler, smaller action units for those unable to master continuous or complex actions. In some cases, actions may be carried out on a stop-and-go basis, rather than with continuous movement. For example, in volleyball, instead of hitting the ball back and forth across the net without letting it bounce, players may be permitted to hit it on the bounce or to catch and then throw it.

Facility adaptation normally would take two forms: (a) modifying the facility so that individuals have access to it and can use it, by providing ramps, properly designed rest rooms, water fountains, and other equipment; and (b) redesigning or laying out the playing space so that it can be used by the disabled. In a game like baseball this might mean reducing the field size or using a larger, lighter ball. In volleyball or badminton, it might mean putting more players into a smaller area to permit better coverage by players who have limited mobility. Swimming pool modifications might include having a warmer water temperature or using special lifts to help individuals get in and out of the pool.

In lead-up activities, relatively complex games or sports are broken down into their component parts, and each of these is presented as a separate game. Thus, baseball might involve separate practice sessions stressing running, throwing, catching and striking. Players might begin to learn how to run bases by playing "kick-ball," or how to catch a batted ball and throw it by playing "one-o-cat." When analyzed, many games can be found to have similar, interchangeable elements that can fit into a progression of skills. Activities should be selected and/or modified so that it is possible for individuals to carry them out successfully as presented, have fun while doing so—and also learn basic skills that can lead them to more advanced levels of play.

Although this section has stressed games and sports, the same principles apply to many other areas of participation. Learning to take a trip in the community, to

---

[8]*Ibid.,* p. 67.
[9]Ronald C. Adams, Alfred N. Daniel and Lee Rullman: *Games, Sports and Exercises for the Physically Handicapped.* Philadelphia, Lea and Febiger, 1975.

clean a room, to draw or paint a picture, to play a rhythm instrument or to cook a meal may involve exactly the same steps. Even learning to be part of a group or to initiate a successful conversation will involve, for a developmentally disabled individual, careful selection and modification of sequential tasks along with repeated encouragement and praise.

GROUP READINESS AND PROGRAM GOALS

A final consideration in the selection, modification and presentation of therapeutic recreation activities has to do with the readiness of groups of patients or clients to undertake certain activities. Just as individuals have their own unique capabilities, so groups have levels of ability and disability. They too need reassurance, opportunities for socializing and successful participation, and sequential learning experiences in a nurturing environment.

In selecting group activities the following questions should be asked:

Will each activity provide a reasonable measure of success for the individuals in the group, and will it contribute to a sense of cohesiveness and cooperation in the group itself?

Does it blend with other activities carried on by the group so that there is a reasonable balance of physical, social, creative and mental activities in the overall program?

Will the activity provide the opportunity for members of the group to play different roles (as leaders or followers) or to learn the kinds of rules or cooperative behaviors that will contribute to their being able to interact favorably?

Will the activity lend itself to mainstreaming the group itself; i.e., will the group be able to engage in it in an integrated, community-based environment or to invite nondisabled individuals to share the activity with them?

Apart from its therapeutic benefits or its potential value in helping the group achieve other collective goals, will the activity provide a "fun" dimension that will enrich the quality of life for all participants?

ADAPTATION OF SPECIFIC ACTIVITIES

To illustrate a number of the general guidelines presented earlier in this chapter, the following are major categories of recreational activities as they may be used with various types of physically or mentally disabled individuals.

Physical Activities: Aquatics, Games and Sports

As indicated earlier, almost all the games and sports played by nonphysically disabled persons can also be enjoyed by those with impairment. It is necessary in many cases to modify playing conditions, rules and equipment, however, so that the disabled player can be successful rather than frustrated. Often, since such participants have had limited experience in physical activities, it is necessary to stress slow, careful, sequential teaching of basic skills.

SWIMMING

This is one of the most useful activities, because it can be adapted to the needs and capabilities of almost every type of disabled person. It is particularly suitable for those who have serious physical impairments. Sherrill points out that even those who usually are confined to bed experience satisfaction in water play; the discipline of physical therapy has long recognized the rehabilitative values of water exercises:

Therapeutic exercise underwater is especially valuable for the nonambulatory individual whose body parts lack the strength to overcome the force of gravity. In the pool, the force of gravity is greatly minimized, permitting some range of movement to limbs which have none when not immersed in water. Children who require crutches and/or braces to walk on land can often ambulate in water.[10]

Swimming provides the disabled child with freedom of movement he or she cannot enjoy out of water. The youngster is free of wheelchairs, special appliances or the support of parents' arms and is able to join his or her friends in a pastime that brings new confidence and pleasure. Swimming also offers the opportunity for the disabled to socialize with their peers.

For persons with most types of disability, water should be heated to a warm temperature to avoid tension or chilling that may discourage the disabled child or youth from entering the water or have an adverse effect on the impairment. There should be a fairly large area with shallow water to permit casual water play for children who have not yet gained confidence in the water. The pool should have a wide surrounding deck with a slip-proof surface. Steps with handrails leading into the water should be built with short risers and a wide step to permit easy entrance and exit. Sometimes rails are fixed across the pool to permit participants to hold on and gain a feeling of security.

Since fear of the water may be present in all nonswimmers, and especially so for the physically disabled, it is important for the swimming instructor to gain the trust of the participants and to help them relax in the water. Working in small groups, with aides helping those children who need support, the first step is to accustom participants to being in the water and help them lose their fear of it. The fun of swimming should be emphasized with simple ball play, such as water dodge ball. In a manual on swimming for the disabled, the Canadian Red Cross outlines the following steps for helping fearful children become used to the water:

---

[10]Claudine Sherrill: *Adapted Physical Education and Recreation: A Multi-Disciplinary Approach.* Dubuque, Iowa, Wm. C. Brown, 1981, p. 313.

1. Talk with the child. Explain to him the pool or beach rules.
2. Take him on tour of the swimming area and if possible show him children his own age swimming in deep water.
3. Getting wet and water entry — initially any way the child wants to, e.g., washing himself, splashing, drowning the instructor. Don't be impatient if a child won't get in the water completely the first day — once he trusts you he will.
4. Different ways of entering the water, e.g., walking, jumping, hopping, slipping, cannon-ball, downstairs, etc.
5. Walking out into deeper water holding hands.
6. Walking out into deeper water unassisted beside instructor.
7. Ducking to shoulders, neck, eyes, hair, completely under, holding breath as long as he can.
8. Jumping into water and submerging holding breath.
9. Blow bubbles on top of water; with face in water; completely submerged.
10. Tow the child on his front and back, head out, and then head in water.
11. Bobbing holding breath, then blowing bubbles.[11]

Artificial floats should be used for beginners; generally, floats are considered preferable to having other persons hold beginners. Children using foam or inflated floats should be closely watched at all times, however, to prevent them from slipping from the supporting surface.

The selection of strokes depends on the specific disability of each participant. For persons with loss of arm function, an asymmetrical stroke, such as the side stroke or trudgeon stroke, is often used. Learners who have had a loss of leg function, either full or partial, usually prefer symmetrical strokes, such as the elementary backstroke, breast stroke or dog paddle. For those individuals who cannot put their heads in the water, their bodies should be held at approximately a 70° angle, with their faces out of the water. If learners do not have use of their arms, a glide and flutter kick may be used; swim fins help to give them added propulsion and to build up leg strength. For more severely disabled persons, the emphasis at the outset may be simply on teaching breathing rhythms and floating. Even if they cannot learn to swim, just being in the water is likely to bring pleasure.

Swimming is particularly useful in working with blind children and adults since it provides a degree of freedom that they do not normally experience on land. A slight elevation around the pool protects blind persons from accidentally falling in while walking around the deck. Swimming areas should be carefully roped off for those of different swimming abilities, and ropes may be used to guard the blind participant from deep areas or to help him find his way to the ladder. No particular stroke is to be preferred for the blind. Since many of them fear to wet their eyes, however, they may prefer to learn a slow backstroke or breast stroke, with their heads above water. A safety precaution that is often helpful is the buddy system. If diving is permitted, the diving area should be carefully roped off from swimming areas to prevent accidents.

---

[11]*Swimming for the Handicapped: Instructor's Guide.* Toronto, Canadian Red Cross, 1974.

ACTIVE GAMES AND SPORTS

Many different types of ball games may be used with the physically disabled. In order to permit such groups as the orthopedically disabled to take part in these activities, Pomeroy suggests a number of ways to simplify ball games:

1. Walking or wheeling may be substituted for skipping or running, when necessary.
2. A bounced throw or underhand toss may be used to replace a regular throw.
3. Positions such as sitting, kneeling or lying down may be substituted for standing positions.
4. The distances of bases or boundary lines, or of the dimensions of playing areas such as horseshoe courts, volleyball fields or baseball diamonds, may be reduced.
5. Lighter or more easily controlled equipment may be substituted for regular equipment.
6. Players may be restricted to a definite position or area on the playing field.
7. Players may be allowed to hit a ball any number of times, or to hold the ball longer in games like volleyball or basketball.
8. In games like baseball, if a child is unable to run, a runner may be used for him.[12]

Other devices may be used, such as increasing the number of players, permitting an extra number of strikes or modifying the rules. Those children who are not able to play, even under these circumstances, may act as umpires, referees or scorekeepers.

Even with such modifications, it is usually desirable to build up the readiness of disabled children through games in which they learn the fundamentals of throwing or catching, kicking, running or dodging—before attempting to play more complex sports. All sports should be designed to emphasize the *abilities* rather than the *disabilities* of those taking part. They should stress maximum physical development, consonant with medical safeguards, and should emphasize the cooperative aspects of play. The pressure to win should be very low-keyed, and care should be taken to equalize teams according to ability.

For youth and adults with paraplegic conditions or amputations, but who are otherwise physically capable, one of the best organized sports programs is the wheelchair sports movement. A number of games and sports have been carried on by players in wheelchairs since World War II. In 1957, Benjamin H. Lipton, director of the Joseph Bulova School of Watchmaking, launched the first National Wheelchair Games in the United States. A year later, the National Wheelchair Association was organized "for the prime function of establishing rules and regulations governing all wheelchair sports in the United States, except basketball, which has its own national association."[13]

Today, thousands of athletes engage in organized wheelchair sports throughout the United States, Canada, and in many other nations. There is a "Paralympics"

---

[12]Janet Pomeroy: *Recreation for the Physically Handicapped.* New York, Macmillan, 1964, pp. 306–307.
[13]Benjamin H. Lipton: "Wheelchair Sports: Its Role in the Rehabilitation of the Physically Disabled." *Therapeutic Recreation Journal,* Fourth Quarter, 1970, p. 9.

that takes place around the time of the regular Olympics at which teams and disabled individuals from various nations compete in wheelchair sports. The events include archery, bowling, track and field (including javelin, shotput and racing), swimming, weight-lifting and basketball. Participants are placed in one of five classes, according to their degree of disability, and competition in each of the sports is classed according to different levels of ability. In each event, modifications or devices may be used to adapt the rules to the needs of wheelchair competitors. Thus, in throwing events such as the shotput, an official shotput circle is used, but a stopboard or attendant may keep the contestant's chair from going outside the circle.

In the 1976 Olympiad for the Physically Disabled, held in Toronto, Canada, just after the Montreal Olympics, 50 countries were represented by about 1600 competitors, including, for the first time, amputee and blind as well as wheelchair athletes.

Realistically, many physically disabled persons are *not* able to compete on the international level. However, many different sports and games can be modified to permit enjoyment for even the most limited players.

Archery. Archers may use lighter bows and shoot from shorter distances. When shooting, a person on crutches should lean forward on one crutch and a person in a wheelchair should turn his wheelchair sideways and shoot from that angle. A person with only one hand or arm may have the bow fixed to a post anchored in the ground.

Bowling. Bowling is enjoyed by many disabled persons. Lighter balls and pins and shortened alleys may be used. Individuals in wheelchairs may be permitted to swing the ball back and forth more than once to give it extra momentum, or they may use a specially constructed metal rack to release the ball. Players on crutches may stand at the foul line. The blind also bowl, using a guide rail to approach the foul line. A sighted person tells the blind player what pins he must shoot for and keeps score. A Blind Bowlers' Association assists in the formation of leagues and conducts tournaments through the mail.

Dual Games. These games, such as badminton, tennis, billiards, table tennis or shuffleboard, which are usually played by two, all may be played by the disabled. In tennis, for example, the court may be smaller and several players may be on the court at a time to make up for their limited mobility. When advisable, players may use shortened rackets or hold the racket higher up the handle; players with one arm begin the serve with the ball on the racket. In this or other racket games, like badminton, even double arm amputees may take part by having the racket strapped to their arm stumps.

Table tennis has been adapted several ways for the physically disabled. Special paddles have been made for poorly coordinated players, such as those with cerebral palsy. Patients with scoliosis who are in a body cast and children with Legg-Perthes disease or with dislocated hips can all play table tennis using high stretchers that support them. Those in wheelchairs can play, provided that there is enough room around the table for them to maneuver. Similar adaptations are made for other dual games.

Golf. A smaller and less demanding course can be developed, with players using an electric golf cart to get around. In some cases, miniature or "putt-putt" courses are used for the disabled. Depending on the disability, players may use lighter or shorter clubs and vary their stance or grip in order to stroke successfully.

In addition to these sports, many other forms of physical activity may be adapted for the physically disabled, including dancing, roller-skating, fishing, quiet games, camping and nature activities. With some types of disabilities, the individual may be able to master the required skills perfectly well, but may have other difficulties that affect successful play. For example, the hearing-impaired may be able to play any sport without difficulty, but cannot communicate as readily with other team members, or cannot hear a referee's whistle or a coach's instruction. It is necessary to develop hand signals or other means of communicating with hearing-impaired participants while the action is going on. Similar adaptations may need to be made for other types of disabled participants, depending on the activity and its requirements.

QUIET GAMES

Quiet games and hobbies are extremely useful with the physically disabled, partly because they may require extremely limited skills and partly because they lend themselves to either individual or small-group participation.

Table games, including cards, chess and checkers, dominoes, Parcheesi and equipment games like Nok Hockey or Skittles, are extremely useful. Special equipment may be designed for those with manual limitations, such as those with cerebral palsy or similar conditions. The equipment may include holding racks for cards, electric shufflers or devices with which to move chessmen or checkers. As crude an instrument as a stick held in the mouth may be used to move pieces. Braille playing cards have been designed for the blind, and board games with raised squares that can be touched are also helpful. Other quiet games include social games and mixers, usually played while sitting in a circle.

Hobbies may be pursued in a variety of settings, such as social clubs, hospital wards in rehabilitation centers and even as individual activities for those confined to their homes. Hobbies usually involve special interests like collecting (stamps, coins, records, dolls, postcards and so on) or the development of a particular skill or craft. Often, group projects lend themselves to hobby shows at which the disabled can exhibit what they have accomplished.

Dance and Movement Therapy

Dance and movement therapy are other forms of physical activity that stress creative expression, socialization and exploration of movement potential—rather than competition, which is the focus of most sports and games. Dance in particular is used in many hospitals for the mentally ill but may also be adapted to the needs of the physically disabled. Essentially, three forms may be presented: (a) *creative dance* in any of its forms, such as modern dance, ballet or children's rhythmics; (b) *social dancing*, also known as ballroom dancing; and (c) *folk* or *square dancing*, which is usually conducted as a group activity. It is an extremely useful form of activity because it combines physical exercise with emotional or artistic expression.

Sherrill comments that creative rhythmic movement can be enjoyed in modified form by the nonambulatory in beds and wheelchairs, by other health-impaired individuals who need mild range-of-motion exercise and by many children and youth who prefer individual or dual activities to team sports. Many physical activities stress group interaction—cooperating, competing, leading and following, but creative movement emphasizes self-discovery and self-expression. Sherrill points out that disabled children in particular need to get a sense of their own bodies and to become confident in movement before they can cope effectively with the demands of the external world. She writes,

---

The additional barriers to self-understanding and self-acceptance imposed by a handicapping condition intensify the need for carefully guided non-threatening movement experiences designed to preserve ego strength, increase trust, and encourage positive human relationships. Gesture, pantomime, dance, and dance-drama can substitute for verbal communication when children lack or mistrust words to express their feelings.[14]

Creative dance may be readily adapted for the physically disabled, depending on the nature of the impairment. Deaf men and women students at Gallaudet College in Washington, D.C., have formed an outstanding modern dance club that performs throughout the year; despite their not being able to hear music, deaf people are able to "feel" the rhythm through floor vibrations and use visual cues to coordinate their movements.

Disabled children also enjoy creative dance, particularly when dancers move freely and spontaneously to music or other rhythmic accompaniment. Blind children, in particular, profit from dance because it encourages them to learn spatial relationships and to move freely and expressively—as opposed to their usual cautious restrained movement.

Simple folk and square dances, in lines, circles or squares, can also be mastered by the physically disabled. Obviously, dances at a high tempo or with complicated foot movements should be avoided. However, the blind, the deaf and other disabled individuals can do a wide range of such traditional dances to find pleasure in the lively rhythm and social involvement. When a group with mixed disabilities is taking part in folk and square dancing, it is helpful to pair them off so their abilities complement each other. In other words, if a deaf teen-ager is partnered with a blind teen-ager, as a *couple* they have both *vision* and *hearing* and can help each other master the dance.

Wheelchair square dancing has become a popular activity for many orthopedically disabled persons. They are able to do many of the same dances that are done by the nondisabled, but certain modifications need to be made. Since a wheelchair is considerably wider than a person and cannot revolve or turn in as narrow a course, it is necessary to enlarge the dance area and to slow down, or allow longer musical sections, in order to perform each part of the dance. Since wheelchairs cannot move sideways, forward-and-back movements should be substituted where appropriate. Other actions, such as the swing, do-si-do and promenade, can all be danced in modified form by wheelchair square dancers.

---

[14]Sherrill, *op. cit.*, p. 289.

MOVEMENT THERAPY

Movement or dance therapy (often the terms are used interchangeably) is used primarily with mentally ill patients. It incorporates psychoanalytic principles that see a close relationship between posture and psychological make-up. Jung explored artistic experience as a means of expressing deep feelings that defied verbal communication, but presented symbolic movement images that could be seen and dealt with. Reich spoke of chronic muscular tensions as being deeply entrenched defense mechanisms that confined the body as a "defensive armor." The dance therapist helps a patient to release these muscles and thus expose repressed feelings. Dance becomes a medium through which the psychiatric patient can communicate his or her feelings, release inner tensions and find a sense of security.

Dance therapy was initially used as a diagnostic tool and then as a therapeutic modality. Espenak, for example, describes typical postures of patients that displayed their inner feelings:

1. The dejected attitude — slumped shoulders, fallen chest, head on chest, fumbling steps.
2. The retiring attitude — shy, inwardly drawn, regressive, shoulders turned in, head between shoulders.
3. The heightened tension — with restricted and ineffectual movement in states of anxiety — shoulders lifted up to ears, head in the neck, elbows tense, hands nervous.
4. The aggressive attitude — strutting chest, swagger of shoulders, accent on heels.[15]

Typically, the therapist would adapt his or her approach to the needs and characteristic movement of the patient. Marian Chace, for example, a leading pioneer in dance therapy, would move lightly back and forth, touching palms lightly with a passive, fearful schizophrenic, gradually increasing the velocity and impact of these initial contacts as the patient gained confidence. With an aggressive, psychotic patient, she might present a passive, submissive pose or perhaps, with hands placed on the patient's shoulders, begin a swinging motion to draw her into a common rhythm. Other physical manifestations of tension in psychotic patients, such as hyperactivity, tics, grimaces, rigidity or postural distortions, might all be dealt with through movement.

At the same time that the patient develops movement expression, verbalization of feelings and group interactions are encouraged; movement sessions take on a decidedly social character. Dance movements as such are not taught, although the leader may express themes, suggest directions, provide music or lead discussions that help to stimulate creative expression on an individual or small-group basis. Ultimately, patients are helped to better accept their bodies, to have a clearer image of themselves and to discover a new medium through which they can communicate their feelings and release inner tensions. In some cases, images of childhood experiences may be evoked as a way of helping patients recognize and express repressed feelings and memories—thus contributing to other psychotherapeutic processes.

---

[15]Lilian Espenak, cited in E. Thayer Gaston: *Music in Therapy*. New York, Macmillan, 1968.

Although primary emphasis is given to the use of movement therapy with psychiatric patients, it has also been used with the physically disabled, the elderly and even the deaf and blind as a way of helping them come to grips with their own body images and become more fully integrated emotionally and physically through nonverbal experience.

Movement has also been used with the mentally retarded or other developmentally disabled children and youth to promote overall growth. Somtimes called "adapted physical education" and sometimes "perceptual-motor" learning, a variety of tests of motor skills may be used at the outset to assess each individual's status, and then a plan may be developed for remedying gross motor deficits. The emphasis is usually on essential movement patterns and on enhancing such elements as strength, balance and agility in an effort to help children avoid being labeled "awkward" or "clumsy." Basic skills, such as standing, hopping, walking, crawling, jumping, climbing, sliding and hitting, are emphasized, as well as concepts of level, direction, tempo, intensity, repetition and movement quality.

On another level, modified dance and movement techniques may be used with older residents in a nursing home, both as a pleasurable form of recreation and as a moderate form of conditioning exercise. Even patients who are in wheelchairs or in bed may perform upper-body and arm movements as a small-group activity to music.

Dramatics

This is another extremely useful and enjoyable recreational experience in which the disabled may take part. It is easily adapted so that those with different levels of ability and almost every type of impairment may take part with great satisfaction. In part, this is because dramatics can take so many forms and be approached on so many different levels. It provides, more than any other medium, the opportunity to play roles, express emotions, ventilate fears and hostilities and find release from tensions. Individuals who normally stammer severely are often able to speak with fluency and ease when playing a dramatic role.

The rehabilitation therapies manual of a large state mental hospital comments on the role of drama in working with psychiatric patients:

It is a method of diagnosis as well as a method of treatment. One of its characteristic features is that role-acting is organically included in the treatment process. It can be adapted to every type of problem, personal or group, of children or adults. . . . The psychodrama is human society in miniature, the simplest possible set-up for a methodical study of its psychological structure. Through techniques such as the auxiliary ego, spontaneous improvisation, self-presentation, soliloquy, the interpolation of resistance, new dimensions of the mind are opened up, and what is most important, they can be explored under experimental conditions.[16]

---

[16]*Program Media.* Manual of Rehabilitation Therapies Department, Spring Grove State Hospital, Catonsville, Maryland, September 1970, p. 6.

Although emotional catharsis is not as significant a part of the need of physically disabled persons, many of them have psychological problems stemming from their disability. Blind, deaf, paraplegic or otherwise severely impaired persons frequently are withdrawn, isolated, lacking in confidence and unable to relate easily to others. Dramatics—because it is *make-believe*—provides a vehicle through which they can *safely* express themselves, making their feelings and needs known to others, and temporarily leave their *own* identities to play other roles.

Dramatics have been especially successful in senior centers and residential care settings serving elderly persons. The particular value of dramatics is that it helps reinforce the self-confidence of the actors, particularly when they succeed in memorizing lines, a task that many of them feel is impossible. Based on a survey of dramatics with the elderly, Gray writes,

---

Participants in dramatics stressed that their participation kept them mentally active at a time of life when opportunities for mental activity were greatly reduced through loss of work roles and physical decrements such as deteriorating eyesight. Another source of great satisfaction to members of dramatics groups was the fact that they succeeded in acting for the first time in their lives. They were delighted to disprove the old adage that "you can't teach an old dog new tricks."[17]

Other benefits are that elderly participants work together as a group, overcoming withdrawal and isolation, and are provided with a rich means of emotional release—often elderly patients in nursing homes are so involved, they forget their aches and pains. Even the audience benefits from dramatic performances because they show vividly what the elderly are capable of, and other residents proudly identify with the performers. Obviously, as in any form of recreation or activity therapy with the disabled, there are problems to overcome. Gray reported a number of the most common problems encountered in working with the elderly in dramatics, as well as the methods used by recreation leaders in working with them (Table 5-1).

Other expressive activities related to dramatics have proved extremely useful in working with the elderly. One technique recently explored among patients in nursing homes, hospitals and prisons is poetry therapy. Like drama, poetry may serve as a means of expressing one's chaotic or hostile emotions or even helping to explore one's own feelings and past experiences. A Yale psychiatrist, Albert Rothenberg, comments that a patient who suddenly discovers the message of a great poet may experience a flash of understanding similar to the dramatic insight that may also come through intensive psychotherapy.[18] Similarly, by writing an original poem, an inhibited, repressed person may tell his or her therapist much that was secret previously. A leading modern poet, Kenneth Koch, has worked closely with patients in nursing homes and achieved remarkable success in involving them enthusiastically and creatively.[19]

---

[17]Paula Gross Gray: *Dramatics for the Elderly.* New York, Teachers College Press, Columbia University, 1974, p. 4.
[18]"Poetry Therapy." *Time,* March 13, 1972, p. 45.
[19]Kenneth Koch: *I Never Told Anybody: Teaching Poetry Writing in a Nursing Home.* New York, Random House, 1977.

Table 5-1   Physical and Psychological Limitations of Participants as Perceived by Recreation Personnel

Problem	Most Common Solution
Inability to memorize, or fear of memorization	Use of improvisation
Hearing disability	Helped by fellow actor
Visual impairment (blindness)	Large-print scripts, and individual coaching
Physical disability (confinement to wheelchair)	Limited action; used ramps to move about
Lack of interest	Individual contact and encouragement
Senility	Gave no lines
Limited reading skill	Individual coaching
Lack of self-confidence	Constant reassurance

From Paula Gross Gray: *Dramatics for the Elderly.* New York, Columbia University, Teachers College Press, 1974, p.7.

Musical Activities

Music is one of the most varied and useful activities for meeting the needs of persons with every type of disability. It can be conducted on every level from the simplest to the most complex and has value both as a "listening" and as a "doing" activity. It may involve single individuals or large groups in choral or instrumental programs. It engenders a feeling of companionship and group solidarity and at the same time is an expressive art that brings emotional pleasure and release. Essentially, there are three phases to the program of music as it may be provided for the physically disabled: (a) listening; (b) singing; and (c) instrumental music.

1. *Music listening.*   This can range from listening to recorded or taped popular or classical music to having visiting performers entertain in a large hospital. Sometimes listening may involve music appreciation sessions, with discussion of the type of music—whether it be classical, jazz or folk.

2. *Singing.*   This may involve informal folk singing or community songfests, as well as choruses, madrigal groups or other performing units. Young children are likely to enjoy action songs, while older persons will prefer songs that were popular years ago. Singing for disabled persons may simply be a casual recreational activity—preferably with an accompanist at a piano or accordion—or it may become an important area of personal growth and emotional release. In general, all those with physical disability, except the deaf, may take part, although some individuals with major speech defects (such as the severely cerebral palsied) may have some difficulty in singing. Singing may actually be used to *improve* voice production.

3. *Instrumental music.*   Obviously, this requires skilled leadership. Often, if the recreation leader is not able to direct instrumental music programs and there is no skilled music therapist available, it is possible to get volunteers from the community who have a high degree of skill in instrumental music. The programs may range from rhythmic sessions with children or beginners, using simple percussion or other rhythm instruments, to instruction on beginning, intermediate or advanced levels for players of all ages. Since the key factor in playing music is the use of hands and arms, and particularly finger dexterity, individuals with other types of disability are usually able to play wind, string or percussion instruments.

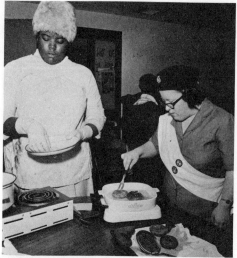

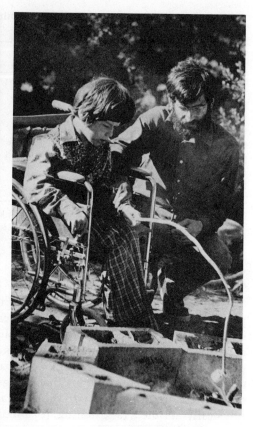

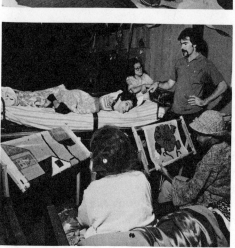

Physically disabled and mentally retarded participants at San Francisco's Recreation Center for the Handicapped take part in crafts, a marshmallow roast and cooking as part of A.D.L. (activities of daily living). (Bill Cogan, Photographer.)

Arts and Crafts

Probably more than any other major category of recreation, arts and crafts lend themselves to adaptation for individuals at all levels of ability. Like hobbies, they may be carried on individually or in groups and may range from the simplest projects to extremely advanced activities. They offer an excellent outlet for creative expression and the constructive use of energy. In addition, since the work produced may be used as decorations in a home or hospital ward, as gifts to friends or family or as exhibits in shows, arts and crafts help to bring about a strong sense of accomplishment.

One major area of activity is the graphic arts: sketching, water-color and oil painting or print-making. For those with adequate vision and manipulative skills, these activities may be approached just as with nondisabled persons. For those with more limited dexterity, it may be necessary to devise special holders for crayons, charcoal or brushes.

Clay modeling, soap carving and papier-mâché work also are useful for the physically disabled. These may be approached on an extremely rudimentary level or may involve advanced projects. They may include carving or modeling animals, dolls, puppets and similar projects. Ceramics is a more advanced medium that may be carried on using the mold process or, for those capable of using their hands effectively, with the potter's wheel or by building slabs or pinch-pots. There are many other craft activities that can be suited to the physically disabled, many of which improve manual dexterity and coordination.

The emphasis in using arts and crafts should be on creative expression rather than on developing useful or impressive products. Participants should be allowed considerable choice in selecting their products and should be able to move at their own rate. Although it may be convenient for the leader to use prestructured craft materials, such as "paint-by-the-numbers" kits, these reduce the value of the activity for participants. As much as possible, they should be creating their *own* works.

Art may also be used as a basic therapeutic technique, particularly with disturbed or psychotic patients. Like other creative or expressive forms, it has the potential for promoting healing psychological processes through essentially nonverbal forms of communication. Edith Kramer, who has worked with delinquents, the blind and the mentally ill, points out that art should be regarded as a form of therapy in its own right rather than as a tool of psychotherapy. The art therapist, she writes, functions as an artist and educator who is capable of modifying his methods according to the patient's pathology and needs:

He is trained to appraise the patient's behavior and production and to interpret his observations to the therapeutic team. He implements the team's therapeutic goals, but he does not ordinarily use his clinical insight for uncovering or interpreting to the patient deep unconscious material, nor does he encourage the development of a transference relationship.[20]

As patients create art, Kramer suggests that the art therapist's response must be geared to their needs and developmental levels. In some cases, they should be helped to relate what they have done to reality or to apply aesthetic criteria to their work. In others, the mere fact that they have been able to make a creative effort is sufficient, and it would be a mistake to apply external standards that might inhibit or discourage them or to force them into a recognition of why they have created the kinds of images they have. Although technique is never an end in itself, the art therapist helps patients explore the elements of art and learn how to use its tools most expressively.

---

[20]Edith Kramer: *Art as Therapy with Children.* New York, Schocken, 1971, p. 25.

Special Events

Special events are an important aspect of recreation programs for the physically disabled in all kinds of settings. They provide an opportunity for working together with others to plan events or simply to enjoy the entertainment offered. Special events may be informal last-minute activities or elaborately planned parties, carnivals, concerts, shows, dances, sports programs, celebrations or trips. In addition to providing recreation for physically disabled persons in a rehabilitation center or community-sponsored program, special events may be used to educate the public about programs serving disabled people. By holding an open house or inviting outsiders to come to a party, carnival or other event, it is possible to show them what disabled persons are like, dispel their misconceptions and build more positive links with community groups.

In Veterans' Administration hospitals, special programs frequently include visits by performing groups from the community who will put on musical, dramatic or dance programs or provide other special entertainment for large numbers of patients. In hospitals in large cities, professional performing companies will often appear on their nights off, and professional athletes may also give talks, demonstrations or clinics. When physically disabled persons plan their own programs, such as carnivals, festivals, large-scale picnics or barbecues or talent shows, these events should be carefully organized. As much as possible, the disabled persons themselves should form committees (such as program, publicity, finance, clean-up or special arrangements committees) and do the actual work of running the event.

An example of a special event may be found in a nursing home that sponsors an annual bazaar to raise money for a charity selected by members of the Residents' Council.[21] This event had the following steps or tasks:

1. Reviewing literature and films about potential agencies to be aided and making a decision as to which one should receive a charitable gift.
2. Establishing a planning committee and setting up subcommittees to handle each aspect of the bazaar: refreshments, publicity, raffle tickets sales and other functions.
3. Preparing products to be sold at the raffle, in crafts groups, sewing, jewelry-making and other sessions conducted by the home's recreation staff.
4. Holding the bazaar itself, as a full day event, on a Sunday before Thanksgiving.
5. Post-event activities, such as an evening of home movies of the bazaar or a special day when the check was presented in a ceremonial award to the recipient agency.

This event, which was well attended by members of the home's staff, volunteers, guests from the community and members of residents' families, raised an impressive sum and was regarded as a major success. One of its positive values was to increase the residents' sense of self-worth by having them participate in a service to people outside the institution. The award was given to a small nonprofit agency in the nearby neighborhood, so that the home's residents had a sense of helping their immediate community. By working over a period of time toward a distinct

---

[21]Rhonda Schuval: Graduate paper at Herbert Lehman College, New York, 1976.

and achievable goal, many of the recreation activities carried on during the preceding weeks and months were given a sense of purpose and high morale. Cooperative relationships were developed among the staff and residents of the home itself, along with a sense of group awareness and improved communication. Finally, family members were drawn into the process in a variety of ways. The home's residents had the opportunity to feel pride in themselves and to welcome their relatives to a positive and significant event.

Many agencies and institutions sponsor such events to raise money, improve morale, strengthen ties to family members and community groups and as a desirable form of public relations. For example, the New Lisbon State School in New Lisbon, New Jersey, sponsors a series of large-scale events throughout the year, including a Memorial Day Program, an Annual Picnic and Governor's Day (attended by the state governor), an Independence Day Celebration, a Circus Day, Labor Day Carnival, annual Parents' Bazaars and other shows, sports events or holiday programs that succeed in attracting thousands of relatives, families and friends to the school. Such programs help to break down the barrier that too often exists between large state institutions for the retarded and the outside world and provide positive and productive ways of involving families and friends of the school's residents in its program. Recreation becomes an absolutely vital service within the overall administration of the institution.

Camping and Nature Activities

Day camping, resident camping and nature activities in general are among the most successful and valuable programs provided for the disabled. Usually, such activities provide an opportunity to live, play and work with others in an environment that promotes good fellowship and an understanding of the outdoors. Group interaction is a strong benefit of camping programs, and participants learn new skills and recreational interests that may serve them in good stead. Particularly for individuals who may be restricted to a hospital or other residential setting with crowded wards, hospital beds and bleak surroundings, the opportunity to experience the out-of-doors can be an enriching and morale-building experience.

There are special camps in the United States today that serve epileptics, diabetics, cardiac patients, the blind, the deaf, the mentally retarded, convalescent patients and other persons with physical disabilities. Such programs usually require a high staff-to-patient ratio and often make considerable use of volunteers. Day camping programs are usually easier to operate; the extensive care that many disabled persons require makes overnight or residential camping much more demanding. Frequently, campers who are given responsibilities for self-care or for helping to do chores for their bunks or in the dining area gain a new degree of independence and social functioning and make dramatic gains in personal adjustment.

Water activities, such as games, boating, fishing or swimming, are usually extremely popular. If a lake or beach is being used, extreme caution must be taken with the physically disabled, since such areas are not as easily supervised as a swimming pool (because of the rapidly changing depth of the water or surf or the difficulty in seeing beneath the surface). Safe swimming areas should be clearly marked off with ropes and closely watched, with a high ratio of staff to participants.

Other special factors involved in selecting a camping area include the desirability of having nearby natural settings suitable for outdoor education or nature-oriented activities or for more advanced hiking, boating or other survival-related programs, when appropriate. If numbers of the campers are in wheelchairs, it should be recognized that it is difficult to move these through low, muddy areas or along sandy beaches without walkways. Camps provided for older persons in particular may require an additional level of warmth, comfort and access to toilet areas.

The ideal camp is one in which the physically disabled are integrated with the nondisabled. For many, however, their limitations are such that they cannot keep up with the full range of activities enjoyed by the nondisabled and are not yet ready for the degree of independent self-care required in such a setting. For them, a segregated camp is preferable, in order to build the necessary skills and help them gain confidence. For some physically disabled children, there may be a progression through the following stages: (a) day camp, in which they begin to gain skills and confidence; (b) resident or overnight camp for the disabled alone; and (c) resident or overnight camp for both disabled and nondisabled children.

A number of examples of special camps for disabled children and youth are described elsewhere in this text. Particularly for adolescents and young adults, an increasing number of programs have begun to include "adventure," "survival" or "wilderness" camping. These have been used particularly with psychiatric patients or groups of clients with drug or alcohol problems or delinquency. Patients or clients are put into situations where they must be largely responsible for taking care of themselves in the wilderness. They are subjected to a degree of physical risk as they meet various challenges in the environment—often based on the Outward Bound program.

Gibson has reviewed the literature on therapeutic wilderness camping programs. Based on this analysis, he concludes,

> While many of the empirical studies are of questionable validity due to methodological shortcomings, it is clear that wilderness programs can and do result in positive changes in the self-concepts, personalities, individual behaviors and social functioning of the program participants. Therapeutic wilderness programs are . . . a potentially powerful, albeit largely unrecognized, alternative to traditional therapeutic interventions.[22]

Information about established camps for the disabled may be gained from major voluntary organizations serving special populations (usually within a specific category, such as the visually or orthopedically impaired), which tend to have chapters in large metropolitan areas.

[22]Peter Gibson: "Therapeutic Aspects of Wilderness Camping: A Comprehensive Literature Review." *Therapeutic Recreation Journal*, Second Quarter, 1978, p. 30.

Trips and Outings

When any sort of trip or special outing is planned for the disabled, careful arrangements need to be made with respect to (a) arranging transportation; (b) getting permission for those who will be traveling (either permission from parents or, when necessary, medical approval); (c) screening all participants to determine whether the trip will be appropriate for them; and (d) making arrangements at the place that will be visited, to be certain that there are suitable accommodations for a group of physically disabled persons.

The value of such programs is that they provide novelty and special interest to the lives of the physically disabled and help to keep their morale high. The trips help the disabled to maintain constructive ties with the community as well as to promote socialization and group involvement. For patients in a rehabilitation center, trips and outings have the very special value of helping them learn to get around in the outside world and to develop the kinds of practical skills they will need when they are discharged.

Over the past several years, a number of organizations have moved more vigorously into planning and carrying out extensive trips for the physically and mentally disabled, often with marked success. The Moss Rehabilitation Hospital in Philadelphia maintains a Travel Information Center, which provides access guides to many large cities and airports, information on cruises and accessible cruise ships, tourist attractions, hotels and motels, and travel by car, train, bus or plane. A Philadelphia-based organization called The Guided Tour has run carefully directed trips for the learning disabled and mentally retarded for the past several years to such places as New York, Washington, Nashville, Nassau, California, Mexico and even Hawaii, with groups of about 25 to 30 individuals, accompanied by a social worker, special education teacher or recreation specialist for every five clients. Another organization promoting travel for the handicapped is the Society for the Advancement of Travel for the Handicapped, a New York–based nonprofit group consisting of more than 200 travel agents and tour operators seeking to promote more travel opportunities for the disabled.[23]

Horseback Riding

The number of children and adults in the United States and Canada who have severe physical or mental disabilities and who participate in programs of therapeutic horseback riding has sharply increased during the past decade. A survey carried out in the mid-1970's indicated that there were 40 such programs, with the number steadily increasing. Mayberry writes,

---

[23]Mike Shoup: "Clearing House of Information to Assist the Handicapped Traveler." *The Philadelphia Inquirer*, February 8, 1981, p. 3-G.

The rapid growth and interest in using horseback riding as a therapeutic adjunct resulted from an unusual alchemy of enthusiasm of handicapped riders, parents, horsemen, educators, therapists, and physicians. This stems largely from observations that persons who are handicapped and participate in well-conducted programs appear to improve in muscle strength, mobility, balance, coordination, and the relaxation of spastic muscles.[24]

While there is no definitive explanation of the value of this form of activity, a number of theories have been advanced: (a) the unique gait and motion of the horse, coupled with the need of the disabled rider to concentrate on controlling his or her mount, results in the relaxation of spastic muscles; (b) there is considerable psychodynamic value for an individual who must normally use a wheelchair or otherwise be severely limited in locomotion to control a powerful and mobile animal like a horse; and (c) riding represents a form of controlled risk and physical challenge for disabled individuals, which all people need today, but which is difficult for them to obtain in other ways. Mayberry warns, however, that riding should be respected as a pleasurable and valuable recreation experience, and that the horse should not be "reduced" to being simply an animated "gymnastic instrument."[25]

PLAYROOM ACTIVITIES IN PEDIATRIC UNITS

As a final example of the selection and modification of activities in therapeutic settings, one might use playroom activities in pediatric hospitals. Unlike a number of the other kinds of treatment settings described in this text, pediatric units serve a wide diversity of patients of different ages and levels of need. In general, recreation is seen as a way of helping children who are removed from their everyday world and placed in a stressful situation maintain a link with their normal daily routine. Narwold suggests that the goals of recreation in such a situation are

. . . aimed at helping children adjust emotionally to the hospital situation, come to terms with their physical handicaps, and accept themselves as worthwhile individuals. . . . Spontaneity and a warm, trusting, nonthreatening atmosphere are stressed.[26]

Within the playroom itself, children who are tense and apprehensive are able to become more comfortable. Parents and the playroom supervisor may become

[24]Robert P. Mayberry: "The Mystique of the Horse as Strong Medicine: Riding as Therapeutic Recreation." *Rehabilitation Literature*, June–July 1978, p. 192.

[25]*Ibid.*, pp. 195–196.

[26]Sally J. Narwold: "Coping with Hospitalization through Play." *In* Larry Neal, ed.: *Leisure Today: Selected Readings.* Washington, D.C., American Association for Leisure and Recreation, 1975, p. 35.

involved with the child's play or craft activity if they wish; normally, a wide range of toys, puzzles or craft projects are available. If children cannot come to the room itself, recreation therapists often make use of a movable cart, brightly decorated and filled with various play and game materials, that can be taken to the patient's bedside. A unique value of recreation in the pediatric setting is that it can be used to help children accept, understand and adjust to the hospital. Using projective dolls and toys, children may act out their fears, play the role of doctors and nurses and become familiar with many of the hospital's instruments and procedures in a positive, rather than passive, way.

Children in the hospital, because of fear of being deserted, often become more dependent, clinging to their parents and sometimes showing regressive behavior symptoms. They have virtually no control over what will happen to them and are subjected to painful and frightening procedures. Since play is a normal part of the child's life pattern and allows him or her to take charge of a "make-believe" world, expressing and communicating feelings about his or her environment, it can be an extremely helpful therapeutic agent. Dramatic play, water play and activities that channel the child's aggressive feelings (such as the punching doll that pops back up, pegs that are hammered into a board or blocks that can be built up and then crashed to the floor) are all helpful forms of expression. Particularly for children confined to their beds or in heavy casts, who tend to become extremely restless and hyperactive, play can provide an extremely important release. Besides games, music, stories told by hospital volunteers and arts and crafts are particularly useful in such situations.

For children who have undergone surgery and are on the road to recovery, play can be provided in close cooperation with physical and occupational therapy. The patient is encouraged to take part in activities that increase strength, maintain or improve motion in a joint or otherwise aid in rehabilitation. Swimming or even such active games as wheelchair basketball or other modified sports are extremely helpful, under the direction of medical staff. Narwold writes, "In this way, children are encouraged to be active, aggressive and noisy. Competition, a normal healthy aspect of growing up, is not lost when the child is hospitalized."[27]

When the problem is more severe and the patient is undergoing a series of difficult operations and treatments, along with a high level of impairment, disfigurement or pain, recreation in the pediatric setting becomes all the more important. Observers note that many children who have been in treatment over a period of time lose vitality and initiative and become sad, depressed and withdrawn. For such patients, it is critical that recreation serve as a vital tool in maintaining morale, interest in life and a positive self-image and outlook toward others.

This chapter has provided an overview of current approaches to patient/client assessment, activity analysis, prescriptive programming and modification or adaptation of program elements. It has also given examples of several of the major areas of recreational activities offered in programs for the disabled, accompanied by examples of how they may be designed to meet specific therapeutic needs.

---

[27] *Ibid.*

Suggested Topics for Class Discussion,
Examination Questions or Student Papers

1. Outline the elements that are typically found in an individualized treatment plan, and show why the individualized treatment plan is an essential tool in meaningful therapeutic recreation programming today.

2. Define activity analysis, and present a number of the characteristics of activity that should be considered in carrying out such an analysis. Then demonstrate how these characteristics would be considered in selecting appropriate forms of involvement for a given patient or client.

3. Describe several approaches to assessing a patient or client's needs, interests or recreational capability, to be used in program development or preparation of treatment plans.

4. Select one of the major forms of activity described in this chapter, and outline a number of specific ways in which it might be adapted, modified or presented in order to meet the needs of a given population or group of participants.

6

Recreation and Mental Illness

As earlier chapters have shown, mental illness is one of the chief areas of disability in which recreation is used as a therapeutic medium. This chapter examines the nature of mental illness, the various approaches that have been used to treat it and the role of therapeutic recreation service in such programs.

Mental illness is a complex form of human disorder. Medical authorities have at best only limited knowledge of the causes and symptoms of mental illness. Indeed, there are no clear-cut criteria for defining this disorder or for characterizing a person as mentally ill. Despite these facts, it is clear that mental illness constitutes a major social problem today. In the early 1970's, it was said to affect one out of every ten persons in the United States. Psychiatric patients occupied almost half of all hospital beds at an estimated cost of about $3 billion a year. However, by the late 1970's, owing to the increased use of medication and the growth of the deinstitutionalization movement, the number of persons in mental hospitals in the United States had declined to approximately 200,000.[1]

Nonetheless, mental illness continues to be a major health concern in our society. A substantial number of persons who are mentally ill are not hospitalized. For example, the National Institute of Mental Health has estimated that between four and eight million Americans each year suffer depressions severe enough to keep them from performing their regular activities or to compel them to seek medical help. In addition, an estimated ten to 15 million have less severe depressions; the majority of both groups, however, are not institutionalized.[2]

There is a widely held belief that mental illness is most prevalent in large cities, owing to the stress of urban life and the high incidence of other social pathologies. A recent report to the American Psychiatric Association based on community mental health statistics gathered by the National Center for Health Statistics, however, found that people in rural areas and small cities reported 20 per cent more symptoms of psychological disturbance than did big-city residents.[3] Indeed, the estimated mental-morbidity rate of a rural Canadian area, to which the researchers gave the

---

[1]However, the number of "patient-care episodes" involving inpatient or outpatient mental health services rose from 1028 per 100,000 in 1955 to 3079 per 100,000 in 1977; see *Statistical Abstract of the United States, 1980*, U.S. Bureau of the Census, 1981, p. 121.
[2]Jane E. Brody: "Mental Depression: The Recurring Nightmare." *The New York Times*, January 19, 1977.
[3]"Mentally, the Urban Life Beats the Rural." *The New York Times*, May 8, 1977, p. E-7.

name Stirling County, was substantially higher than that of midtown Manhattan in New York City. Mental illness affects all ages, classes and geographical areas. Statistical evidence has shown that it is closely related to economic factors—whenever the economy declines, with resultant unemployment, psychiatric admission to mental hospitals rises dramatically. Depression in particular is subject to economic factors, as evidenced by recent studies by the National Institute of Mental Health in California, New Jersey and Missouri.

CONCEPTS OF MENTAL ILLNESS

In modern psychiatry, there are two conflicting approaches to characterizing mental illness.

The older approach, which might be characterized as the *disease model*, suggests that the psychotic behavior of a disturbed individual unfolds inevitably from a defective psychological or neurological system that is essentially contained within the person. Symptoms of mental disorder are not caused by the social system in which the individual exists; mental illness is considered in the same manner a virus infection or other physical illness might be.

The more recent approach, which might be described as the *maladaptive model*, takes into account the social environment—including the family, neighborhood and larger community—of those persons who are described as mentally ill. The mentally ill, according to this viewpoint, should not be thought of or treated as diseased persons but rather as individuals with severe problems of adjustment. Disturbed behavior is seen simply as maladaptive and often caused by stresses of the social environment and the inability of the individual to meet these stresses—rather than by pathology as such.

There is no clear line of distinction between so-called normal and abnormal behavior. Unlike physical illness, in which the norm is the structural or functional integrity of the body and in which medical science has little trouble identifying "illness," it is difficult to identify, along the range of possible actions, the point at which human behavior shifts from a normal to an abnormal form of expression.

For example, it was recently reported by the National Institute of Mental Health that violence was surprisingly endemic in American families. Should such violence be classified as a sign of mental illness? Surprisingly, the reported mayhem was found in intact families, among "apparently normal, average Americans, and took place as often among the well educated as among those with little schooling."

Lee Meyer puts the question bluntly:

. . . are deviations from "normal" therefore indicative of mental illness? One problem is the difficulty in determining the appropriateness or inappropriateness of someone's behavior in a given situation due to the variations in social norms and values that exist and the range of possible responses. Usually, digressions from the normal are not regarded as mental illness unless they are persistent or so extreme that no other explanation is possible.[4]

---

[4]Lee E. Meyer: "Recreation and the Mentally Ill." *In* Thomas A. Stein and H. Douglas Sessoms, eds.: *Recreation and Special Populations*. Boston, Holbrook, 1977, p. 138.

Medical science has, however, suggested certain criteria for identifying the mental health of individuals. These criteria are rather broadly stated as personal adjustment, personality integration, personal maturity and growth and social or group involvement. The actions of persons, in terms of whether or not they are able to function effectively in terms of family, vocational responsibility or other interpersonal relationships, are used to determine whether they are mentally healthy.

Physicians have established two major divisions in the classification of the mentally ill: disorders associated with organic brain disturbance and disorders of psychogenic origin.

Chronic brain disorders, which result from severe, lasting damage to cerebral tissue, may impair judgment, memory or orientation. Epilepsy is an example of a brain disorder usually caused by physical injury to a tiny but critical part of the brain. Temporary injury to brain tissue may result in acute behavioral malfunction from which the patient recovers. These two examples fall within the realm of organic brain disturbance.

In contrast, disorders of psychogenic origin have no apparent physical cause. Temporary personality disorders may be triggered by acute stress and tend to involve previously normal individuals who have a good potential for recovery. Another form of disorder is the presence of neurosis or psychoneurosis that is related to acute anxiety and partial inability to function effectively; this ordinarily does not require hospitalization, although psychotherapeutic treatment may be helpful. Psychosomatic illnesses, such as migraine headaches or hypertension, are often connected to such neuroses. Other forms of character disorders may result in various symptoms, such as alcoholism, drug addiction or severely antisocial behavior.

Functional psychosis is the most severe and disabling psychogenic disorder, and it is to this category that the term mental illness is most frequently applied. Functional psychosis usually involves a severe degree of personality disorganization and a progressive loss of contact with reality. It is customarily classified under one of four headings: *schizophrenia, manic depression, involutional states* and *senility*. These represent the major disabilities of patients in mental hospitals today. It must be recognized, however, that such diagnostic terms should not be viewed as precise or permanent labels. For example, more than one set of symptoms may be present at a given time, and patterns of behavior may shift from one diagnostic category to another. Despite such reservations, there is fairly widespread agreement as to the following major diagnostic categories, both in the literature and in professional practice. (It should be noted that in a revised classification system approved in 1981 by the American Psychiatric Association, four primary disorders were identified: schizophrenia, paranoid reactions, involutional psychotic reactions, and affective disorders. Manic depression was described as one of the paranoid reactions, and clinical senility as an affective disorder.)

Schizophrenia

Schizophrenics are characterized by a striking withdrawal from society and from emotional ties with other persons. This may be caused by the general social alienation of the person or loss of the ability to think in meaningful and logical terms. Five common characteristics of schizophrenics are (a) withdrawal from reality; (b) autism; (c) emotional distortion; (d) delusions and hallucinations; and (e) abnormal or bizarre behavior.

Persons suffering from schizophrenia often have a history of social inadequacy. They tend to be disorganized persons who have never developed adequate roles or self-concepts. In the face of emotional difficulties or disappointments, they tend to withdraw into a fantasy world. They no longer communicate meaningfully with others, and their thought processes become disorganized and unreal. As a consequence, schizophrenics are unable to relate to or understand others, take meaningful social roles or function well in their families or in society.

Brody describes schizophrenia as a "weird, seductive, baffling form of madness that has long been a source of fear, fascination and contempt." Although other forms of mental illness have faded from prominence or yielded to scientific discovery, she writes, schizophrenia continues to afflict about 1 per cent of the American population:

As a worldwide problem and the westernized societies' most common severe mental disorder, schizophrenia has little respect for race, creed, intelligence, wealth or breeding. In the United States, schizophrenics comprise half the patients in mental institutions. Many more live in society, but must return occasionally to hospitals for treatment. On the average, one-third of the schizophrenics get better, one-third get worse, and one-third stay the same indefinitely.[5]

Schizophrenia has often been referred to as evidence of a "split" personality, with a sharp contrast between the outer and the inner self of the individual. Based on recent studies, it is now evident that schizophrenia has a strong genetic component. A child with one schizophrenic parent, even if adopted and brought up by others, has a ten times greater chance of becoming schizophrenic than does the general population; with two schizophrenic parents, the risk is 40 times greater.

Schizophrenic disturbances can be categorized into the following groups.

SIMPLE SCHIZOPHRENIA

Persons suffering from this disorder are not always confined to mental hospitals but may simply lead undemanding, socially withdrawn lives. Simple schizophrenics are generally isolated, have few friends, and have jobs requiring only superficial contact with others; they often have peculiar habits of dress or speech.

HEBEPHRENIC SCHIZOPHRENIA

This condition frequently emerges at puberty, a time of physical change and emotional stress. The individual's thoughts become confused and his language

---

[5]Jane E. Brody: "Schizophrenia Is Unyielding." *The New York Times*, May 19, 1974, p. 6-E.

unintelligible; he may be prone to hysteria or uncontrollable laughter or rage. Hebephrenic schizophrenics often report hearing voices or other forms of hallucinations. They may ritualize their lives in great detail, apparently as a means of controlling their environment and avoiding ambiguous or threatening situations.

PARANOID SCHIZOPHRENIA

Persons with this common disorder often have a strong sense of persecution. They may feel that their entire environment is hostile and threatening, that people are plotting against them and even that they are inhabited by, or controlled by, other persons. Paranoid schizophrenics tend to be suspicious of others and to resist social communication or emotional contact.

Manic Depression

Many persons experience mild depressions. These deepen markedly in the psychotic form of this disorder. The patient feels sad and lonely; his thought processes and behavior slow down. He refuses to respond to others, and the entire functioning of his mind, memory and thought processes is retarded. Depressive persons may become suspicious and irritable and have frightening hallucinations, but, most commonly, they become slow and drowsy, sitting or lying in one spot for hours on end. Ultimately, the patient may become suicidal as a result of his feelings of hopelessness and lack of worth.

It is the nature of the manic-depressive patient to have violent mood swings from extreme elation to severe depression. In the manic, or "high," state he may feel great optimism and become extremely energetic and overexcited, talking incessantly. He may develop unreal, grandiose images of himself. His judgment becomes faulty; he is easily distracted and may readily fly into sudden rages. When exhausted, he may then swing into a state of severe depression.

Many individuals do not experience the manic phase of this form of mental illness and instead appear to vacillate between a relatively normal state and a mild or acute state of depression. Depression can be caused by many factors, including stressful events, organic diseases, drugs or even childbirth or the completion of a major creative effort. In addition to being a severe problem itself, when the depressed individual becomes almost totally incapacitated and withdrawn, depression may also lead some victims to seek escape through excessive drinking, marital infidelity, gambling or other forms of compulsive behavior—which in turn create further problems.

Involutional Psychosis

This disorder is similar to the extreme state of depression found in those with manic-depressive psychoses. It tends to occur for the first time in later middle age, along with general physical and intellectual decline. Patients complain of insomnia, excessive anxiety, restlessness and concern about unimportant matters; often they fall into spontaneous periods of weeping. Suicidal impulses and delusions of hypochondria are also frequently seen in involutional states. Those with involutional psychosis tend to remain in the depressive state and do not recover spontaneously, as sometimes occurs with manic-depressive individuals.

Senility

In senile patients, progressive mental deterioration occurs as a result of the degenerative brain changes and arteriosclerosis that affect many older persons. Withdrawal from social contacts, a narrowing of interests and a general lessening of alertness and awareness of the environment are typical of senile patients. Often they become extremely confused, with severe memory impairment, even of recent events. Today, it is recognized that, in addition to organic causes, social isolation and the lack of environmental stimuli may also lead to senility.

Other Behavior Disorders

In addition to these diagnostic categories, the American Psychiatric Association has identified seven categories of behavior disorders which are not as serious as psychoses or major personality disorders, but which nonetheless are stable, internalized and resistant to treatment. Frequently these disorders have been referred to as "emotional illness" or "emotional disturbance." However, a more widely used term today is "behavioral disorder." Sherrill sums up the seven categories recognized by the American Psychiatric Association:

1. Hyperkinetic behavior marked by overly short attention span, restlessness, easy distractability.
2. Chronically anxious behavior marked by unrealistic fears, difficulty in sleeping, and nightmares.
3. Flight reaction among children and youth, who seek escape from threatening situations by running away from home.
4. Withdrawal syndrome, marked by extreme shyness, over-sensitivity, and difficulty in forming close personal relationships.
5. Aggressive and hostile reaction marked by quarrelsome and destructive behavior, temper tantrums, or other unsocialized forms of "acting out."
6. Deviant social behavior involving delinquent group affiliation, acceptance of anti-social values, and specific forms of rebellion against adult mores and controls.
7. Other reactions which do not fit under the preceding headings, but which are more serious than temporary situational disturbances, and less so than the major forms of psychoses, neuroses and personality disorders.[6]

---

[6]Claudine Sherrill: *Adapted Physical Education and Recreation: A Multi-Disciplinary Approach.* Dubuque, Iowa, Wm. C. Brown, 1981, p. 462.

PERSONALITY DISORDERS

This term is generally used to apply to deeply ingrained behavior patterns that are either antisocial or seriously self-destructive, such as alcoholism or drug abuse. Many individuals who have such difficulties are able to function to some degree in society. For example, many alcoholics hold good jobs and maintain reasonably acceptable relationships with others. Some, however, require psychotherapeutic or other forms of assistance to maintain themselves in the community. Still others may suffer from such extreme disorders that they are unable to deal at all realistically with life, and must be institutionalized. Typically, such disorders become more acute at a critical stage of the developmental process, such as adolescence; many young people undergo crises that require hospital care or intensive intervention within the community.

NEUROSES

The term "neurosis" applies to less severe forms of personality disturbance, such as obsessive ideas or compulsive and ritualistic acts, chronic fatigue, hypo-chondria, an excessive level of anxiety or depression. In general, neuroses are not regarded as serious forms of mental illness, although they may become so severe as to be almost crippling to the individual's day-by-day functioning.

CAUSES OF MENTAL ILLNESS

The term "mental illness" has never been precisely defined in terms of personal behavior or psychological states. Diagnostic categories such as those just presented are frequently modified or changed in the literature.

In past centuries, physicians tended to accept the view that all mental illness resulted from anatomical lesions of the brain or nervous system. This view, which dominated the practice of neurology and psychiatry in the United States until the turn of the twentieth century, held that only the body could become diseased; the mind could not. As a result, only those who had suffered organic brain damage were regarded as legitimately mentally ill. All other disturbed persons were held to blame for their actions and often prosecuted as willful criminals.

Sigmund Freud was responsible for the view that mental illness should be regarded as a functional maladjustment, without discernible anatomical basis. He conceived of the role of the psychiatrist or psychoanalyst as a practitioner of the science of the mind rather than of the brain and nervous system. According to Freud, all persons—even those who are considered mentally healthy—tend to adjust to life's problems by creating subtle delusions of reality and employing defense mechanisms to deal with stress and problems of human relationships.

Freud sought to eliminate the sharp differentiation between neurotics and so-called normal people. It was his view that abnormal psychology merely represented an exaggerated picture of processes at work among all human beings; the mentally ill were seen as caricatures of their more smoothly functioning brethren; and the state of the disturbed constituted a mirror held up to human nature.[7]

Despite the influence of Freudian theory in discouraging the doctrines of nineteenth century pathology, the view that mental illness is the result of biochemical imbalance or disturbance has been presented repeatedly during the twentieth century. Pavlov, the Russian physiologist, drew a connection between schizophrenia and physiology in the overdevelopment of the process of cortical-based inhibitions that resulted in the individual's withdrawing from the outside world.

Recent scientific research has indeed demonstrated that biochemical and electrochemical disturbances accompany certain clinical manifestations of mental illness. Scientists have found that the brain encompasses a complicated system of nerve connections between arousal structures in the brain stem and the many areas of the cerebral cortex. Specific chemicals are employed in these connections to transmit impulses. They either arouse or retard the operation of brain processes, and their proper functioning is the basis of balanced behavior, including the generation of moods, appetites, desires and drives. Other pathways in the brain are concerned with countering such arousal activities by diminishing or inhibiting their effects.

In cases of severe psychosis, it has been shown that the excitatory pathways and their chemicals have sharply increased their activities. This results in an increased state of arousal, which becomes difficult to handle. The patient becomes distracted and confused and often overwhelmed by hallucinations, rages and other disorders of mental functions. In contrast, in depressed states, the patient does not appear to be properly aroused, with the likelihood that the arousal pathways in his brain are not sufficiently stimulated. In short, it is hypothesized today that both the explosive thought processes and behavior of the manic patient and the extreme withdrawal of the severely depressed individual are caused by physiological malfunctions.

It has still not been determined whether biochemical malfunctions of this type are the *cause* or the *result* of functional mental disturbance. Certainly, there is a strong body of medical opinion that holds that the primary cause of mental illness lies in environmental and social factors and that psychosis results not from a chemical malfunction but from inability to handle the stresses of daily living.

Those who take this position emphasize that mental illness is a problem all persons have to some degree. It is not seen as a disease in the classic sense but rather as the result of the inability to cope with life according to social norms. Since all persons deviate occasionally from what is considered normal behavior, some authorities have argued that it is wrong to classify such deviation as mental illness. Meyer writes,

---

We are all in fact, at times mentally ill. Most, however, are never so far down on the continuum, or for long enough periods of time as to require professional assistance. The number requiring professional assistance varies by definition. If you define mental illness as needing 24-hour-a-day

---

[7]Donald Fleming: "The Meaning of Mental Illness." *The Atlantic Monthly,* July 1964, p. 73.

residential care, the number is indeed small. If you define mental illness as a condition which interferes with maximum performance and a reduction in happiness and self-fulfillment, you are talking about a massive number of people, perhaps 50 to 75 per cent of our total population.[8]

Some authorities, critical of current psychiatric treatments, hold that there is no such thing as mental illness in a medical sense. Thomas Szasz, for example, characterizes mental illness as the impersonation of society's stereotype of madness by individuals whose real impairment concerns a problem in living. Mental illness, unlike a physical disease or defect, is perceived as an individual's strategy to help himself cope with a psychological crisis or to get help from others. Since the behavior norm upon which the diagnosis of mental illness is based is a psychosocial and ethical standard, Szasz argues that it is illogical to attempt to "cure" it by medical means. Carrying the argument further, Szasz calls mental illness a false concept that serves to hide certain real problems in human needs, aspirations and values. It is his position that it is wrong to diagnose cases of "mental illness" as forms of disease that should be treated. He argues vigorously against treatment by forced custodial care in mental hospitals. Szasz regards mentally ill persons as those who have broken out of their normal social roles and tried to define their own identities; he sees the normal process of psychiatric treatment as forced repression by an organized society of individuals who are socially deviant.[9]

Other authors have presented similar points of view. Thomas Scheff, for example, suggests that most chronic mental illness represents a form of role playing in response to stereotypes that are established by society. He points out that at times of stress, severe depression or so-called psychological "crisis" states, many persons tend to be unsure of their own feelings and to behave in ways that deviate from normal behavior. They tend to be in a highly suggestible state and are vulnerable to the suggestion by others that something is wrong with them, that they are "sick" or "going mad."

To support this argument, Scheff points out that the images of insanity in our society are continually reaffirmed and stereotyped through childhood games, mass media imagery and ordinary social interaction. The process of becoming a confirmed deviant, of being "mentally ill," is completed when the traditional imagery of insanity becomes part of the disturbed person's own orientation and he accepts it as a basis for guiding his own behavior.

Scheff suggests that the assumption of the role of being "crazy" is used as a means of adjustment by the patient, because he is just as confused about his own behavior as are the observers. The patient prefers the role of insanity as a replacement for his normal self-image, which has broken down under stress; the label of "I'm going mad" is preferable to the feelings of nothingness that the severely depressed person feels. Scheff concludes that the mentally ill person has in a sense

---

[8]Martin W. Meyer: "Recreation and Mental Health." In *Dialogue with Doctors*, North Carolina Recreation Commission, Bulletin No. 41, April 1968, p. 18.
[9]See Thomas S. Szasz: *Law, Liberty, and Psychiatry: An Inquiry into the Social Uses of Mental Health Practices.* New York, Macmillan, 1963.

become a forcibly type-cast actor, forced into this role by society's reaction to his personal crisis. Ultimately, he cannot control his behavior; chronic mental illness is on the border between the volitional and the nonvolitional.[10]

The arguments made by Szasz and Scheff have been strongly supported by other authorities. Erving Goffman, for example, writes,

---

. . . I want to stress that perception of losing one's mind is based on culturally derived and socially engrained stereotypes as to the significance of symptoms such as hearing voices, losing temporal and spatial orientation, and sensing that one is being followed, and that many of the most spectacular and convincing of these symptoms in some instances psychiatrically signify merely a temporary emotional upset in a stressful situation, however terrifying to the person at the time. Similarly, the anxiety consequent upon this perception of oneself, and the strategies devised to reduce this anxiety, are not a product of abnormal psychology, but would be exhibited by any person socialized into our culture who came to conceive of himself as someone losing his mind.[11]

Another eloquent spokesman for this point of view is R. D. Laing, who has gone the furthest in criticizing the disease model of mental illness and has implied that there is nothing really wrong with the person described as "mentally ill." Instead, Laing holds, it is the environment that has somehow gone wrong.

Laing argues that madness is not a disease to be cured but results from the conflict between an outer "false" self and an inner "true" self. He suggests that this split is begun in childhood, when children have certain needs and feelings that they wish to express but are taught by parents to suppress or change in order to be socially acceptable. By sheer social force, Laing argues, this inner self is compelled to become isolated from the false outer state that arises in compliance with society and gradually becomes alienated from relatedness to the outside world. In what is frequently referred to as a "nervous breakdown," the individual experiences the sudden removal of the veil of the false self, which served to maintain an appearance of outer normality but did not reflect the true feelings of the inner self. In Laing's view, getting a person to behave in a conforming way, acting adaptively to the norms of society, is not a "cure" for what is disturbing him. He suggests that the traditional mental hospital approach attempts merely to restore the split between the true, inner and the false, outer self. Although it produces an outward compliance in the individual and an apparent "cure," it has merely denied the validity of the inner self.

In response to traditional treatments, Laing developed a radical new approach that was carried out in an English institution called Kingsley Hall. The treatment involved an experiment in communal living, in which residents, all of whom had come from traditional mental institutions, were permitted to make up their own rules of operation instead of accepting old ones. The purpose of the Kingsley Hall experiment was to see what would happen if disturbed people were allowed to com-

---

[10]Thomas Scheff: *Being Mentally Ill—A Sociological Theory.* Chicago, Aldine, 1966.
[11]Erving Goffman: *Asylums: Essays on the Social Situation of Mental Patients and Other Inmates.* New York, Doubleday, 1961, p. 132.

pletely abandon their outer selves and let their "inner selves," which emerge during psychosis, take over. They were urged to follow their impulses completely rather than attempt to curb them, so that they could live and grow through their own "madness." No attempts at all were made to urge them to return to "normality," and no restrictions were placed on the behavior of members.

Kingsley Hall yielded some remarkable results. Many of its members, who had not been "cured" by years of treatment in traditional programs of psychiatric therapy and who had been locked up for sustained periods in mental wards, were able to leave therapy and lead emotionally happy lives.[12]

The arguments offered by Szasz, Scheff and Laing—that mental illness is essentially a form of deviant social behavior or unwillingness to accept societal norms, or a form of semi-volitional self-labeling, which society controls by forced treatment in mental hospitals—have considerable appeal. Several years ago, a Stanford University psychology professor, David Rosenhan, reported a study in which several perfectly sane researchers had themselves committed to 12 different mental hospitals in five states over a three-year period by temporarily faking one symptom of mental illness, hearing hollow-sounding voices.[13] At none of the institutions did the staff suspect the sanity of any pseudopatient, although other patients frequently did. The hospitals were of several types, large and small, public, private and voluntary, but in all cases the researchers were treated the same—in a totally depersonalized way. When they sought to ask reasonable questions about their status, staff members refused to talk to them, often without even making eye contact. The stereotypical view that they were insane *because* they were in mental hospitals was invariable, and although the researchers stopped reporting hallucinations as soon as they were admitted to the hospitals and behaved perfectly normally, it took them from seven to 52 days to get out. The very fact that the researchers (themselves skilled social scientists) began to insist that they were really sane was taken as convincing evidence that they were insane. When the staff of one research hospital heard that they had so consistently misjudged patients and that a follow-up study would be made, they went on the lookout for new pseudopatients—with the result that of 193 patients legitimately admitted, staff members tagged at least 41 as faking.

In addition to the consistent finding that mental patients were not treated as human beings but were dehumanized and ignored in the 12 hospitals investigated, the study also came to the conclusion that any diagnostic process that could be so easily fooled and then sustained in its massive error by an immovable and unresponsive bureaucratic structure could not be a very trustworthy one.

Despite the arguments of Szasz, Scheff and Laing and such evidence, however, there continues to be widespread agreement that there *is* such a phenomenon as mental illness—and that it is a disorder that prevents or inhibits happy and effective living in society. While treatment approaches vary considerably, an increasing number of therapists today are moving toward a "behaviorist" view of mental illness.

---

[12]See R. D. Laing: *The Politics of Experience*. New York, Ballantine Books, 1967.
[13]David L. Rosenhan: "On Being Sane in Insane Places." *Science Magazine*, January 19, 1973, pp. 250–257.

The Behavioral Psychology Viewpoint

The behaviorist holds that all human behavior is the result of learned associations of stimulus and response that the individual has been conditioned to adopt. Behavior generally is seen as coming about as a response to external pressures rather than coming from within as a coherent unfolding of the personality.

In this approach, human behavior is seen as adaptive; the actions of even the "strangest" individual are perceived as the long-term result of social influences to which he or she has learned to adapt. Therefore, behavior is neither normal nor abnormal, neither right nor wrong; it is simply how the individual has *learned to* act. The goal of behavior therapy today is to get the mentally ill person to readapt to society's norms by learning to act in ways that are considered normal. Only the part of the person's self that comes into contact with the outside world is important for the behaviorist. The so-called inner self is not observable and therefore is meaningless.

The behavioral therapist rules out any introspective report by the patient on his or her own mental processes and instead is concerned solely with observable, external behavior. It is the behaviorist view that if the symptoms of abnormality can be arrested, the person has been cured. Neurotic or even psychotic behavior is seen as the product of defective learning and can be unlearned by intensive reconditioning and reeducation.

Freudian psychotherapists see this approach as superficial—dealing only with the surface manifestations of underlying neurosis. They argue that if the therapy succeeds in removing or repressing a specific symptom, it will be replaced by another symptom until the neurosis itself is uncovered and dealt with. Freudians see behavior therapy as a form of symptomatic relief that removes the outward evidences of disturbance without attacking the essential personality disturbance or giving the patient any real insight into his or her own needs.

In contrast, William Glasser, a leading proponent of "reality therapy," stresses that each patient must learn to face reality and assume responsibility for his or her own behavior in the present:

The past has certainly contributed to what he is now, but we cannot change the past, only the present . . . Why become involved with the irresponsible person he was? We want to become involved with the responsible person we know he can be.[14]

The emphasis is not on blaming others or asking where things went wrong but rather on what is happening now. Within this treatment framework, Glasser suggests, there are three separate but intimately interwoven procedures. First, the patient must begin to face reality with the therapist's help and see how his behavior is unrealistic. Next, the therapist must reject the patient's unrealistic behavior, while at the same time accepting the patient as a person and maintaining a trusting rela-

---

[14]William Glasser: *Reality Therapy: A New Approach to Psychiatry.* New York, Harper & Row, 1965, p. 32.

tionship with him. Finally, the patient must begin to learn better ways of fulfilling his needs within the confines of reality—rather than by denying it, which in Glasser's view is the key element in all mental illness.

Erikson's Life-Cycle Approach

A final approach to understanding mental health and mental illness which is of particular relevance to the field of therapeutic recreation service may be found in the "Eight Ages of Man" theory of human development put forth by Erik Erikson, a leading contemporary psychiatrist.

Erikson suggests that there are eight important developmental stages in the maturation process. If there is significant failure at any stage of the process, serious difficulty in one or more later stages can be anticipated. The stages themselves are (a) *trust versus mistrust,* which corresponds to the oral stage in classic psychoanalytical theory (usually extending through the first year of life), in which the infant gains a sense of security and trust in the world and those in his or her environment; (b) *autonomy versus doubt,* corresponding to the Freudian anal stage (spanning the second and third years of life), in which the child begins to master physical skills and gains a sense of competence and autonomy; (c) *initiative versus guilt,* linked to the genital stage of classical psychoanalytical theory (covering ages 4 and 5), in which the child gains confidence in initiating his or her own adventures and explorations of the environment or personal skills; (d) *industry versus inferiority,* corresponding to the latency phase (ages 6 through 11), during which children develop great curiosity about how things work and become capable of organized effort and commitment to a task and of obedience to rules and societal expectations; (e) *identity versus role confusion,* the adolescent period in which classical theory holds that children overcome their "romantic" attachment to the parent of the opposite sex and relate to opposite-sex partners of their own generation (ages 12 through 18) and, beyond this, bring together all the things they have learned about themselves and achieve a clear sense of psychosocial identity and personal direction; (f) *intimacy versus isolation* (young adulthood, comprising roughly the period of courtship and early family life), in which the individual succeeds in relating to others, sharing and caring deeply without fearing loss of himself or herself in the process; (g) *generativity versus self-absorption* (middle age), in which the adult becomes concerned with others beyond his or her immediate family, particularly with helping young people and striving to make the world a better environment for them; and (h) *integrity versus despair* (later middle age and the early retirement period), during which the individual's major work tasks are nearing completion and he or she has time for reflecting on the past and enjoying grandchildren, if any.[15]

Particularly in the early stages of development, play provides an indispensable channel for healthy development. For example, during the *initiative versus guilt* period,

---

[15]For a useful summary of Erikson's analysis, see David Elkind: "Erik Erikson's Eight Ages of Man." *In* E. Mavis Hetherington and Ross D. Parke: *Contemporary Readings in Child Psychology.* New York, McGraw-Hill, 1975, pp. 350–360.

Children who are given much freedom and opportunity to initiate motor play such as running, bike riding, sliding, skating, tussling and wrestling have their sense of initiative reinforced. Initiative is also reinforced when parents answer their children's questions (intellectual initiative) and do not deride or inhibit fantasy or play activity. On the other hand, if the child is made to feel that his motor activity is bad, that his questions are a nuisance and that his play is silly and stupid, then he may develop a sense of guilt over self-initiated activities in general that will persist through later life stages.[16]

Essentially, the value of Erikson's theory with respect to recreation in the treatment of mental illness is that it provides a medium through which the patient or client can relive earlier experiences and master important challenges that were not dealt with appropriately at an earlier stage. Erikson stresses that failures at any stage of development can be rectified by successes at later stages; indeed, his emphasis on the problems of adolescents and adults in today's world has helped balance the traditionally limited emphasis on childhood as the beginning and end of personality development. Instead of the earlier dogmatic view that one's personality is essentially fixed at a very early age, he reaffirms that individuals can become more healthy and productive throughout their lives.

Before examining the specific approaches to the treatment of mental illness that are widely accepted today, it is helpful to gain perspective on past methods of treatment.

TRENDS IN PSYCHIATRIC CARE

Humanitarian attempts to care for and heal the mentally ill began about 150 years ago. Prior to that time, mental illness had been considered a result of witchcraft or possession by spirits, and its treatment had been carried on by such primitive measures as flagellation, confinement in dark cells and severe contrivances for mechanical restraint, shock treatments and purging the sick person through emetics or bleeding.

The first half of the nineteenth century saw a new philosophy of treatment called "moral therapy." This method emphasized kinder treatment of the insane, as well as the view that they should become involved in occupational and recreational activities. Moral therapy also emphasized the need to keep institutions small so that personal contact between the patients and the supervisor could be maintained. During this period, cure rates as high as 90 per cent were reported for hospitals that had adopted this approach.

By the 1870's, a new approach replaced the moral therapy method. Mental institutions became largely custodial in nature. Recoveries and discharge rates declined to less than 10 per cent in many hospitals during the first two decades of the twentieth century. Many psychiatrists believed that fewer than 5 per cent of schizophrenics could be expected to recover. Tourney attributes the growing therapeutic ni-

---

[16]Ibid., p. 353.

hilism—as this period has been termed—to "personnel problems, budgetary difficulties, hospital overcrowding, the large proportion of chronic cases, and a dogmatic depersonalized theoretic approach to insanity."[17] However, a number of the basic principles underlying modern care for the mentally ill were first developed then. Individual patient treatment, open-door policies, patient freedom, voluntary admissions, home and after-care services and sheltered or specially arranged employment for patients were all experimented with during this period.

Before the end of the nineteenth century, owing chiefly to the efforts of Sigmund Freud, attention was given to the effectiveness of the new method of psychotherapy in treating the mentally ill. This approach emphasized the direct relationship between the physician and the patient rather than reliance on medical or surgical procedures. Techniques of dream analysis, exploration of the unconscious, free association and the use of transference were developed, based on a growing body of theory of psychoneurosis as the cause of mental illness. Psychotherapy tended to be offered chiefly in clinics and private practice and to devote itself to the treatment of psychoneurosis. Its success with psychotic patients in mental hospitals was limited.

During the 1930's, new approaches in the field of somatic therapies were employed, including the use of insulin coma, convulsive therapy and lobotomy. Tourney writes,

---

Two broad schools of psychiatry emerged, the organic-physical treatment oriented, and the psychodynamic-psychotherapeutic group. The former focused on psychotic patients, and the latter largely on the psychoneurotic and characteriologic problems.[18]

Somatic therapy as developed in the 1930's survives today in the use of electroconvulsive therapy for the treatment of depression. However, it aroused interest in the use of physical therapies and drugs in the treatment of psychotic patients; this paved the way for the two most recent and promising developments in psychiatry, *psychopharmacotherapy* and *community psychiatry*. To some degree, these two schools of psychiatry illustrate a somewhat broader "split" that has developed as part of what Restak describes as an identity crisis in psychiatry.

Restak suggests that the continuing debate about what mental illness is and what psychiatrists ought to do has been markedly affected by clinical and laboratory research demonstrating that hereditary disturbances in brain function may be as important as psychodynamic factors in some illness. The impact of research dealing with biochemical aspects of depression has been, in part, to help separate psychiatrists into two camps. One analysis suggests that many psychiatrists trained before 1970 tend to be politically liberal, committed to psychotherapy as a key treatment and convinced that environmental and other psychosocial influences are major causes of emotional illness. In contrast, many psychiatrists entering the field after

---

[17]Garfield Tourney: "Psychiatric Therapies: 1880–1968." *In* Theodore Rothman, ed.: *Changing Patterns in Psychiatric Care*. New York, Crown, 1970, p. 12.
[18]*Ibid.*, p. 35.

1970 tend to be more politically conservative, better trained in brain sciences, research-oriented and persuaded of the influence of heredity and biological factors in causing mental illness.[19]

Psychopharmacotherapy

The revolution in modern drug-based psychotherapy began in 1951 when the French scientist Laborit synthesized chlorpromazine (Thorazine). This drug became widely used as a tranquilizer and accounts for the major portion of drug treatment today. Along with drugs such as reserpine, chlorpromazine is used to treat anxiety states, agitated depressions, manic states and schizophrenia. The effect of these drugs is to calm the overly aroused nerve systems in the brain.

The second phase of the psychopharmacological movement began in 1954, when iproniazid (Marsilid) was found useful with severely depressed patients. This drug and other "psychic energizers" that stimulate the arousal pathways in the brain began to replace convulsive therapies—particularly electro-convulsive treatment—in the care of depressive illness.

Since the mid-1950's, the increase in the use of drugs in the treatment of the mentally ill has been tremendous. As an example, the total number of psychopharmaceutical tablets dispensed by the Boston State Hospital grew from 113,503 tablets in 1955 to 1,675,190 tablets in 1965—a more than tenfold increase. The use of tablets in outpatient care also has grown tremendously.

Many investigators regard psychopharmacology as palliative rather than curative. They claim that although drugs are useful in the reduction of symptoms, they do not attack the basic causes of mental illness. The value of psychopharmacology appears to lie chiefly in its use with other therapeutic methods. It has made a great number of patients more accessible and amenable to treatment and has been used in combination with psychotherapy, milieu therapy and other specific treatments. "An immediate and outstanding value is the control of tension and of disturbed behavior, reflected in the virtual elimination of restraint and seclusion in the department's institutions."[20]

The psychopharmacologic revolution has done much to change the nature of mental hospitals and of psychiatric care in general. In recent years, there has been a marked shift from large, impersonal mental hospitals devoted chiefly to custodial care, to smaller institutions based on the therapeutic community model and, most recently, to the development of community mental health centers.

Within institutions, because it is no longer necessary to confine many patients, a new emphasis on activity therapy is possible. In general, there is a stronger push toward treating patients and getting them out of the hospital—or avoiding institutionalization in the first place. Fewer patients are neglected, and the total resources of the hospital may be used for therapeutic purposes. Emphasis is placed

---

[19]Richard M. Restak: "Psychiatry in Search of Identity." *The New York Times,* January 12, 1975, p. E-9.
[20]*Treatment in the Modern Mental Hospital.* Albany, New York State Department of Mental Hygiene, 1966, p. 1.

on helping patients return to community life by a combination of resocialization, living skills and work readiness experiences.

It should be made clear that medical opinion is still somewhat divided regarding drug therapy. Some psychiatrists regard psychopharmacotherapy as a "chemical strait jacket" that simply serves to make patients more docile, allowing overburdened hospital staffs to control them easily. In their view, doctors simply do things *to* patients rather than work meaningfully *with* them. Beyond this, there has been growing concern that excessive and continued use of common antipsychotic medications has resulted in serious organic damage for many patients. Gochman sums up some of the findings in this area:

Twenty to thirty years after the widespread administration of such medications, clinical observations and studies of mental patients have increasingly indicated an extraordinarily large proportion of iatrogenically organically damaged persons . . . The more years the patient was in treatment, the more likely it was that there were clinical signs of organic damage not noted at the time of hospital admission.

The infirmities of tardive dyskinesia, reflecting motor and other diffuse brain damage due to medication, are common effects among mental patients. They follow earlier common effects, such as loss of sex drive, dry mouth, loss of appetite, visual problems, leg-tingling sensations and imbalances, Zombie-ism.[21]

One major effect of the increased use of such medications has been the sharp decrease in the number of patients confined on a long-term basis in large, isolated, custodial-type asylums and the corresponding increase in the use of community mental health centers or small local hospitals or units in general hospitals for short-term treatment. Many other individuals have not been hospitalized at all but have been served on an outpatient basis while living in the community, as part of the major thrust of the late 1960's and 1970's toward deinstitutionalization.

Community Psychiatry

This represents the most important and promising recent trend in psychiatric care. Its purpose is to prevent hospitalization by maintaining disturbed patients in the community or to reintegrate them after hospitalization as rapidly and effectively as possible. Deriving its principles from the idea of social causation of mental illness, community psychiatry stresses the need to understand the familial, social and cultural milieu of each patient. The community psychiatry approach also defines mental illness broadly and includes, as part of its concern, delinquency and crime, sex offenders, addicts and alcoholics, as well as mentally retarded and isolated senile persons.

---

[21]Stanley I. Gochman: "On the Road to 1984: Twenty Questions on the Psychology of Social Action." *Journal of Community Psychology*, September 1981, p. 111.

Community psychiatry works through decentralized mental health centers to prevent hospitalization or, when it is necessary, to get patients back into the community as rapidly as possible. Emphasis is placed on using a variety of groups or resources in the community, such as family, friends, employers, health and welfare agencies or sociorecreational organizations to support and work with patients. The problems of isolation and resistance to treatment that often occur when patients are institutionalized a great distance from home may be minimized.

Emphasis is placed . . . on treatment in the community, the utilization of clinic resources, day and night hospital units, crisis-oriented therapy, rehabilitation and aftercare, hospitalization in psychiatric units in general hospitals, earlier discharge, use of halfway houses, and the establishment of special programs for the mentally retarded, aged, alcoholics, and addicts. The education of the public regarding mental illness becomes paramount in helping change community attitudes toward the mentally ill.[22]

The community psychiatry movement was given a strong impetus by the Mental Retardation Facilities and Community Mental Health Centers Construction Act of 1963. This legislation stipulated that, in order to qualify for federal funds, a community mental health center must provide at least five essential services: (a) inpatient services; (b) outpatient services; (c) partial hospitalization services, including at least day-care; (d) emergency services 24 hours per day within at least one of these three categories; and (e) consultation and education services available to community agencies and professional personnel. In addition, adequate services were defined as including such other components as diagnostic services, rehabilitation programs (including vocational and educational activities) and pre-care and after-care services (including foster home placements, training and research and evaluation). In many states, new legislation and reorganization of mental health treatment services made it possible to release large numbers of patients for treatment in community mental health centers. Many community mental health centers today maintain social groups to which patients can be referred, either by hospitals, psychiatrists, outpatient community clinics or other social agencies. In most cases, such clubs serve as an intermediate step for the patient in moving from a treatment center to a more active social life. Another technique of helping patients in their return to community life is the halfway house, where discharged persons can live in the company of professional staff members and other former patients. The halfway house provides a means of helping them adjust to community life before attempting to live independently. It offers an alternative to living alone in a run-down hotel or having to return to unsympathetic or overanxious relatives.

In addition to such programs, many communities have developed other types of neighborhood-based services dealing with such problems as family violence, alcohol abuse and suicide threats. These agencies, sometimes called "alternative counseling centers," are part of the total spectrum of community mental health ser-

---

[22]Tourney, *op. cit.*, p. 32.

vices.[23] The success and failure of the community psychiatry movement and its current directions are discussed later in this chapter and in Chapter 10.

RECREATION IN PSYCHIATRIC TREATMENT

Although it has not been possible to develop valid scientific evidence to show that recreation can either prevent or cure mental illness, it has been widely accepted that recreation makes an important contribution to psychological well-being. Meyer writes,

---

Basically, recreation is an experience which leaves one refreshed, rejuvenated, fulfilled, happy, content and at peace with oneself and the world. It reinforces companionship, group belonging and esteem, mutual interests, concern for our fellow human beings. It is a happy, productive, creative and positive experience, fostering a feeling of well-being. It does not leave us isolated, withdrawn, anxious, apprehensive, suspicious, hostile, fearful and totally sick inside. The outcomes of recreation, the very experience itself, are so closely related to positive mental health that one may consider them as almost synonymous.[24]

Individuals with poor mental health often have exaggerated feelings of worthlessness and deficiency in body structure, athletic ability, intellectual performance and other personal characteristics. Unable to achieve normal relationships, they frequently become supersensitive to social slights and apprehensive about failure or rejection, and they ultimately withdraw from social contacts.

Recreation can help such individuals be successful and develop feelings of self-worth. It provides a socially acceptable release for violent or hostile emotions. Recreation may be used to strengthen or develop such defense mechanisms as repression, displacement of emotions, substitution, sublimation and compensation. Although it may be argued that these mechanisms do not deal with the fundamental problems that affect emotionally unstable persons, the fact is that they make it possible for many such individuals to live with themselves and others in a reasonably happy and constructive way.

Thus, recreation provides a means of dealing with one's antisocial or unhealthy impulses. Meyer writes,

---

A classic example is the "substitution" of dangerous aggressive impulses, such as the desire to destroy or kill, to a more acceptable, but none-the-less aggressive activity. Kicking a ball, striking at a punching bag, chopping wood, throwing a rock at a target, can serve as initial substitutions.

---

[23]C. Alec Pollard and Stephen E. Fair: "Community Psychology and the Alternative Counseling Center." *Journal of Community Psychology*, January 1982, pp. 48–52.
[24]Martin W. Meyer: "Recreation, A Positive Force for Mental Health." *American Recreation Journal*, September-October 1964, p. 140.

These impersonal and socially harmless acts can be further redirected or refined to more meaningful releases, with rules established as controls, such as in the organized sports of soccer, handball, archery, football and tennis. As aggressive impulses are brought under control or redirected . . . important defense mechanisms can thus be established which may serve as a safety valve when dangerous aggressive impulses are ready to explode. . . .[25]

Art, music, dance and similar activities may also serve as desirable forms of release or sublimation. The kinds of pathological high-risk, destructive play described earlier can be made less appealing by providing more constructive and self-enhancing activities.

Typically, recreation programs in psychiatric institutions have been designed to improve patient morale, provide constructive outlets, promote resocialization, redevelop capacities for creative self-expression and the enjoyable use of leisure and promote the patient's capability for independent community living following discharge from the hospital.

Activity Therapy Approach

As described in Chapter 3, the activity therapy approach includes various types of rehabilitative therapies, such as occupational therapy, physical therapy, recreational therapy, educational therapy and work therapy. The basic premise underlying this method is that by prescribing a diversified program of manual and creative activities, patients are given incentives, outlets and the means for creative satisfaction. Pertinent data are provided to the psychiatric treatment team regarding the patients' reactions, aptitudes, interests and social adjustment.

Woloshin and Tamura point out that within the rehabilitative-adjustive model, support is given for productive instead of inappropriate behavior. Essentially, the method is geared to the behavioral viewpoint described earlier:

The message that should be clearly communicated is that staff respects the patient enough to expect something of him. He is expected to participate in his program and activities, to contribute to his community, and be productive rather than "crazy." . . . the rehabilitative-adjustive approach is based upon those things which are tangible and easily seen. . . . The staff and patient can chart progress more readily through tangible accomplishments . . . than through therapeutic gains in a one hour interview. If a person indeed can be productive and see the results of his productivity, it is an assumption that behavior modification takes place. Deep insight need not occur within this model for behavior modification to begin. An enhanced self-image and a greater belief in one's ability to be productive, to trust oneself and to trust others can result in further ego strengthening and social growth.[26]

---

[25]*Ibid.*
[26]Arthur Woloshin and Robert Tamura: "Activities Therapy in a Community Mental Health Center." *Therapeutic Recreation Journal,* First Quarter, 1969, p. 31.

This approach has generally been accepted throughout the country. As an example, in 1964, the Joint Information Service of the American Psychiatric Association and National Association for Mental Health, in conjunction with the Division of Community Psychiatry of Columbia University and the Department of Mental Health of the American Medical Association, published a survey titled "The Community Mental Health Center—An Analysis of Existing Models." Ten mental health centers in the United States and one in Saskatchewan, Canada, were studied in depth. All of these centers were reported as strongly emphasizing occupational and recreational therapy, with considerable emphasis on the resocializing aspects of these programs.

Within the activity therapy program, the primary thrust today is toward the maximum "push" in helping "rapid-recovery" patients move toward discharge. Because of the use of drugs, many patients are able to move freely around hospital grounds or even to go into the community on trips or work sessions; this would not have been possible in the past. Almost every aspect of programs in many of the newer mental hospitals is geared directly toward developing competence for community living. Chapters 4 and 5 described the use of therapeutic recreation as a treatment geared directly to achieving specific objectives for individual patients, based on a carefully worked out patient assessment, treatment plan and activity analysis. In contrast, in many psychiatric treatment programs, the trend has been away from *treating* patients with recreation and toward *making use* of recreation as a medium for social interaction. The major value of recreation with mental patients is seen not as the opportunity to provide individualized psychodynamic prescriptions of activity, but rather the opportunity to play and create in a manner that allows the patient to recapture his or her own sense of individuality and purpose. This approach has been stressed as part of "milieu therapy" in particular.

Milieu Therapy

It has become widely accepted that a psychiatric disorder is integrally related to the social milieu in which it has developed. Consequently, the conviction has grown that the community in which he is *treated* must be a healthy and constructive one if the patient is to regain a positive relationship with his family and community. This viewpoint is the basis of "milieu therapy," which stresses the importance of the total physical and social climate in which the patient is treated. Stanton has written,

---

The onset, symptoms, and recovery rates of major psychiatric illness are decisively influenced by the environment within which the patient is observed and treated. . . . There is no patient "untreated" by his environment—only patients "treated," well or ill.[27]

---

[27]Alfred Stanton: In V. Cumming and E. Cumming: *Ego and Milieu.* New York, Atherton Press, 1969, p. v.

Milieu therapy, or, as it is often referred to, the therapeutic community approach is concerned with *all* aspects of the hospital environment, including its physical structure, the opportunity for patients and staff to interact with each other in emotionally supportive ways and the provision of a wide range of important experiences and activities that support meaningful change. In short, the total philosophy of the hospital must be therapeutic, and in every aspect of hospital life, therapeutic agents must be at work:

The concept of the therapeutic or curative community may be described as an arrangement in which all of a patient's time in the hospital — not just the time he spends in therapy — is thought of as treatment. The milieu in which he finds himself — i.e., the hospital, is seen as exerting a powerful influence upon his emotional life and behavior. Every contact, every casual conversation with a fellow patient, a nurse, even a kitchen helper, is regarded as potentially therapeutic. Milieu therapy . . . is an attempt to take into account what psychiatrists have called "the other 23 hours in the day" — to treat mental illness through a careful restructuring of the social environment.[28]

Interest in the patient's environment as an important element in treatment was heavily influenced by the British social psychiatrist, Maxwell Jones, who in 1947 established what was later to be called the "therapeutic community." Instead of the authoritarian, hierarchical structure that had been common in mental hospitals, Jones encouraged a treatment system with permissive, democratic and communal values. "Everybody in the community, both staff and patients, was encouraged to maximize his therapeutic potential. Furthermore, all ward activities were deliberately integrated so as to be part of the total treatment program."[29]

Maxmen, Tucker and LeBow point out that the terms "milieu therapy" and "therapeutic community" have been used synonymously with a number of similar terms, such as "sociotherapy," "social psychiatry" and "psychotherapeutic community." Although the specific examples of this approach may vary considerably in practice, the concept is defined as

---

. . . a treatment modality which attempts not only to utilize maximally the therapeutic potential of the entire staff, but also to place a major responsibility upon patients to serve as change agents. In other words the unit's structure facilitates patients having a significant therapeutic role in the rehabilitation of other patients. Thus, all staff and patients meaningfully participate in the unit's decision-making processes about patient care as well as in the implementation of these plans.[30]

The therapeutic community concept represents a radical departure from the traditional view of a mental hospital as a custodial institution or "asylum." The asy-

---

[28]Maggie Scarf: "In the Therapeutic Community Patients Are Doctors." *The New York Times Magazine,* May 25, 1969, p. 109.
[29]Jerrold S. Maxmen, Gary J. Tucker and Michael LeBow: *Rational Hospital Psychiatry: The Reactive Environment.* New York, Brunner, Mazel, 1974, p. 17.
[30]*Ibid.,* p. 25.

lum was deliberately located at a place far from the community to afford the patient protection from the stress of daily life or the problems that had beset him and probably also to "remove" him from the family as a source of grief or shame. Within such hospitals there was little sense of community life or interaction; patients were not expected to make decisions, exercise judgment or function responsibly.

The proponents of milieu therapy claim that removing patients from social stress and meaningful community roles serves to make their return to society more difficult because of the prolonged period of dependence they have experienced. Their social skills and ability to face the outside world may have atrophied during hospitalization, and they may understandably fear that there is no longer a place for them among family and friends and in the vocational world. Milieu therapy, therefore, is committed to making a patient's stay in the hospital a replica of the social interactions of ordinary life—in terms of social and recreational activities, work, civic or community responsibility, human relationships and other significant aspects of life. Within the therapeutic community, patients, while being treated for their illness, are encouraged to function as fully as possible in settings that are realistic and make real demands on them.

CURRENT TRENDS IN THERAPEUTIC RECREATION IN MENTAL HEALTH CARE

What has been the total impact of the milieu therapy and decentralized mental health centers movements upon therapeutic recreation service? First, it should be made clear that theoretical statements of philosophy, or of idealized programs, do not always portray the reality of what goes on in institutions. The reality is that many institutions are badly overcrowded and that chronic wards or "extended-care" facilities still exist for many older, highly regressed patients, while newer, smaller centers situated in and around cities represent the big push for patients with more hopeful prognoses.

The very notion of the therapeutic community, where every staff member, every aspect of living, every physical or social element of hospital life serves as a supportive therapeutic agent, belies the reality of crowded wards, overworked personnel who may be moonlighting because of poor salaries, and lack of cooperation among disciplines or difficulty in developing meaningful relationships with community groups. Nonetheless, the new approaches are exciting ones. They have had a significant impact on therapeutic recreation service in the following ways.

Shifting of Emphasis in Activities

In the traditional psychiatric hospital recreation programs, in addition to numbers of special events or other mass activities, there were normally a variety of regularly scheduled sports and games, arts and crafts, music, dance or other social programs that patients were, in effect, assigned to as part of regular ward or building

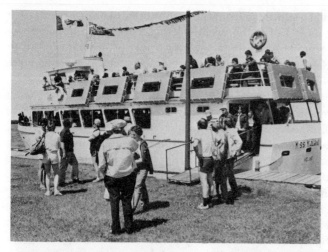

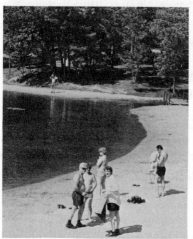

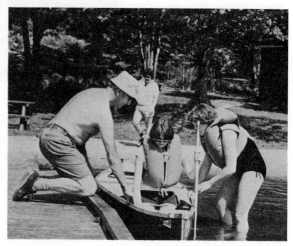

Water sports and boating are popular outing activities at the Penetanguishene, Ontario, Mental Health Centre.

unit schedules. Today, the emphasis has shifted away from this type of clearly recreational activity, frequently in the direction of activities that have an informal, less structured, social-learning kind of orientation.

Instead of having patients learn dances, games or crafts or play sports or music—with the emphasis on the activity involvement—many departments are today providing activities in which patients become involved in self-discovery processes that are heavily based on "encounter" or "sensitivity group" activities. As an example, one such program in a New York State Department of Mental Hygiene mental hospital schedules the following kinds of activities throughout the week:

grooming (male)   newspaper group
grooming (female)   coffee and conversation
bowling   hootenanny

open shop   self-expression
dance therapy   exercise group
drama and poetry   small groups
cooking   ward clean-up
small crafts   movies
"psychogymnastics"

Such activities are more personally involving, demand fewer skills and permit much freer expressive behavior than more traditional recreational activities. Whether they are more or less valuable in terms of the fundamental goals of therapeutic recreation than the traditional kinds of activities is not easy to measure.

Another example of an innovative program in psychiatric treatment is therapeutic camping. More and more state and private mental hospitals, for example, have experimented in recent years with camping programs, even for extremely sick and unresponsive patients. A leading example is Oregon State Hospital, which has taken as many as 50 patients at a time on wilderness camping trips involving white-water boating, rock climbing and survival-ecology activities. In a similar program involving a modified version of Outward Bound, the private psychiatric division of the Massachusetts General Hospital in Belmont, Massachusetts, has involved patients in activities such as long distance bicycling, rock-climbing, cross-country skiing, a confidence-building ropes course, group initiative tests and two- to five-day backpacking expeditions in the White Mountain National Forest. Such ventures have challenged mental patients to deal with reality, test their own capabilities and act as mature, responsible adults, with surprisingly positive effects in most cases.

Unitization and the Blurring of Professional Roles

In a number of large mental hospitals, patients are grouped in terms of housing and treatment services, according to their original residence or "catchment area." The purpose of this is to strengthen community affiliation and, presumably, to facilitate planning for return to the community, recreation counseling and community-patient interaction. What it has meant in a practical sense is that patients with all degrees of illness or recovery stages, and of various ages and backgrounds, are lumped together in hospital units rather than housed according to age and type or severity of illness, as in the past. In this type of structure, staff members no longer serve their hospitals on a system-wide basis, planning overall hospital activities and acting as specialists within their areas of competence. Instead, they are attached solely to their units and assume roles that contribute generally to the therapeutic community process—but in which they do not specialize in their fields of particular training or skill.

In an increasing number of hospitals, staff members working in such programs are no longer identified according to their professional specialties but are simply called activity therapists. The implication is that they no longer will be presenting specific areas of activity in which they are highly competent leaders but instead will simply be promoting group process and the therapeutic interaction of patients and staff. The notion of recreation *as* recreation appears to have suffered a decline in such settings. Instead, the group process and the experience of living, planning and making decisions together appear to be the primary emphases.

Development of Community-Based Facilities

The community mental health movement has broken down the rigid walls that have separated psychiatric patients from community life in the past. Recreation has become a part of special day-care and night-care programs. In many communities, it is now provided as part of day-center programs that, operating as satellites to a hospital or existing independently in the community, meet the needs of discharged mental patients who require a protected setting or are living at home and are receiving psychiatric clinical counseling for part of the day.

Particularly when foster communities are developed—in which patients, rather than return to their original homes and families, are located in residential "halfway houses" or helped to set up apartments with other discharged patients—it has been found that continuing social and vocational assistance is needed to help them move effectively back into the community. This is particularly true of ex-patients who are placed in "welfare" hotels, S.R.O. (single room occupancy) units or similar environments and who run a high risk of being totally isolated if special services and programs are not designed for them.

MENTAL HOSPITAL PROGRAMS

This chapter concludes by providing descriptions of the activity therapy or recreation programs in a number of hospitals in the United States and Canada. In each case, some of the more interesting aspects of the program are provided, along with examples of rating or evaluation forms, personnel assignments and program schedules.

Athens Mental Health Center, Athens, Ohio

This center provides both inpatient and outpatient services, assisting persons in a 15-county area of southeastern Ohio who have a "major" mental illness and less severely ill persons in a five-county area. Multi-disciplinary teams of mental health workers operate through four major treatment units: (a) Community Services, for outpatients and acutely disturbed inpatients; (b) Adolescent, for inpatients up to 18 years of age; (c) Geriatric, for inpatients 65 years of age and older; and (d) Continued Care, for patients requiring long-term hospitalization.

The history of this hospital reflects changing trends in psychiatric care throughout the United States. Founded in 1874 as the "Athens Lunatic Asylum," its name changed to the "Athens Asylum for the Insane," the "Athens State Hospital" and finally the "Athens Mental Health Center." Its treatment procedures also shifted through the years, from a primary emphasis in the 1950's on farm work and hydrotherapy, to a heavy use of lobotomies and finally to the use of psychiatric drugs coupled with a strong emphasis on the activity therapies and the therapeutic community approach. The inpatient population has been reduced from 1800 to about 600; in addition, several hundred outpatients are treated monthly.

The treatment staff is organized into several departments (Fig. 6–1). Of these, the Activity Therapy Department includes the following services: Volunteer Services, Patients' Library, Beauty Shop, Recreation Therapy, Music Therapy, Physical Therapy, Education Therapy, Industrial Therapy, Arts Therapy and Occupational Therapy (including Arts and Crafts Shop and Home Management).

A key element in this program is the evaluation committee responsible for appraising patients (based on past history, medical record admission information and personal interview), determining the needs and interests of clients and assigning them to appropriate placement groups of patients. This committee also is responsible for reporting periodically on each patient's progress and for recommending changes in assignments. The goals of all elements of the Activity Therapy Program are clearly outlined.

Recreation is offered in conjunction with other creative activities, such as art, music and drama therapy. Activities are divided into two classes, based on the nature of participation required:

1. Passive participation
   a. Movies
   b. Theater
   c. Church services
   d. Art exhibit
   e. Bus rides
   f. Concerts
   g. Trips to Columbus Zoo
   h. Spectator sports
2. Active participation
   a. Club activities (press club, garden club, cooking club, literary club, drama and radio club)
   b. Adapted sports (softball, basketball, shuffleboard, horseshoes, touch football and bowling)
   c. Glee club and choir activities
   d. Individual music lessons (voice, piano, organ, guitar and brass instruments)
   e. Music appreciation groups
   f. Art therapy groups
   g. Social recreation (dances, parties, teas and picnics)
   h. Tournaments (pool, checkers, bowling, Ping-Pong, table shuffleboard, cards and horseshoes)
   i. Camping (overnight and day camping)
   j. Library (regular lending services, literary and current events groups, for both leisure and educational purposes)

The facilities used include an extensive variety of shops, studios and other recreation areas at the hospital itself, as well as other resources in the community, such as schools and colleges, hobby groups, service clubs, fraternal organizations, families and friends.

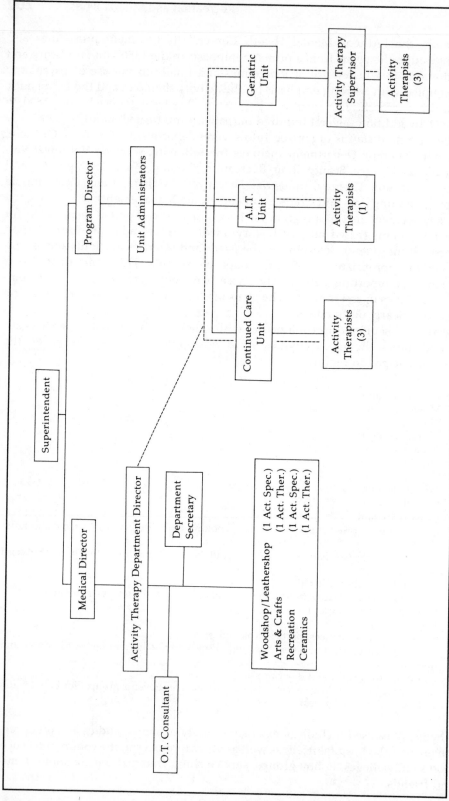

Figure 6–1. Table of organization of Activity Therapy Department, Athens Mental Health Center, Athens, Ohio (1982).

Mt. Sinai Medical Center, New York, New York

The psychiatric unit within the Mt. Sinai Medical Center in New York City provides an excellent example of activity therapists employed as fully integrated members of the psychiatric treatment team. The rationale for this role is stated in the departmental manual:

> The Activity Therapist is responsible for full-time in-patient psychiatric care. The patients involved are not confined to bed; yet they must remain within the hospital for an average stay of 35 days. The patient generally spends only one-and-a-half hours a week with his resident psychiatrist; if he has a private psychiatrist, he will usually spend five hours a week with him at best. The balance of the patient's time, a considerable part of the day and the entire evening and weekend time, the patient's treatment plan is implemented by his Activity Therapist. There is considerable need for this care; in psychiatric illness, the constructive use of this time is of the utmost importance toward the patient's recovery. An Activity Therapist must be professionally trained for this responsibility. His activities must facilitate the patient's recovery, and bring him back to healthy functioning, by restoring an interest in life and constructive action; and guiding the patient to an awareness of his unhealthy mental habits, pointing the way to a positive change toward healthful balanced attitudes. This must be done with the cooperation of the nursing staff, regarding medication and medical problems; and the programs must complement the doctor's long-range treatment goals for the patient.[31]

The time of Activity Therapists at Mt. Sinai is about equally divided between servicing an inpatient unit and working on the ninth floor of the hospital, where activities and programs are provided on an all-hospital basis. They have the following specific responsibilities for their own units:

1. Supervision of patient government meetings.
2. Leading activity planning sessions for events that will take place on weekends or evenings when Activity Therapists are not present.
3. Attendance and participation in daily morning group meeting with patients and staff and follow-up discussion meetings with medical and nursing staff.
4. Attendance and participation in twice- or thrice-weekly unit conferences with medical, nursing and social work personnel at which new admissions are interviewed and discussed.
5. Staff meetings with medical, nursing and social work personnel to bring out and discuss inter-staff problems.
6. Meetings between the chief resident and Activity Therapists, and the unit chief and Activity Therapists, to keep each of these individuals aware of patients' progress.
7. Meetings with nursing staffs of individual units to exchange information regarding patients.

In addition, Activity Therapists attend weekly staff meetings of their own group, in which they deal with the mechanics of running the program, such as

---

[31]*Departmental Manual.* Mt. Sinai Hospital, New York, 1971.

Patient's name: _____ Date: _____
Unit: _____

I. Evaluation summary: Performance deficits and strengths related to
    A. Self-concept and identity
    B. Need-drive adaptation
    C. Interpersonal and social relations
    D. Cognition and problem solving
    E. Perceptual-motor functions
    F. Life tasks skills and vocational adjustment
II. Program focus and recommendations:
    A. Program focus
        1. Remedial:
            a. deficits in performance skills around which program is to be structured
            b. essential characteristics of remedial activities
        2. Supportive:
            a. existing skills, capacities and interest which should be sustained and/or
                protected
            b. essential characteristics of supportive activities
        3. Life tasks skills and vocational adjustment
            a. areas and level of daily life tasks skills and vocational adjustment needs toward
                which rehabilitation program should be directed.
            b. activity and/or task assignment recommendations
Staff: _____

Figure 6–2.   Performance evaluation summary and program recommendations.

scheduling, planning of special events, problems relating to equipment, supplies and similar matters. They also meet in regular in-service seminars concerned with evolving new types of programs designed to best serve psychiatric patients today. Essentially, Activity Therapists are responsible for three types of group experiences: leisure-time groups, prevocational groups and rehabilitative groups. In each situation, they must serve as resource persons (with emphasis on skills involved in the activity) and as facilitators of group process. The team approach to the use of the Activity Therapist is illustrated in the listing of meetings to which he is committed, as well as in the following statement:

Since his function is that of a professional within the Department of Psychiatry, it is necessary for the Activity Therapist to have a working double professional vocabulary; one relating to activities, and one involving psychodynamics, psychopathology, and psychopharmacology. The foregoing knowledge is essential when writing in nursing report books on the individual units, and in filling out evaluation sheets on patients in . . . ninth-floor activity groups, and in verbally sharing information on patients with the medical staff. . . .[32]

---

[32]*Ibid.*

Each form of activity is seen as providing a particular kind of challenge and a special opportunity to observe and evaluate patient skill and response. In general, the emphasis is on open-ended, creative kinds of activities or projects and on experiences that are rooted in feeling and fluid group relationships and that provide opportunities for self-discovery. Various forms are used in evaluating patient performance and in making recommendations for activity. An example of such a form used in the Mt. Sinai psychiatric treatment program is shown in Figure 6–2.

Inventories, forms or rating scales are used as part of the evaluation and counseling process in activity therapy at Mt. Sinai. For example, this department has patients fill out (if they are not able to do so independently, they are assisted) a comprehensive background profile. Excerpts from this form are shown in Figure 6–3.

A final example of program development taken from the Mt. Sinai program is a sample schedule for a period of several weeks in February and March 1972, listing activities and the times they are offered, the location and the criteria for admission

I. Identification: Name _____ Address _____
   Age _____ Family Members _____
II. Education (includes dates, diplomas or degrees, type of program, courses most enjoyed and most disliked, etc.)
III. Avocational experiences:
   Hobbies: What activities or hobbies do you enjoy doing during your leisure time? Please list. How did you become interested in each?

   Check your special skills, talents or outstanding abilities and state whether skillful or average in each case:

   Singing _____   Woodworking _____
   Debating _____   Painting _____
   Dancing _____   Sports
   Photography _____   Teams: Baseball _____
   Sewing _____   Volleyball _____
   Arts and crafts _____   Individual: Tennis _____
   Playing instrument _____   Skiing _____
   Needlework _____   Swimming _____

IV. Family occupational inventory: (includes questions about age, educational background, major area of work or occupation, interests and hobbies of father, mother, sisters, brothers, spouses or other close relatives)
   (The profile also asks specific questions regarding:)
   Hobbies, work or other activities as part of early background of patient or shared with family.
   Total vocational experience record. Attitudes toward various jobs, qualities of employer, special vocational skills and work experience.
   Personal ambitions and self-perceived abilities, strong points, weaknesses and interpersonal relationships.

Figure 6–3. Educational, vocational and interest profile.

			Monday

TIME	GROUP	ROOM	CRITERIA FOR ADMISSION TO GROUP
Morning			
10:15–11:15 A.M.	Painting group	Room 3 OT area	By referral only
10:15–11:15 A.M.	Sewing workshop	Room 1 OT area	By referral only
Afternoon			
1:30–2:00 P.M.	Body awareness		
2:00–3:30 P.M.	Current events	Music room gym area	Voluntary
	Discussion group		
2:00–4:00 P.M.	Clay workshop	Room 4 OT area	By referral only
2:30–3:30 P.M.	Gym for pediatrics	Gym	Pediatrics only
5:00–6:00 P.M.	Planning for leisure time	Room 2 OT area	By referral only
Evening			
7:00–8:00 P.M.	Gym for child psychiatry	Gym	Child psychiatry only

			Tuesday

TIME	GROUP	ROOM	CRITERIA FOR ADMISSION TO GROUP
Morning			
10:15–11:30 A.M.	Crafts workshop	Room 3 OT area	By referral only
10:15–11:30 A.M.	Food a la carte		By referral only
10:15–11:30 A.M.	Production lines	Room 4 OT area	Two separate groups—tie dye workshop and candlemaking workshop. By referral only
Afternoon			
2:00–3:30 P.M.	Painting group	Room 3 OT area	By referral only
Evening			
6:00–7:00 P.M.	Gym-free time	Gym	Voluntary
7:00–8:00 P.M.	Gym for child psychiatry	Gym	Child psychiatry only
8:00–9:00 P.M.	Gym—volleyball, basketball, table tennis	Gym	Voluntary

Figure 6–4.   Department of Psychiatry, Mt. Sinai Hospital, Therapeutic Activities Division: February–March activity schedule. (Figure continued on opposite page.)

to the group. The schedule is prepared for the entire week; however, only a portion of it is presented here (Fig. 6–4).

RECREATION SERVICE IN HEALTH-CARE AGENCIES

Mt. Sinai also provides an excellent example of recreation provided as a general service to the total population of a large health-care agency, much as many large industries offer recreation programs as a personnel service to their employees and

Wednesday			
TIME	GROUP	ROOM	CRITERIA FOR ADMISSION TO GROUP
Morning			
10:00–10:45 A.M.	Social dance instruction	Gym	By referral only
10:15–11:30 A.M.	Crafts workshop	Room 3 OT area	By referral only
10:15–11:15 A.M.	Food nutrition group	Room 5 OT area	By referral only
10:15–11:30 A.M.	Production lines	Room 4 OT area	By referral only
Afternoon			
2:00–4:00 P.M.	Sewing workshop	Room 1 OT area	By referral only
2:30–3:30 P.M.	Gym for pediatrics	Gym	Pediatrics only
Evening			
5:30–6:00 P.M.	Coed body movement and exercise group	Gym	Voluntary
6:00–7:00 P.M.	Volleyball instruction	Gym	Voluntary
7:00–8:00 P.M.	Men's physical fitness group	Gym	By referral only
8:00–9:00 P.M.	Gym—volleyball, basketball, table tennis	Gym	Voluntary

Figure 6–4. Continued

their families. This medical center has some 7000 staff members, including 1000 medical students from many lands, a medical faculty of about 1200 and 800 residents and interns. It also has many recreational facilities, including gymnasiums, auditoriums, meeting rooms and various other recreational opportunities in New York City.

The recreational program is intended to improve communication and relationships among students, volunteers, employees and management of the Mt. Sinai Medical Center and to assist in maintaining the physical and mental health of employees and students. It has a number of unique emphases, including an extensive ticket program, through which 40,000 tickets to cultural, sports and other events are distributed each year to participants in the program. In addition, consumer information and discount buying opportunities are part of the plan. Recreation activities are largely directed by volunteers and include a symphony orchestra, bowling, basketball and softball teams and numerous hobby and other leisure skills classes, along with special events and trips.

Although not an example of therapeutic recreation as such, the program does provide leisure counseling and presents recreation as an important component of an overall "wellness" approach within the large medical center complex. The center's management is convinced that recreation improves the morale of participants, increases productivity, reduces absenteeism and contributes to an overall preventive medicine approach.[33]

---

[33]Inez Greenstadt: "Medical Center Activities Program." In *Handbook of Health Care Human Resources Management*. Rockville, Maryland, Aspen Systems Corporation, 1981.

Friends Hospital, Philadelphia, Pennsylvania

Another leading psychiatric hospital in the eastern United States with a long tradition of using recreation and related activity therapies as part of its treatment program is Friends Hospital in Philadelphia. At this institution, four different but related disciplines—Creative Arts Therapy, Horticulture Therapy, Occupational Therapy and Recreation Therapy—are administered through a Department of Adjunctive Therapies. While the four disciplines use different materials and techniques, they all have the same objective: helping the patient regain health and successful return to family and community.

Programs are developed to meet the physical, cultural, social, recreational and rehabilitation needs of patients. Each patient is evaluated and placed in a treatment program consisting of a combination of therapies designed specifically to meet his or her needs. Treatment programs are reviewed and revised according to the changing needs of the patient population. The essential purpose is to move patients along a continuum from directed or prescribed activity to truly voluntary recreation. Prescribed activity is mandatory because the capacity for making sound choices may not be possible for some patients who are brain-damaged, disabled or ill to the degree that cognitive functioning and/or social skills are seriously impaired.

The Friends Hospital Recreation Program has three important elements, which provide the basis for patient involvement, scheduling, staff assignments and other managerial functions. Directed by Ann C. Durante, it includes:

Recreation therapy groups—consisting of mandatory involvement directed toward specific treatment goals (to assess functional ability, promote interaction and socialization and increase patients' energy level)

Leisure awareness activities—consisting of leisure counseling and leisure education, designed to promote favorable leisure attitudes and skills and resource utilization

Leisure-time program—based on fully voluntary participation designed to promote self-actualization, self-expression and enjoyment.

PATIENT ASSESSMENT

All patients undergo an adjunctive therapies evaluation before being scheduled for a treatment program. The purpose is to evaluate the patient's level of functioning in a number of different areas so that an appropriate treatment program can be established. The assessment includes two essential parts: (a) an evaluative task is used to assess cognitive functioning, observe behavior and gather other diagnostic information; and (b) an interview is conducted for additional information. Specific areas of performance, history, behavior and mental status are recorded in this adjunctive therapies evaluation process.

Based on the evaluation, a treatment plan is developed that notes the patient's strengths and problems and outlines an initial treatment using activities provided by the adjunctive therapies department. The program itself includes a number of group and individual activities designed to meet the specialized needs of patients, including the following:

Initiatives.   An "initiative" is some physical task with a certain amount of psychological risk. A small group of patients pool their resources to cope with the challenge it presents. Its purposes include the facilitation of peer relationships, independence and autonomous decision-making and the improvement of concentration span, self-image and self-confidence.

Physical Conditioning.   This is an "open hall," co-ed activity which provides social interaction along with independent and group physical exercises designed to meet the needs of individual patients of varying ages. Its goal is to promote awareness of the importance of exercise, diet and conditioning in relation to physical, social and emotional integration.

Recreation Therapy.   Patients scheduled into the recreation therapy group must be able to follow multi-step verbal directions, cooperate with other patients and tolerate competition. The activities encourage spontaneous interpersonal interaction, promote fun and relaxation, and contribute to the patient's skills and awareness of leisure activities that may be utilized upon discharge.

Each program area or specialized service has defined criteria for patients assigned to it, as well as clearly outlined goals and methods (see Fig. 6–5, as an example).

At the evening leisure-time program, patients may choose whether to participate in activities which contribute generally to the therapeutic objectives of the Adjunctive Therapies Department. The activities differ each evening of the week and include physical games, slimnastics, arts and crafts, New Games, informal sports lessons, bingo, cake bakes and other hobby activities. Another special program initiated by the department in the early 1980's is a therapeutic work program, designed to provide a supportive environment in which work is used as a therapeutic tool.

Therapeutic Work Program.   This program serves patients whose self-esteem is directly related to their ability to work and feel productive. The work program includes patients who lack confidence in their functional capacities, need to identify work-related problems more clearly or have difficulty holding jobs. Patients in the individualized therapeutic work program work one hour a day, five days a week, in the dietary, grounds and maintenance, purchasing, business, community relations and adjunctive therapies departments of the hospital, as well as in the gift shop. Singer writes,

They perform tasks such as delivering mail, filling purchase requisitions, cleaning dining room tables after meals, assisting in greenhouse maintenance, and typing. . . . Each job is analyzed to assess the demands of the placement. Patients' interests, skills, and individual goals are primary in setting up each program . . . Both the supervisor and the patient complete an evaluation weekly and daily, respectively.[34]

---

[34]Susan B. Singer: "A Therapeutic Work Program in a Short-Term Hospital." *Hospital and Community Psychiatry,* September 1981, p. 637.

CRITERIA

1. Patient should be a drug or alcohol abuser.
2. Patient should be able to tolerate an interactional group situation.
3. Patient should be able to follow multi-step directions.
4. Includes patients of any age.

METHODS

—Discussion of problem areas as related to drug and alcohol abuse and social self-confidence.
—Interaction games.
—Leisure and discharge planning.
—Questionaires and handouts.
—Relaxation exercises.

GOALS

—Explore present lifestyle and alternatives to substance-abuse related to coping and leisure.
—Develop repertoire of constructive activities to help decrease addictive behavior and promote more healthy use of leisure.
—Develop a social support system for sobriety by creating awareness of appropriate available leisure resources.
—Build confidence in interaction skills, increase socialization and validate abilities in a substance free environment.
—Provide relaxation experiences for release of tension and anxiety.
—Help increase self-esteem.
—Increase awareness of self-image and begin to develop a more positive image of self and social self-confidence.
—Provide trust building experiences to explore trust patterns and relationships.
—Assist patient in exploring more healthy leisure pursuits in relation to discharge planning.

Figure 6–5. Recreation therapy for substance abusers.

Within the overall adjunctive therapies program, individual therapists work under the close supervision of a qualified psychologist. Counseling and training sessions sharpen their psychological understanding and perceptions; they sometimes become group therapists. At Friends Hospital, recreation therapy is respected as a valid type of treatment. At one time, the voluntary leisure-time program was not given a full measure of support, primarily because it was regarded by some in the hospital's administration as merely "fun and games," not as a significant part of the patient's rehabilitation. Today, there is full acceptance of its therapeutic value, and it plays an important part in the adjunctive therapies effort.

Saskatchewan Hospital, Weyburn, Saskatchewan, Canada

For a period of years, this hospital was one of the major institutions for psychiatric care in western Canada, with a patient count in the late 1950's of well over

1500. As part of the shift to smaller, community-based institutions and more flexible treatment services, the patient load was reduced to 350, chiefly extended-care (long-term, chronic) patients. The following section describes the recreation program of the hospital *prior* to its shift in focus. It is deliberately included here to show how large, traditionally conceived mental hospitals operated in the past and, in a limited number of cases, continue to do so today. A number of the elements in its program, such as the "voucher" system (token economy), evaluation of patients' interests and participation, and role of the patient council, illustrate principles presented earlier in this and preceding chapters.

Compared with a municipal institution like Mt. Sinai, the Saskatchewan hospital had extensive facilities which made possible an extremely varied program. These areas and buildings included a curling and skating rink, poolroom, shuffleboard areas, music rooms, hobby rooms, game rooms, sports field, auditorium, gymnasium, picnic areas, miniature golf course, lawn bowling courts, croquet courts, horseshoe pits, library and other specialized facilities. In addition, the recreation department used buses and rented camps to provide vacations for both in- and outpatients.

The recreation department emphasized three major goals: (a) retraining in social and recreational skills; (b) fostering independence; and (c) exposing the patient to the community. It structured its operation so that it was similar to the normal model of citizens living in the community. During the hours of 9 to 5, patients engaged in occupational therapy or in work assignments, either in a sheltered workshop manufacturing wood products or in hospital departments such as the laundry, gardens or plumbing shop. Recreation was provided after 5 P.M. or, by prescription with special patients, between 9 A.M. and 5 P.M.

PROGRAM ORGANIZATION

This was carried out in the following ways:

1. By assigning several facilities and activities to each patient unit of the hospital.
2. Through the general function or core program, which was scheduled five nights a week for those patients who were able to attend them independently.
3. Providing equipment and activities for unit-building living rooms (day rooms) to serve patients who were too sick to leave this area.
4. Services for outpatients. The recreation staff of the hospital was also active in planning and setting up programs for youth, the physically disabled or elderly people in the adjacent community, by providing consultation, offering workshops and helping to establish youth coffeehouses and sports programs, nursing home activities and other events.

EVALUATION OF PATIENTS

Both in the assignment of patients to activities and in the evaluation of their continuing participation and progress, a five-point rating scale was used by staff. The patients were rated with respect to their attendance and participation in recreation and social activities on the following scale:

5. Attends willingly and participates in activity as it would be expected of someone in a similar situation in the community. _____
4. Attends willingly but is mostly a passive observer. _____
3. Will attend, but only after protesting about it. _____
2. Usually refuses to attend. _____
1. Considered too ill to attend. _____

Patients were rated each week on these points, and their status was charted on a graph that extended over several weeks or months, thus providing a longitudinal view of their progress as seen by recreation therapists and nurses.

In addition, two other devices were used to ascertain patient needs and interests and to evaluate systematically their participation in recreation activities. The first was a Recreation Interest Questionnaire (Fig. 6-6), and the second was an Evaluation Form for Patient Participation and Interaction (Fig. 6-7).

The second form was used to measure patient involvement in three types of activities: group activities, spontaneous or individual activities and "voucher activities." This refers to activities the patient attended, for which he or she paid with vouchers received as a reward for work. The entire hospital operated with a system of such vouchers or "chits" through which the patients purchased merchandise, candy, clothing and similar articles or gained admission to special events at the hospital. The purpose of this device was to encourage appropriate spending. Patients were expected to spend a certain minimum amount each month in recreation activities as evidence of social involvement.

PROGRAM ACTIVITIES

This included a substantial number of activities, both inside and outside the hospital. In a recent year-end report, the following were listed (partial listing):

Social Activities

Coffee groups in city
Dances
White Cross socials
Seasonal parties
Whist tournaments
Scavenger hunts
Darts tournaments
Barbecues
Wiener roasts
Music listening
Bingo in hospital and city
Checker tournaments
Pool and pool tournaments
Picnics
Ping-Pong tournaments

Education and Cultural Activities

Films
Art contests

Magazine subscriptions
Weekly newspaper
Library services
Craft sessions
Musical sessions
Talent shows
Cooking contests

Physical Activities

Archery
Curling
Broomball
Shuffleboard
Miniature golf
Fishing
Ice fishing
Bowling in city
Gymnasium activities
Lawn bowling
Horseshoes
Croquet

Date:

Name _____ Age _____ Occupation _____

Home Address _____ Town _____ Rural _____

In your community,

do you have: *did you ever:*   *would you like to learn:*

_____ a rink   _____ curl

_____ a bowling alley   _____ bowl

_____ a theater   _____ attend shows,

_____ a pool hall   _____ dances, bingo

_____ a swimming pool   _____ play pool

_____ a golf course   _____ swim

_____ a community hall   _____ golf

Do you belong to any clubs such as:

_____ a homemakers club   did you ever_____ would you like to_____

_____ a square dance club

_____ a Legion society   Do you have any hobbies?

_____ a church organization   What games or instruments have you enjoyed playing?

_____ a craft club (What?)

What types of activities would you enjoy (Yes, No, Don't know):

Quiet Games   *Active Games*   *Social Activities*

_____ playing cards   _____ volleyball   _____ community singing

_____   _____ darts   _____ tours

_____   _____ shuffleboard   _____ picnics

_____   _____ croquet   _____ parties

_____ table games   _____ horseshoes   _____

_____   _____ ring toss   _____

_____   _____   _____

_____   _____

Entertainment   *Hobbies and Clubs*

_____ bands   _____ drawing and painting

_____ plays   _____ leathercraft

_____ slides   _____ wood carving

_____ variety shows   _____ rug making

_____ television   _____ needlework

_____ sports events   _____ gardening

_____ speakers   _____ cooking and baking

_____ discussion groups   _____ reading

When you return to your home would you like help from anyone to join in any activities or clubs there may be in your town?_____

Comments:

Figure 6-6.   Recreation interest questionnaire.

NAME	ATTENDANCE			PARTICIPATION AND INTEREST					VERBAL INTERACTION DURING ACTIVITY				WARD___
Date	Refuses	With Persua-sion	Will-ingly	Does Not Partici-pate	Spec-tator (Shows Inter-est)	Partici-pates with Persua-sion	Partici-pates Freely	Assists in Starting Activity	Assists Others	None	Some When Spoken to	Some Sponta-neous Inter-action	Inter-acts Freely	Comments
Group Act. (1) Spont. Act. (2) Voucher Act. (3) Activity													

Figure 6-7. Evaluation form for patient interaction and participation.

Volleyball	Curling matches in city
Floor hockey and tournaments	Band performances
Badminton	Caroling
Soccer	Hockey games in city
Tobogganing and sleigh riding	Television sports watching
	Softball in city
Audience Activities	Fair in city
	Karate performances
Weekly movies (popular)	Tours of city sites of interest
Weekly educational films	

Many hospital patients also were taken on one-week vacations, based on satisfactory performance in the industrial therapy (work) program, satisfactory social behavior and payment of vouchers at an approved level. In addition, a selected group of outpatients were taken on trips to scenic sites, parks, picnic areas and spectator events in various parts of southeastern Saskatchewan.

PATIENT COUNCIL

A final interesting aspect of the Saskatchewan Hospital was its patient council, which functioned in the following ways: (a) as a patient union to deal with patient employment problems in the industrial therapy program; (b) to help plan and critically evaluate the recreational services in the hospital; and (c) to deal with patient complaints regarding individual treatment programs or general ward affairs.

The officers of the patient council were elected from the general patient population every three months, or whenever a presiding officer was discharged or regarded as too ill to hold office. General meetings were held weekly and dealt with a variety of problems; reports were also heard from various patient committees set up to deal with aspects of hospital life. Once a month, 25 patient representatives of all the units in the hospital met with the recreation staff to discuss and critically evaluate recreation activities. Their suggestions were implemented, unless they were regarded as detrimental to hospital or treatment goals. Reports were made regularly to the general meeting of the patient council.

As mentioned earlier, the Saskatchewan Hospital has been converted from an institution serving the general mentally ill population to a "level four" facility, designed to serve older patients (chiefly in the 45- to 70-year age range). As described in the official guidelines,

---

This level of care is for persons of all ages who do not require acute hospital care and treatment but do require regular and continuous medical attention, highly skilled technical nursing provided under appropriate supervision on a 24-hour basis, and, in addition, special techniques for the improvement or maintenance of function. Patients at this level require initial and continuing medical assessment involving investigation and diagnosis for which appropriate facilities must be readily available. The aims of treatment are to control the disease process, to achieve maximum recovery of function, to prevent further disability, to retard deterioration, and to alleviate pain and distress.[35]

---

[35]*Annual Report.* Saskatchewan Hospital, Weyburn, Saskatchewan, Canada, 1971.

Realistically, these patients are regarded as poor-prognosis, long-term care patients, who have little or no prospect for recovery and will probably spend the remainder of their days within the facility. It is believed that when such patients are permitted to become completely passive, they deteriorate sharply, both physically and mentally. However, "where there is a therapeutic environment in which there is motivation and stimulation for patients to be as independent as possible, even those with poor prognoses may improve."

Obviously, as some large institutions (like the Saskatchewan Hospital) have been transformed into smaller settings for chronic-care patients, others have been created or strengthened to provide more active treatment programs and strong community linkages for patients who are regarded as candidates for quick recovery and discharge.

Penetanguishene Mental Health Centre

An excellent example of such a facility is the Mental Health Centre at Penetanguishene, Ontario, Canada, operated by the Province of Ontario. This institution places special emphasis on a strong program of leisure counseling (see p. 146). The rationale for this program is described by James Montagnes, formerly Director of Vocational, Recreational and Volunteer Services in the Penetanguishene Mental Health Centre.

Since the beginning of our department in 1968 we have been moving toward developing a Recreational Service which offers both a treatment modality and rehabilitative avenue for a patient's avocational time upon discharge. It has been our experience . . . that regardless of the abilities an ex-patient has upon discharge, it is generally the hours during which he is not working when difficulties arise and he is no longer able to cope. In order to overcome this problem we have developed a number of programs . . . which assist us in overcoming these difficulties. Not only do we provide for the avocational needs of the patients while they are in the Centre, but actively utilize both institutional and community facilities to reintegrate and rehabilitate the patients to community leisure activities.[36]

There are two units within the facility: a Regional Hospital with 258 beds to serve residents of three contiguous counties or districts, and a 292-bed maximum security psychiatric hospital that serves the entire Province of Ontario. There is a recreation staff of 16 full-time workers, all with extensive experience or professional training in the field, as well as additional summer staff leaders. It should be noted that, in many institutions, recreation staff members feel they are not sufficiently valued or supported by administrative or medical directors; in others, they are an important element in the treatment team. Recreation staff members at Penetanguishene clearly belong in the second category. Montagnes writes,

---

[36]Letter to author from James M. Montagnes, Director of Vocational, Recreational and Volunteer Services, Penetanguishene Mental Health Centre, January 16, 1974.

Our services are well recognized by the Senior Management of the Centre and I believe this is what makes us somewhat unique within the Province of Ontario, if not the country of Canada. I know of no other institution . . . where acceptance by the total professional group within the Centre is such that referrals are made consistently and recommendations followed very closely by the Clinical Teams in their dealings with our recreational professionals. . . . We have a well-established assessment and counseling program which not only provides service to the inpatients of our institutions, but is also available upon request to local community facilities. In order to do this, we have used the expertise of many professionals in psychology, social work, and vocational services, as well as recreationists. At the Senior Management level we are regarded as a senior department within the Centre and therefore have our equal say in matters pertaining to the total institution and its philosophy.[37]

In this, as in other psychiatric treatment centers in which therapeutic recreation service has achieved a significant and respected place as a treatment modality, the key factors seem to be the following: (a) having a solid philosophical base; (b) developing an intelligent, well-organized and professionally staffed service; (c) being able to develop effective cooperative relationships with members of other rehabilitative disciplines in the institution; and (d) using varied communication media to influence and inform team members, the overall institutional staff, provincial officials and the public and community groups. The value of effective communication in defining a service's goals and describing its programs cannot be overestimated.

COMMUNITY SERVICES: AN APPRAISAL

This chapter describes the trend in the late 1960's and 1970's of using community-based programs to serve the mentally ill who are capable of a reasonable level of independent living, while keeping only the most severely ill patients in custodial settings. The question must be asked—how effective are the services that are provided for the mentally ill in community life?

First, it should be made clear that many of the sweeping reforms and innovations proposed during the 1960's were either naive or uncritical in their assumptions. For example, the "open door" policy, under which many large state institutions unlocked all or almost all gates inside and outside their buildings, turned out in some cases to be a disaster. Patients with various degrees of illness roamed through buildings, in some cases committing violent acts or stealing; others fled from hospitals, frequently creating problems in nearby communities or neighborhoods. In many hospitals that initiated "open door" policies at that time, the practice has now been largely curtailed.

It also became apparent that the assumption that patients could, after discharge, readily assume or reassume roles of responsibility at work or within their own families was often based on tenuous ground. It was increasingly evident that many psychiatric patients were not simply people who had undergone a mental breakdown and who, after treatment, were "cured" and ready to assume a normal life.

---

[37]*Ibid.*

Instead, it was recognized that many such individuals are not really psychotic as such but rather simply disorganized, weak and unable to cope with the demands of community living, particularly in neighborhoods that are dangerous and exploitative. In a study of recidivist patients, investigators of the New York State Department of Mental Hygiene found that many patients return chiefly because they are familiar with the hospital and feel comfortable there.

Such patients, report Rosenblatt and Mayer, are not primarily seeking psychiatric treatment. Instead,

---

These patients are weary sojourners in a hostile world. They want a place to rest. For example, one patient began sleeping under a bridge because his family refused to shelter him any longer. He gave this account of his return to the hospital:

"I returned because I had no place to sleep. I had nowhere to stay. And I was hungry and wanted something to eat. I tried to sleep in the emergency room (but this didn't work). I thought to myself that if I go to the hospital I will eat."[38]

Another patient, who was receiving welfare benefits, could not find a safe place to live; he was in an old building about to be torn down, and he feared drug addicts in the new place he would be sent. With his life in danger, he returned to the hospital. Another patient, separated from her husband and worn by the hassle of raising children alone, said, "I needed a rest period in the hospital. Maybe I would have done better on a vacation, but, then, I couldn't afford one. . . ." Still other patients return in part because they have pleasant memories of the social life and recreational program in the hospital. One returned individual explained, "I went swimming and picnicking. We went on trips to the movies and to the zoo. . . . I felt that it was good being in the hospital." Another said, "I liked the hospital. I enjoyed it very much. I used to go to the game room and play a lot of pool. And there were parties. I really enjoyed myself when I was there." Still another stressed the social life and friendships found in the hospital: "It's beautiful the way we get along together. We eat together. We sit down. We have conversations. We express ourselves—no arguments. I think it's wonderful how a group of people on the ward can get together and live together from day to day and there's no confusion."

The message from this study is clear. In part, it is that hospitals cannot afford to let themselves simply become safe refuges for society's weaker members—providing food, shelter and an enjoyable, problem-free recreational life. The goal of discharging patients into the community cannot be realized unless the community is prepared to accept them and unless adequate housing, therapy, medication and other supportive services, including vocational and activity therapy, are provided. The after-care centers and social clubs described earlier in this chapter are all too few. At a 1976 conference of mental health authorities in Washington, it was pointed out that because of sharp federal cutbacks only a fraction of the mental

---

[38]Aaron Rosenblatt and John E. Mayer: "Patients Who Return: A Consideration of Some Neglected Influences." *Journal of Bronx, New York, State Hospital,* Spring 1974, pp. 73–74.

health centers that had originally been scheduled for construction were actually built.

Residential plans for outpatients, which were intended to include such varied accommodations as dormitory housing with "live-in" therapists, supervised apartment units and unsupervised apartment units, also were greatly limited in their development. Consequently, many discharged mental patients have been "warehoused" in single-room occupancy units or in welfare hotels that provide only the bare necessities of living—a shameful exploitation of this population. Often discharged patients live in dangerous slums where they are preyed on by the criminals around them.

In the late 1970's, *Newsweek* commented that the bright hope for a new era in mental health had dimmed. While it was true that many state hospital wards had been emptied,

> . . . vast numbers of their former inmates are worse off than they were before. Because of poor planning at all levels of government, lack of funds and the hostility of the healthy members of communities, ex-patients wander desolately in inner-city ghettos and live in squalid single rooms or nursing homes that are ill-prepared to render the care they need. For some of them, "deinstitutionalization" has been tragic.[39]

Although the number of patients in state hospitals dropped sharply, resulting in a considerable financial savings, this was offset by the disturbing fact that about half the patients were readmitted to state hospitals at least temporarily, within a year after their release. Some mental health authorities have described the system as a "revolving door," with little coordination among the agencies responsible for community services. When efforts have been made to place discharged patients in group homes in neighborhoods where cheap housing or substandard hotels are available, there is often sharp resistance from community residents. In examining the reduced use of mental hospitals in Massachusetts, Scholberg, Becker and McGrath found that

> Abstract expression of support for the policy of deinstitutionalization rapidly evaporates when citizens become aware of plans to establish halfway houses or family type residences in their midst; formidable opposition coalesces overnight when a specific site is suggested. Fears of physical or sexual assault are invariably expressed, along with anxiety about bizarre behavior in the neighborhood, a lowering of property values, noisy disruptures, destruction of property, panhandling, prostitution, and so forth. . . . Public outcries have mounted against the dumping of helpless persons and (one town) has even passed a constitutionally questionable ordinance (later overturned in Federal court) barring former patients from residing there.[40]

---

[39]Matt Clark: "The New Snake Pits." *Newsweek*, May 15, 1978, p. 93.
[40]Herbert C. Scholberg, Alvin Becker and Mark McGrath: "Planning the Phasedown of Mental Hospitals." *Community Mental Health Journal*, Spring 1976, pp. 9–10.

In some communities, such as Long Beach, New York, large seaside hotels that once catered to summer vacationers now provide housing for many discharged psychiatric patients from the chronic wards of state mental hospitals. Anderson, writing about such hotels as "the new snake pits," describes the attitudes of the owners of such hotels:

This neglect arises from the fact that the facilities to which most former patients are transferred are privately operated and, for the most part, subject to few legal controls in terms of accountability. For most owners, each new resident merely represents a potential profit. The less that is spent on him in the way of food, therapy, recreation, medical and psychiatric care, the greater the profit will be.[41]

The original plan for remodeling state or provincial mental health services throughout the United States and Canada was based largely on the assumption that huge mental institutions had outlived their usefulness and that for those who might require long-range or lifetime care, smaller, more specialized facilities were needed. For most mental patients, it was thought that rehabilitation would best be effected by placing them back in the community, in small, well-staffed intermediate facilities, such as halfway houses, sheltered workshops and evening hospitals. With the lack of such facilities, however, and with a disagreement between state and local agencies as to the responsibility for such populations, many patients are left in limbo, in exploitative or inadequate facilities as described above, and with almost no meaningful rehabilitation.

A recent study of mental health services in a major American city (Philadelphia) found that thousands of mentally ill individuals were left to fend for themselves—often as "bag men" or "women," sleeping on the streets or above manhole covers for warmth, through the dead of winter. Other thousands moved through the revolving door of state and municipal hospitals, often rebuffed as patients because they were too seriously disturbed. Many such individuals were able to find shelter and emergency care only in the city's prisons.[42]

The need is clear. If the community mental health concept is to be made workable, it will have to be supported with a large-scale development of effective neighborhood or community centers. These, in turn, will have to provide badly needed rehabilitative services, including not only medication, which helps mental patients live in the community at a reasonable level of functioning, but also educational, counseling, vocational and recreational service.

Within this spectrum of needed services and programs, therapeutic recreation specialists employed by a variety of institutional and community agencies must play an increasingly important role. It is a harsh fact that while many hospitals have provided excellent recreation service to psychiatric patients, it is far rarer to find

---

[41]George M. Anderson: "Ex-Mental Patients and the New Snake Pits." *America*, September 4, 1976, p. 90.

[42]Donald C. Drake: "The Forsaken." Seven-part series in *The Philadelphia Inquirer*, July 18–24, 1982.

effective leisure programming in community mental health centers. Clearly, planning these community programs is an important priority for the profession in the years ahead.

Suggested Topics for Class Discussion, Examination Questions or Student Papers

1. What are the special values and appropriate methods of therapeutic recreation service as presented in programs operating under the *therapeutic community* or *milieu therapy* approaches?

2. Outline an imaginative and comprehensive recreation program for a modern psychiatric hospital or community-based mental health center, showing how the treatment needs of different groups of patients or clients are met.

3. The development of new drug therapies has been a key factor in making many psychiatric patients more manageable and in permitting their deinstitutionalization. What are some of the negative aspects of such drug treatment approaches?

4. Appraise the positive and negative aspects of the break-up of large custodial institutions and the establishment of community-based residential and health care programs, in terms of the range of therapies being offered and the specific implications for recreation service.

7

Recreation for the Mentally Retarded and Learning-Disabled

This chapter provides an understanding of the scope, causes and effects of mental retardation and of recreation's role in institutional or community programs designed to meet the needs of the mentally retarded. Emphasis is placed on the role of recreation in promoting social independence and job capabilities for the mildly or moderately retarded and in minimizing disability and enriching the lives of *all* retarded children, youth and adults.

A section of the chapter deals with the role of recreation in working with the learning-disabled. It should be made clear that the learning-disabled are *not* mentally retarded; indeed, many of them may have a high level of intelligence. However, because this disability often evidences itself in poor academic performance or dysfunctions in communication, it is dealt with in this chapter.

THE NATURE OF MENTAL RETARDATION

Although mental retardation has traditionally been defined as a function of intelligence (with an I.Q. below 75 identifying the retardate), this is an unfortunately narrow view. A more sophisticated definition of the mentally retarded, who encompass a complex population, would be likely to include the following elements:

1. It is generally agreed that mental retardation is a condition that *originates during the developmental period*, i.e., before the age of 18 years.
2. The key concept in many definitions is that of *mental or cognitive subnormality*. This is not the sole criterion of mental retardation, however, and a second significant element must be *social inadequacy*—the inability of the mentally retarded person to function effectively in a social setting.
3. Although there has been a traditional belief that mental retardation must have an *organic cause*, such as a defect in the brain or some other significant pathology of the central nervous system, it has been accepted more recently that *environmental factors* are responsible for a substantial amount of mental retardation.

4. It is believed that mental retardation *cannot be cured* in the sense of a total reversal of the impairment. With appropriate education and supportive services, however, its effects can be markedly reduced; many individuals who are classified as mentally retarded are able to enter community life, hold jobs, raise families and live as responsible citizens.

Recognizing the difficulty of defining the term, the *Manual on Terminology and Classification in Mental Retardation* of the American Association on Mental Deficiency offers the following definition: "Mental Retardation refers to significantly subaverage general intellectual functioning existing concurrently with deficits in adaptive behavior and manifested during the developmental period."[1] In this definition, *significantly subaverage general intellectual functioning* refers to scores that are more than two standard deviations below the mean of either the Stanford-Binet or the Wechsler intelligence test (I.Q. scores of 67 or 69, respectively). *Adaptive behavior* refers to the individual's ability to function independently in the family, neighborhood, school or community. It includes a set of appropriate functional areas at each age level; for example, during infancy and early childhood, adaptive behavior would encompass sensory-motor skills development, communication skills, self-help skills and socialization. If a person has a low I.Q. but is socially adequate, he is not to be regarded as mentally retarded. If a person lacks social competence but has a high I.Q., he is similarly not to be considered mentally retarded. Only when both elements are present is a person considered mentally retarded.

The mentally retarded today are classified on several levels: *mild, moderate, severe* and *profound* (see p. 231). There is a tremendous difference between those at either end of this continuum. For example, the mildly mentally retarded can develop social and communication skills, may be well-coordinated and often are not distinguished from normal children until a later age. School-age retardates may be capable of academic skills up to approximately a sixth-grade level by their late teens. Adult retardates can usually develop social and vocational skills adequate for minimum self-support but may need guidance or assistance when under social or economic stress. In contrast, the profoundly mentally retarded at all ages have much more serious impairments. They have minimal motor and speech capabilities and usually require nursing care.

In describing the lives of mentally retarded individuals, H. Carl Haywood, President of the American Society of Mental Deficiency, points out that by definition they have problems making successful adjustments to the physical and social environments in which they must live, grow, work and carry on the activities of daily life:

Mentally retarded persons have relatively higher social vulnerability than do nonretarded persons. Since social and environmental forces act upon persons, either enhancing or retarding their personal and social development, in relation to the ability of those persons to cope with the demands of environments, retarded persons are acted upon more often by negative environmental forces than are nonretarded persons.[2]

---

[1]See Herbert J. Prehm: *In* Larry L. Neal: *Recreation's Role in the Rehabilitation of the Mentally Retarded.* Eugene, University of Oregon, 1970, pp. 9–11.
[2]H. Carl Haywood: "Reducing Social Vulnerability Is the Challenge of the Eighties." *Journal of Mental Retardation,* August 1981, p. 190.

Haywood goes on to point out that in many ways society compounds the difficulty of the retarded individual by providing limited life opportunities and supportive services or, more destructively, by victimizing mildly and moderately retarded persons who live in the community. Such victimization may include personal, financial and sexual exploitation. Because of their limited ability to understand and deal effectively with such destructive influences, the mentally retarded often have difficulty living independently. Clearly, improving the ability to deal realistically with life and its demands in the community is an important goal of therapeutic recreation service for the mentally retarded.

Numbers and Types of Mentally Retarded

A 1976 report of the President's Committee on Mental Retardation estimated that there were about six million retarded persons in the United States. Past estimates have indicated that half of the retarded are children and youth below the age of 20. Mildly retarded are 89 per cent of the total number, and moderate retardates are about 6 per cent. Only about 5 per cent of the overall number are considered to be severely or profoundly impaired.

The life expectancy of the mildly retarded is about the same as that of normal persons. Although the development of antibiotic drugs that reduce fatal pulmonary illness in the severely and profoundly retarded has resulted in more of these individuals living to adulthood, their life expectancy is still shorter than that of the overall population. Once he or she has lived to the age of 5 or 6 years, the retarded child can be expected to live to adulthood. Following the school years, many mildly retarded individuals gain an adequate level of socially adaptive behavior and a degree of economic independence and are able to blend into community life. Thus, a proportion of persons who were identified as mentally retarded in childhood are no longer classified in this way as adults.

The causes of mental retardation are many. They include the following: (a) genetic or hereditary factors; (b) problems incurred during pregnancy or childbirth; (c) illness, disease or accident; and (d) social or environmental deprivation. Among the hereditary and genetic factors is the chromosomal imbalance that causes Down's syndrome, commonly known as mongolism, which affects one out of 600 children. There are several other metabolic or chemical factors inherited from the mother that can cause retardation; a mixture of incompatible Rh factors may also be responsible. Other illnesses, such as meningitis, or injuries incurred in childhood may lead to mental retardation. Lead poisoning and malnutrition are believed to be frequent causes of retardation among young children in poverty-stricken areas.

There is an increased awareness of the role of the social environment in causing mental retardation. Lack of stimulation and cognitive input from the family means that a much higher proportion of children in extremely poor neighborhoods are classified as mentally deficient than those in middle- and upper-class families. This differentiation becomes increasingly marked during the elementary grades, as does the actual percentage of children classified as mentally retarded.

Categories of Retardation

There are a number of different systems under which the mentally retarded may be classified. Prehm points out that these include (a) the *legal-administrative* system found in the laws of most states and cities that judges which children, youths or adults are eligible for educational, residential or other forms of special social services; (b) the *educational* system, which customarily classifies the retarded into three groups—educable, trainable and custodial (totally dependent); and (c) the *psychiatric* classification system.[3] In the past, the psychiatric system divided mental retardates into categories called *morons, imbeciles* and *idiots.* Today, these demeaning terms are seldom used.

Instead, the most common classification systems are those that relate to educational potential and capability for independent living. Generally, these two factors appear to be highly correlated. In terms of potential for independent living, as a wage-earner, member of a family or resident in community life, adaptive capability is an extremely important factor. The following terms are widely used today to classify the retarded[4]:

Levels	Degree of Impairment	Educational	I.Q. Range	Percentage of Retarded Population
I	Mild	Educable	52–67	89.0
II	Moderate	Trainable	36–51	6.0
III	Severe	Custodial	20–35	3.5
IV	Profound	Totally dependent	Under 20	1.5

Of these groups, it has been estimated that approximately 95 per cent, mostly mild and moderate retardates, live in the community, primarily with their families. The 5 per cent who are classified as severely or profoundly retarded are heavily dependent on others for even the most basic forms of care (most cannot dress or feed themselves or attend to toilet needs without help) and are often institutionalized. A study carried out by the National Association of Superintendents of Public Residential Facilities for the Mentally Retarded reported that in the early 1980's there were 278 such facilities throughout the United States, with a total bed capacity of approximately 156,000. It should be noted that 70 per cent of the residents of these institutions were over 21 years of age. Seventy-seven per cent of residents were severely or profoundly mentally retarded, and about 60 per cent were multiply handicapped, with one or more significant physical impairments.[5] Not included

---

[3]Prehm, *op. cit.*, p. 13.
[4]Adapted from Larry L. Neal: "Recreation for the Mentally Retarded." *Therapeutic Recreation Journal,* First Quarter, 1968, p. 11.
[5]R. C. Scheerenberger: "Public Residential Facilities: Status and Trends." *Journal of Mental Retardation,* April 1981, p. 59.

in this study were a substantial number of residential facilities operated by private, religious or other voluntary agencies.

Hayes points out that it is often extremely difficult to establish distinct categories within this overall population for the following reasons: (a) mental retardation is not a single disease or syndrome but instead is a general state of impairment; (b) individuals with the same medical diagnosis and comparable I.Q. and adaptive behavior levels may still vary widely in specific abilities; (c) mental retardation may be difficult to distinguish from autism, emotional disturbance or learning disabilities; (d) mental retardation may coexist with other forms of mental or physical disability, particularly in more severely impaired individuals; and (e) there is no consistent terminology and classification among different professional groups and in different countries.[6]

Adaptive Characteristics of the Retarded

Heber suggests that each retardate should be evaluated with respect to the following behavioral impairments[7]:

---

1. **Personal-Social Factors**
   a. Impairment in cultural conformity, involving dependable or reliable social behavior, as opposed to behavior which is persistently anti-social or asocial.
   b. Impairment in interpersonal relations, implying inadequate ways for relating to peers and/or authority figures, or for recognizing the needs and feelings of other persons in interpersonal situations.
   c. Impairment in responsiveness and consistent motivation, involving typical inability to resist short-term gratification of needs, and to strive for long-range goals.
2. **Sensory-Motor Skill Impairment**
   a. Motor skills, involving disability in large and fine motor movements.
   b. Speech skills — including such disabilities as stuttering, lisping, or other poor vocalization patterns.
   c. Auditory limitations, in understanding and responding to the speech of others, beyond what might be expected on the basis of measured intelligence.
   d. Visual limitations, involving inadequate response to visual stimulation, beyond what might be expected on the basis of measured intelligence.

In concluding this section, it should be pointed out that the mentally retarded are sometimes referred to today as the "developmentally disabled," particularly in school systems where they are being served in special education classes. In some cases, they may be confused with or served jointly with the learning-disabled. The learning-disabled, however, are a distinctly separate population (see p. 260).

---

[6]Gene A. Hayes: "Recreation and the Mentally Retarded." *In* Thomas A. Stein and H. Douglas Sessoms: *Recreation and Special Populations.* Boston, Holbrook, 1977, pp. 70–72.
[7]See Larry L. Neal: "Recreation for the Mentally Retarded," *op. cit.,* pp. 16–17.

NEEDS OF THE MENTALLY RETARDED

Often, the retarded person is set aside from the rest of society and is heavily dependent on his or her family. It is clear, however, that with intensive training, care and personal attention, a high proportion of retarded persons can develop a reasonable level of adaptation and, in some cases, even academic skills, and can function as useful, contributing citizens.

In the past, the mentally retarded were cruelly treated by society, locked in attics, hidden away from the world, confined in prisons and madhouses or—too often—completely ignored. Even today, many parents view their retarded children with a mixture of apathy and shame. Particularly among families in disadvantaged areas, the signs of retardation are ignored until it is too late to provide remedial services that might have minimized disability. Often, needed educational and community services are not provided.

However, over the past 15 or 20 years, there has been a growing realization of the scope of this problem, as well as the fact that retardation is a disability stemming from identifiable causes and may be minimized and dealt with constructively.

It is now widely understood that the mentally retarded have the same basic needs as all other human beings. They have very strong human needs for love and understanding. They require food, shelter, work (if they are capable of it), and meaningful activity that provides a sense of accomplishment. Although those who do not know the mentally retarded sometimes fear them or believe that they are capable of wild or irrational acts, those who have observed mentally retarded individuals who have been brought up with affection and care have seen that they are usually gentle and friendly, capable of giving and receiving love.

Programs Serving the Retarded

For many years, the only programs serving the retarded were those of custodial institutions—either publicly operated homes and schools for the most severely impaired or private homes or schools. In recent years, a number of public and voluntary organizations have been established to promote needed services for the mentally retarded. These organizations include the following:

1. The National Association for Retarded Children, a private organization involved in a comprehensive program, including research, education, counseling, recreation and promoting public awareness of the needs of the retarded. This body operates both on a national level and through local or regional chapters.
2. The American Association for Mental Deficiency, a voluntary, nonprofit organization involved primarily in research concerning causes and effects of mental retardation.
3. The federal Department of Health and Human Services, which, through a Mental Retardation Branch, promotes research and professional training in special education and other services for the retarded and provides financial assistance to special projects.
4. The Division of Mental Retardation of the Council for Exceptional Children, which promotes research, education and special community services for the retarded.

5. The Kennedy Foundation, a philanthropic organization that operates institutions for the retarded, supports research and demonstration projects and promotes innovation in the field of institutional care and community services.

6. The American Alliance for Health, Physical Education, Recreation and Dance, which has designed tests for the retarded and promoted broad programs of adapted physical education and recreation for this population. With federal funding, it has sponsored a Project on Recreation and Fitness for the Mentally Retarded and published a newsletter, *Challenge*, which presents developments in this field.

In addition to these national organizations, there are many state and municipal groups that have promoted a variety of services and programs, including education, vocational rehabilitation, sheltered workshops, recreation and legislation to serve the needs of the retarded. They have focused on research for the causes and prevention of mental retardation, on the development of new forms of rehabilitation that might succeed in helping retarded persons live independently in the community and on providing programs of public relations that might improve public understanding of this problem.

A major breakthrough came in 1962 when the President's Panel on Mental Retardation, instituted by President John F. Kennedy, recommended a new, comprehensive program to serve the mentally retarded. This program made specific recommendations dealing with research, manpower, treatment, education, vocational preparation, legal protection and the development of federal, state and local programs for the mentally retarded. This was the first large-scale national effort to deal with mental retardation. During the next decade many of the goals that private organizations had been working toward over a period of years were realized.

RECREATION IN THE REHABILITATION OF THE MENTALLY RETARDED

One of the significant outcomes of the President's Panel on Mental Retardation was the recognition of the vital role played by recreation in the lives of the mentally retarded. Many professionals had already recognized that recreation served a variety of useful purposes with the retarded, but the panel was the first influential national organization to affirm this value:

The retarded child, like other children, needs opportunity for healthy, growth-promoting play. The adolescent's vital need for successful social interaction and recreational experience is frequently intensified by isolation resulting from parental overprotection, the numerous failures he experiences in school and occupational pursuits, and by his exclusion by normal groups from everyday play group and social activities. For the retarded adult, opportunity and constructive use of leisure time may prove a major factor in maintaining community adjustment.[8]

---

[8]President's Panel on Mental Retardation: *A Proposed Program for National Action to Combat Mental Retardation*. Washington, D.C., U.S. Government Printing Office, October 1962.

During the 1970's, formal recognition was given to this need through legal authorization of recreation services as part of overall community services for the mentally retarded within federal developmental disabilities legislation. Similarly, the *Standards for Community Agencies Serving Persons with Mental Retardation and Other Developmental Disabilities* manual states that if adequate community recreation is not available for disabled persons, public agencies are required to offer consultation and training to special agencies to develop and implement recreation programs.

The specific values of recreation for retardates lie in four major areas: (a) physical development; (b) social maturity and group adjustment; (c) contribution to vocational adjustment; and (d) constructive use of leisure time.

Physical Development

With the exception of the mildly retarded, many of whom approximate their nondisabled peers in height, weight and motor coordination, the physical appearance, strength, stamina, motor skills and overall physical development of the mentally retarded are often inferior. Frequently they are unable to master even the basic skill of self-care. Since physical development is important not only because it contributes to the health of the individual but also because a person's physical status contributes to a positive self-concept, it is essential that retarded individuals be given a full opportunity to improve their motor skills and enjoy leisure pursuits.

In the past, few mentally retarded children and youth were involved in school-sponsored physical education programs; many were also excluded from sports programs serving youngsters in the community. Because of federal legislation like Public Law 94–142, today there is a much wider effort to provide such experiences for the retarded.

An important goal of recreation should be to provide games, sports, aquatics and conditioning programs that help the mentally retarded reach their full potential of physical development. Many retarded children and youth who do develop skills are able to compete with nonretarded youngsters on an equal basis in team and individual sports. Others are able to live fuller and more satisfying lives at their own levels of development.

Social Development

Many retardates are isolated from the mainstream of community life. Perceived by others as "different" because of their appearance and behavior, they are often excluded from peer groups and find it difficult to establish meaningful social relationships with others. Often they are not motivated to become socially involved and are over-protected by their families. Childish and immature behavior is frequently considered to be an inevitable part of their make-up. Often they are tremendously insecure in groups—partly because of repeated failures and rejection by others. Carefully planned recreational activities, in either segregated or integrated groups (in which they share social contact with the nondisabled), may do much to overcome these limitations.

Vocational Adjustment

Many retardates find it difficult to function well in a regular educational environment. They are often able to function more effectively in special vocational classes that are geared to their capabilities and that equip them to hold either regular jobs or jobs in sheltered workshops. As an example of the success the retarded may achieve at a regular job, the Franklin County Program for the Mentally Retarded in Columbus, Ohio, entered into a joint project with the McDonald's restaurant chain to train and employ a number of mildly and mentally retarded young adults in 15 different restaurants. After working at various jobs for a year, all participants (with minor exceptions) were rated as reliable and capable workers. Their turnover rate was substantially lower than that of nondisabled employees.[9]

However, even when a retarded youth is successful in mastering a job, he or she may fail to function independently and happily in the community. Francis Kelley, formerly Superintendent of the Mansfield, Connecticut, State Training School and Hospital, has stated,

It has been confirmed that many young retarded people have not been able to adjust in the community and have had to be placed in institutions because they have not been able to adjust during leisure, rather than because they failed to perform satisfactorily on the job, or . . . in the home. . . . As we provide for the education, vocational training, occupational and spiritual needs of the retarded, it is equally imperative that we do not overlook (their) recreational rehabilitation and social needs. . . . The presence of this "plus factor" often makes the difference between a happy life in the community or commitment to an institution.[10]

In addition, recent studies have shown that most work maladjustments of educable mentally retarded adolescents stem from poor interpersonal and social skills.[11] Though recreation alone will not overcome this difficulty, it does provide an excellent means for helping the retarded learn to get along with others and to improve their social skills.

[9]Michael Brickey and Ken Campbell: "Fast-Food Employment for Moderately and Mildly Mentally Retarded Adults: The McDonald's Project." *Journal of Mental Retardation,* June 1981, pp. 103–106.

[10]Francis P. Kelley: "Recreational Services for the Retarded—An Urgent Need." *Recreation in Treatment Centers,* September 1964, pp. 12–13.

[11]Gilbert Foss and Susan L. Paterson: "Social-Interpersonal Skills Relevant to Job Tenure for Mentally Retarded Adults." *Journal of Mental Retardation,* June 1981, pp. 103–106.

Constructive Use of Leisure

One of the major problems of the mentally retarded is the use of the leisure time that, for many, constitutes the entire day. For many retardates, the empty hours in their day are characterized by lethargy, frustration and a feeling of uselessness. Too often, they spend their waking hours sitting alone or watching television endlessly. Higher-performing adolescent retardates may become involved in delinquent behavior because of a lack of other stimulation. Carefully planned recreation programs can do much to provide a useful and pleasurable existence for the retarded.

Finally, recreation may greatly promote the *mental development* of retarded children and youth. Recreation may involve creative activities, hobbies, learning experiences, trips and similar experiences that broaden the range of knowledge of participants. Since retardates are so often deprived of the normal range of developmental experiences, it is essential that their lives be enriched in this way.

Even programs of physical activity may do much to improve the mental performance of the mentally retarded. A British researcher, Dr. J. N. Oliver, reported dramatic results from a physical activity program for the retarded. All subjects improved significantly in physical ability, fitness and strength, and 25 per cent showed marked gains in intellectual performance.[12]

Realistically, it is difficult to identify any single type of outcome and to demonstrate that it is the result of a single form of recreational involvement. Most recreation activities involve various kinds of personal growth. Burmeister, for example, describes the multiple values of cultural activities, such as music, drama and dance, with the mentally retarded:

> . . . the cultural arts may be viewed as a therapeutic medium, a multi-faceted, audio-visual, kinesthetic teaching modality, a means of promoting socialization and normalization, and a safety valve for psychological and physiological catharsis. Objectives should be stated for mentally retarded persons participating in cultural arts programs. Broad objectives might include freedom of expression, increased independent functioning, the development of individual skills, and cognizance of the cooperation required of individuals working together as a group.[13]

Substantial evidence has been gathered demonstrating the value of physical activity and other forms of recreation for the mentally retarded. In addition to the Oliver study cited earlier, a number of studies showing the positive effects of play and exercise programs on trainable and educable mentally retarded children were summarized in a publication of The Pennsylvania State University.[14]

---

[12]J. N. Oliver: "The Effect of Physical Conditioning Exercises and Activities on the Mental Characteristics of Educationally Sub-Normal Boys." *British Journal of Educational Psychology*, 28:155–165, 1958.
[13]Julie Gleason Burmeister: "Leisure Services and the Cultural Arts as Therapy for the Mentally Retarded Individual." *Therapeutic Recreation Journal*, Fourth Quarter, 1976, p. 141.
[14]Herberta M. Lundegren, ed.: *Physical Education and Recreation for the Mentally Retarded.* State College, Pennsylvania, Penn State HPER Series No. 7, 1975.

Goals of Recreation Programs for the Retarded

Summed up, then, the goals of recreation programs for the mentally retarded are the following:

1. To improve physical growth and development, enhance motor skills and lend confidence to participants by improving body build and physical fitness.
2. To minimize or prevent social isolation by helping the mentally retarded gain friends and adjust to social situations, minimizing atypical behavior and appearance and teaching social interaction skills.
3. To teach skills for the creative and constructive use of leisure and to provide regular opportunity for hobbies, pastimes and other leisure involvements, either at home, in institutions or in the community.
4. To contribute to the retardate's ability to function independently in the community and to hold down a job, where other ability levels permit this.
5. To improve language skills and develop other cognitive abilities and to broaden the range of knowledge and environmental contacts of the retarded.
6. To provide practice in self-care activities, enhancing the individual's capability for independent living.
7. To improve the morale and quality of family living by helping to make the retardate less of a burden and a more capable and autonomous individual.

PLANNING SERVICES FOR AGE AND FUNCTIONAL LEVELS

Obviously, the kinds of recreational programs that may be provided for the mentally retarded must be geared closely to their capabilities. These, in turn, may be classified on the basis of chronological age, as described here, and in terms of functional performance levels, as described in Chapters 5 and 12.

Planning on the Basis of Chronological Age

There is a temptation, in working with the retarded, to give excessive weight to demonstrated levels of social immaturity or limited mental development and to treat 10- or 12-year-olds as if they were children of primary-grade age. However, as much as possible, it is desirable to carry on activities suitable for each age level, with whatever modifications may be necessary to allow participants to be successful in them.

PRESCHOOL AGE

During this period of early childhood, it is essential that children who have been diagnosed as mentally retarded be given as wide a range as possible of the developmental play experiences that normal children receive. The emphasis should be on providing equipment, settings and structured leadership in games, environmental play, music, dance, drama and other creative experiences, simple arts and crafts, hobbies, group activities, neighborhood trips and similar program elements. The emphasis is on providing activities which will build on the existing capabilities of the child and prevent further disability and which will provide a healthy self-concept.

In a recent review of research on play and the retarded child, Li points out that mentally retarded youngsters differ from most children in that they generally prefer structured rather than imaginative activities, and they engage less in symbolic and social forms of play. Although the play repertoire of retarded children is more restricted than that of nondisabled children, both the amount and the richness of various forms of play can be increased if the retarded are given encouragement and instruction.[15]

ELEMENTARY SCHOOL AGE

This is generally considered a key stage for helping the retarded child realize his or her full potential and for developing a healthy and well-adjusted personality. Play programs should be designed to promote physical vigor and well-being, a range of leisure interests, and satisfying and confidence-giving social adjustment and to make the retarded child as independent as possible. All the activities normally provided for children in this age range may be offered, although many may be modified.

ADOLESCENCE

It is essential that teen-age retardates be helped to adjust to the fact of their disabilities and to gain a realistic picture of their strengths and weaknesses. A considerable amount of emotional and practical support should be given to this age group, whose members face the problem affecting all teen-agers—making the transition from childhood to adulthood—complicated by their unique status in society. Although they require adult guidance, adolescent retardates may lead many of their own recreation and social activities.

EARLY ADULTHOOD

Recreation programs established for young adults in community settings should continue to offer skills instruction and general participation in activities, including remedial help in developing appropriate behavior, appearance and social skills. As much as possible, however, the emphasis should be placed on informational and counseling services, which help young retarded adults develop their

---

[15]Anita K. F. Li: "Play and the Mentally Retarded Child." *Journal of Mental Retardation*, June 1981, p. 121.

own leisure activities and social groups. Not infrequently, a community center will act as host to such a group, with an advisor provided by a local chapter of the voluntary association serving the mentally retarded.

Planning on the Basis of Functional Level

In addition to chronological age, another useful way of developing program services is by assessing the degree of social independence of the children who are to be served. Avedon and Arje outline four descriptive categories that provide a basis for making such determinations. These categories are as follows: *socially independent, semi-independent, semi-dependent* and *dependent.*

For those in the first two classifications, it is essential to provide the kinds of counseling and community involvements which strengthen the retarded individual's capability for living and working in the community, thus preventing social isolation. Semi-dependent children, who generally are not able to hold jobs, even in sheltered workshops, should be given the opportunity for community contacts through trips and other forms of recreation. For dependent children, who are usually in institutions, there should be a strong stress on physical development and self-care programs. Although past practices have been almost completely custodial, it is important to provide intensive treatment services which may improve functioning. In some situations, when even severely retarded children have become involved in intensive programs of physical recreation, they have progressed to the point that they were able to be reassigned to higher-functioning levels.[16]

INSTITUTIONAL RECREATION PROGRAMS

It is curious that, in contrast to many communities in which very limited special programs are provided for the mentally retarded, many state or privately operated residential schools and homes for the mentally retarded offer an impressive range of leisure programs. Examples of such programs follow.

State Training School and Hospital, Southbury, Connecticut

This state-sponsored institution provides excellent recreation facilities, including outdoor ponds and pools, sports fields, a large auditorium, gymnasiums, a bowling alley and play areas or rooms in each of its cottages. Emphasis is given to program activities that improve socialization, teach skills, motivate interest and

---

[16]Elliott M. Avedon and Frances B. Arje: *Socio-Recreative Programming for the Retarded: A Handbook for Sponsoring Groups.* New York, Teachers College, Columbia University, Bureau of Publications, 1964, pp. 15–18.

increase body awareness and balance. Among the major program areas are the following:

Intramural activities, such as checkers, regular and wheelchair bowling (as indicated earlier, many of the most severely retarded individuals have multiple disabilities), pool and kickball.

Special events, such as a Fourth of July parade, Easter egg hunt, amateur night, athletic banquet and soap-box derby race.

Visiting entertainment by outside groups that provide circuses, rock or country and western bands, variety shows, plays and snowmobiling.

Scouting, including Boy Scout, Girl Scout and Sea Scout troops and participation in the New England Scout Jamboree.

Camping and outdoor activities, according to season, including boating, fishing, picnicking, swimming, miniature golf, sledding, skating and tent camping.

Excursions into the community for activities such as plays, movies, athletic events, Connecticut River boat rides, circuses and carnivals.

In addition to four full-time and two part-time recreation workers, many attendants in the cottages are involved in program leadership and bus transportation of residents to community recreation activities. Crafts, sports and hobbies, along with various leagues and tournaments, compose much of the program on the cottage level. Intensive training in small-group recreation skills, along with self-care management, has been presented to small groups of severely retarded adults with the aid of personnel skilled in behavior modification techniques.

It is worth noting that not all institutional programs for the mentally retarded are as diversified as this. Many have tended to be minimal and restricted to higher-functioning residents. Ulrey and Schnell point out that, as a result of federal Public Law 94–103, which required that all residential facilities develop and implement an individual habilitative plan for each client, regardless of age or level of disability, many institutions have sought to upgrade their medical and other habilitative services.

In a number of cases, institutions have developed close relationships with nearby universities. The universities have established innovative training programs for staff, provided consultation or taken direct responsibility for operating entire services, such as medical or physical therapy. Among such university-affiliated programs are Temple University's Developmental Disabilities Center in Philadelphia, the John F. Kennedy Center in Baltimore, the Developmental Disabilities Center at Roosevelt Hospital in New York and the Developmental Evaluation Clinic of Children's Hospital Medical Center in Boston.[17] In a number of cases, the universities have provided assistance to an institution's recreation or activity therapies program.

LEISURE COUNSELING FOR THE RETARDED

It is critical that the mentally retarded be provided with adequate leisure education and counseling sessions to enhance their awareness of the role of recreation

---

[17]Gordon Ulrey and Richard Schnell: "A Program for Developing Professional Services at a Residential Institution." *Journal of Mental Retardation,* August 1981, pp. 163–166.

in their lives and to assist them in making appropriate choices. In many institutions, counseling has become a significant aspect of therapeutic recreation service for the mentally retarded. At the Parsons State Hospital and Training Center in Kansas, for example, Hayes succeeded in having each resident's involvement in recreation made the concern of the institution's vocational evaluation committee. This included such activities as

> . . . weekly individual and group leisure education and counseling sessions, day-long trips to discharge locations which included a variety of experiences pertinent to community leisure living, and cooperative efforts with other staff members in the education, vocational rehabilitation, social work, and nursing services.[18]

Without such preparation, it is all too probable that the discharged individual will be unable to make use of available community recreation resources. Ramm describes the problem of many mentally retarded children who live at home, including the mildly and moderately retarded:

> The retarded child living at home has little recreation opportunity. He may make friends with the children in his special class at school, but unlike the normal children who can play with their school chums in the neighborhood after school hours, retarded children are transported from their homes in different parts of town and have few friends in their own neighborhoods. A similar situation exists with mentally retarded adults who work in a centrally-located sheltered workshop, or who do not work at all. These people are victims of enforced leisure. They have a six-to-eight-hour time block each weekday and more on weekends or holidays during which little or no activity is available to them. Many just sit and watch television.[19]

Recognizing this need, an increasing number of city and county recreation departments provide extensive recreation services for the mentally retarded, often in cooperation with voluntary organizations or parents' clubs concerned with this population.

Too often, retarded persons living in the community have a consistent record of failure; they have few friends, if any, and have been rejected in many areas of life. Even when they enter training centers as young adults, they tend to feel lonely and inadequate, unable to cope with the pressures of the interpersonal experience; they expect further rejection and failure. The purpose of recreation in the community is to help the mentally retarded individual develop interests to improve his or her social relationships and provide a sense of social competence and acceptance. In a study of 24 mentally retarded children and adults taking part in a summer

---

[18]Gene A. Hayes, in Jerry D. Kelley, ed.: *Expanding Horizons in Therapeutic Recreation II.* Champaign-Urbana, University of Illinois Office of Recreation and Park Resources, 1974, pp. 35–37.
[19]Joan Ramm: *Challenge: Recreation and Fitness for the Mentally Retarded.* Washington, D.C., American Association for Health, Physical Education and Recreation, 1966, p. 1.

program provided by the Anaheim, California, Parks and Recreation Department, Seaman found significant improvement in such areas of behavior and in the self-esteem of participants.[20]

Examples of Community-Based Programs

A number of communities throughout the United States and Canada have established comprehensive recreation programs for the retarded. In Washington, D.C., for example, a program was initiated several years ago to develop comprehensive recreation programs for the retarded and to develop guidelines for multi-agency cooperation.

To implement this program, the city was divided into nine areas, each with a center where a variety of activities are provided for the retarded, such as arts and crafts, music, bowling, nature pastimes, golf, trips, self-help classes and aquatics. The program is staffed by members of the city's recreation staff, who have received in-service training at the University of Maryland and who are assisted by volunteers in serving approximately 450 retardates. The program receives the cooperation of community agencies, parents' clubs and departments of the federal government. The program is carefully assessed to determine its effectiveness and has succeeded in arousing a high level of community concern about the needs of the retarded.

Another leading program developed to serve the retarded in the community is the Recreation Center for the Handicapped in San Francisco. This nonprofit corporation has been influential in bringing happiness and companionship to mentally retarded and physically disabled children, youth and adults of many races and creeds in its metropolitan area.

With assistance from both private and public agencies and with appropriations from the city and federal grants, the Recreation Center for the Handicapped operates both integrated and segregated services for the mentally retarded. It also operates a laboratory for training of college students and others in the field of therapeutic recreation. As an example of its work, in a recent year, out of 500 children served, 225 had made sufficient progress to be accepted in city schools for the retarded or in special classes in regular schools. The center also provides educational talks, films and lecture series designed to educate the public about mental retardation.

One of its special projects is Camp Spindrift, which is sponsored by the Kennedy Foundation and other community organizations. Operating in a wooded environment as a day camp, Camp Spindrift stresses living skills and social independence. Many of the campers who had formerly been extremely dependent on their families are now able to camp overnight; others have shown remarkable progress in varied activities and in being able to communicate effectively, take social responsibilities and make friends.

In some cases, camping programs for the retarded have been sponsored by school systems or by state schools or hospitals for the retarded. For example, San

---

[20]Janet A. Seaman: "Effects of Municipal Recreation on the Social Self-Esteem of the Mentally Retarded." *Therapeutic Recreation Journal*, Second Quarter, 1975, pp. 75–78.

Diego, California, has been one of the pioneers in school camping for elementary-age children. For a number of years the city has included a special unit for retarded boys and girls in its program at Camp Cuyamaca. Within an integrated social structure, it was found, many of the anticipated problems did not exist, and retarded youngsters were able to function effectively in the camp.

Camping is of particular importance because it changes the environment of the retarded child radically and puts him in a situation where he is much more dependent on his own efforts. Camp Confidence, a year-round camp for the retarded operated in connection with Brainerd State Hospital in northern Minnesota, stresses the need for young retardates to develop self-confidence, social adjustment and specific skills in camp living, nature and crafts, sports and conservation education. The keynote of the camp is "learning by doing." Endres writes,

If our primary objective . . . is to develop social adjustment within the individual, the camp setting and outdoor education [offer] a natural laboratory. . . . The mentally retarded do not basically learn best by being "told" or "shown" what to do. They must physically experience a given situation to attain comprehension and understanding. Within the aesthetic setting of a camp, they are able to experience things first hand, through outdoor education classes. Such a relaxed atmosphere usually allows for better individual and group counseling. Nature has a way of relieving our tension and anxieties and as such we are better able to live with ourselves, as well as being more considerate of our fellow man.[21]

A fuller description of this and other camping programs for the mentally retarded is provided on pages 254–256. Whatever the setting, it is essential that recreation activities be carefully geared to the needs and capabilities of participants. In selecting activities, it is wise to bear the following principles in mind:

1. The mentally retarded have the same basic needs as other individuals for self-respect and a feeling of accomplishment.
2. Whenever possible, activities chosen should be appropriate for the chronological age of retarded participants.
3. Retardates tend to have a short attention span; activities should therefore be diversified and should have a time limit determined by the behavior of the individuals taking part.
4. The mentally retarded also tend to have a low level of frustration. Therefore, games and other activities should be simplified, where necessary, and the teaching process should be done in stages.
5. The mentally retarded usually do not respond well to "talking about" an activity but learn better from direct participation.
6. Repetition is essential for retardates in learning most activities and skills.
7. Recreation can serve as an important stabilizing factor in the lives of the mentally retarded and should be organized in an orderly fashion, following a familiar schedule.
8. While the leader may have other social or educational goals in mind, activities must provide fun and a sense of enjoyment for participants.

[21]For a description of Camp Confidence, see Richard Endres: "Northern Minnesota Therapeutic Camp." *Journal of Health, Physical Education and Recreation,* May 1971, p. 75.

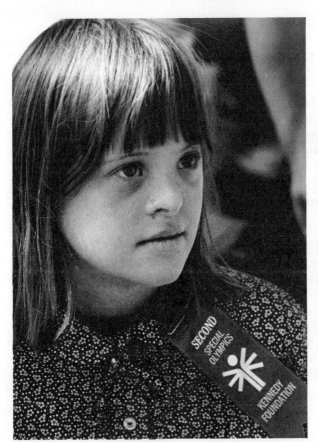

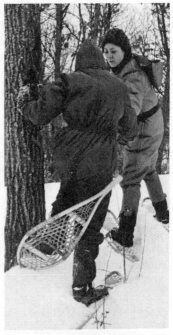

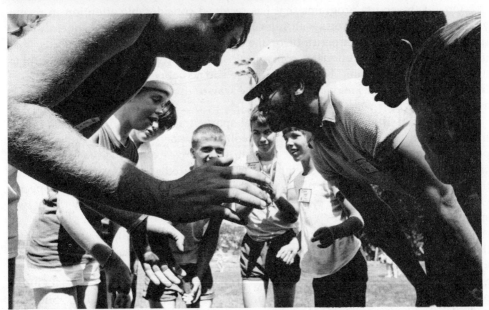

Young mentally retarded athletes enjoy Special Olympics at Parsons State Hospital in Winfield, Kansas. Others take part in winter sports at Camp Confidence in Brainerd, Minnesota.

USEFUL ACTIVITIES FOR THE RETARDED

Recreation programs for the mentally retarded have tended to emphasize the following areas of activity: (a) sports and physical fitness; (b) creative experiences: arts and crafts, music, dance and drama; (c) games; (d) social activities; (e) training in living skills; (f) special events and trips; and (g) camping.

Sports and Physical Fitness

Some of the most successful programs for the retarded include such activities as bowling, skating, swimming, volleyball and track and field. In addition to the physical benefits of sport, these activities provide the opportunity to engage in healthy competition, to strive toward a goal, to gain a sense of accomplishment and to be part of a group.

In general, when a given sport is presented to a group of retardates, it is necessary to teach the basic skills much more painstakingly than with other children of the same age. It may be necessary to simplify the rules and even to modify the structure of the game to ensure success and enjoyment for the participants.

SPECIAL OLYMPICS

One of the sports programs that has received considerable attention in recent years is the Special Olympics—an international program of physical fitness, sports training and athletic competition for mentally retarded children and adults. It is unique because it accommodates competitors at all ability levels by assigning them to "competition divisions" based on both age and actual performance. Even athletes in the lowest divisions may advance all the way to the International Games, which are held every four years.

The Special Olympics offers 16 official sports: track and field, swimming, diving, gymnastics, ice skating, basketball, volleyball, soccer, softball, floor hockey, poly hockey, bowling, Frisbee Disc, downhill and cross-country skiing and wheelchair events. Almost all other Olympic sports are offered as demonstration sports in the Special Olympics. Because of the popularity of basketball and soccer, the Special Olympics offers both team play and individual skills competition in these two sports.

Mentally retarded individuals 8 years of age or older are eligible to participate; there is no upper age limit. Participants usually have I.Q. scores of 75 or less. Individuals who are members of regular intramural or interscholastic teams are not eligible to take part. The Joseph P. Kennedy, Jr. Foundation created the Special Olympics as a nonprofit charitable organization. It is based in Washington, D.C., but state and other local organizations administer the year-round Special Olympics programs within their geographical boundaries.

In recent years, the Special Olympics program has expanded to Canada, France, Switzerland, Mexico and a growing number of other foreign countries. As of the early 1980's, almost one million mentally retarded individuals were taking part in the program, assisted by more than 300,000 volunteers who serve as " . . . coaches, guides, huggers, organizers, publicists, fund-raisers, parade marshals, entertainers, sports officials and other workers."[22]

OTHER SPORTS EMPHASES

Although a strong case can be made for the positive physical, social and psychological outcomes of programs such as the Special Olympics and for the contribution they make to the normalization of the mentally retarded, some authorities have warned of the dangers inherent in overemphasizing competitive sports. Critics charge that the emphasis is on serving more highly skilled performers to the detriment of the less skilled, perhaps a result of our national obsession with "winning at all costs." Many recreation agencies and physical education programs therefore have shifted from an exclusive emphasis on competitive sports, toward a greater support for cooperative games, co-recreational games, games serving different generations simultaneously and innovative programs like New Games.

A report issued by the American Association for Health, Physical Education and Recreation in the late 1960's commented,

Undue emphasis is often placed upon participation in complex and complicated sports or athletic events in physical education and recreation programs for the mentally retarded. Frequently the retarded are placed in sports activities they don't understand, and in which their chances for success are minimized because of the intellectual function required by the activities themselves. An inadequate foundation of fundamental motor skills combined with too-early introduction to complicated sports skills also promotes failure for the retarded.[23]

Recognizing this danger, many institutions and community programs stress only informal and casual sports, usually for higher-functioning retardates. Many activities are approached in an exploratory, "fun" way or emphasize the mastery of a single, fairly basic skill. For example, resistive weight training has been tried successfully with severely mentally retarded youth. Based on six different exercises (presses, pulls, curls and so on) on a single-unit adult-station multi-purpose weight training machine, various adaptations helped students perform the exercises correctly: (a) since none of the students was able to count, or understood the concept of numbers, loud rhythmic music was used to mark the length of time an exercise or lifting period should last; (b) instructors gave manual assistance, with minimal pressure, to help participants fully extend arms or legs in certain exercises when they did not understand the need to do this; and (c) progress was noted by marking

[22]*Fact Sheet on Special Olympics.* Joseph P. Kennedy, Jr. Foundation, September 1980.
[23]*Guidelines for Programming in Recreation and Physical Education for the Mentally Retarded.* Washington, D.C., American Association for Health, Physical Education and Recreation, 1968, p. 13.

scores in colored ink so the participants could understand when they were making progress.[24]

Other activities typically used with the retarded are bowling, skating and swimming. To demonstrate how such activities are presented in an institution serving the retarded, the following activity objectives are excerpted from the leadership manual of the Plymouth, Michigan, Center for Human Development.[25]

Roller Skating

Objectives. Roller skating is used to help develop the balance and motor coordination of the residents. Their sense of accomplishment is increased with mastery of skating skills, and they have a way to use their leisure time constructively. Residents need to learn the following skills:

1. Feeling comfortable with skates on.
2. Standing and moving about with a skate on one foot and the other foot on the floor.
3. Using side rails or rolling stand to initiate movement around the gym or day room.
4. Propelling themselves around the room.
5. Balancing themselves well enough to walk or glide around the room on two skates.
6. Using alternate leg movements to move about on skates.
7. Attempting to skate to music.
8. Participating in a skating party with residents from other buildings.

Structure. Most ambulatory residents can learn and enjoy skating. From ten to 15 residents can be in a group for instruction. Fifty to 75 residents can participate in a skating party. Instruction is scheduled for twice a week for one hour at a time.

Swimming

Objectives. The swimming program for the physically handicapped (many retarded residents in institutions have physical handicaps as well as mental) is planned to meet the following objectives:

1. Build or maintain organic strength and vigor.
   a. Increase the range of movement within joints.
   b. Lengthen periods of sustained activity.
   c. Improve circulation.
   d. Promote deeper breathing.
   e. Improve control of body movements.
   f. Relax the body (sedative effect of immersion).
   g. Promote better elimination.
2. Improve the morale of the participants by:
   a. Socializing in fun activities with persons not physically handicapped.
   b. Developing a feeling of satisfaction in achievement.
   c. Satisfying their desire for physical activities (buoyancy effect of water enhances movement).
   d. Projecting thoughts beyond themselves to concentrate on the movement task.
   e. Reducing the appearance of the handicap.

All residents except the severely physically handicapped receive recreational benefits from swimming. The wide and varied range of swimming skills challenges even the more physically capa-

---

[24]Richard A. Ness: "Weight Training for Severely Mentally Retarded Persons." *Journal of Health, Physical Education and Recreation.* April 1974, pp. 87–88.
[25]*Activity Therapy Manual.* Plymouth State Home and Training School, Northville, Michigan, 1971, pp. 7, 19, 21.

ble residents. Competitive swimming offers an opportunity for them to socialize and increase their ability to take the win or loss in a sportsmanly manner.

Structure. Therapeutic use of the pool is appropriate for any resident recommended by the doctor in charge. Swimming instructions are appropriate for all residents who are able to follow simple instructions and are somewhat mobile. Competitive swimming is appropriate for those residents with swimming skills on a competitive level and the desire to compete.

Each resident in the program should participate for one hour, including dressing time, and should be scheduled at least once a week. Therapeutic swimming can be provided for those residents who need one-to-one assistance in numbers no greater than 15 scheduled for the pool area at one time. Swimming instruction should be given to groups of ten or less per instructor. Competitive swimming should be in groups of six or less.

In order to carry out the program, a series of 21 specific skills are identified, along with their objectives (desired outcomes) and precise descriptions of acceptable performance. Several of the simpler ones follow, as illustrations of the overall sequence:

Swimming Pool Skills	Objective	Acceptable Performance
1. Locate the steps into pool	Orientation and pool safety	To locate and use step properly when instructed to do so
2. How to enter pool from steps	Pool safety	Enter, walk forward using handrail
3. Walk in waist-deep water assisted	Confidence and adjustment to deeper water	Walk in waist-deep water 20 feet with assistance of instructor
4. Walk in waist-deep water unassisted	Confidence and adjustment to deeper water	Walk in waist-deep water 20 feet without assistance
5. Bob in water assisted	Confidence, breathing and coordination	In waist-deep water, feet on bottom, stand and squat four times in succession, breathing in while standing, breathing out with face in water

Creative Experiences: Arts and Crafts, Music, Dance and Drama

A second major area of recreation programming for the mentally retarded is cultural and creative activities. These can be adapted to meet the needs of residents at all ability levels in institutions or to provide engrossing and enjoyable hobbies for the mentally retarded in community life. In general, the same kinds of activities that normal children would engage in are provided for the retarded. As in the case of sports, however, it is necessary to teach them at a slower pace, to keep projects simpler and to provide a fuller level of supervision.

Arts and crafts may range from the use of crayon and paper in drawing, finger painting, play with clay and similar unstructured activities to more elaborate forms of painting or crafts, such as block-printing, leatherwork, weaving and metalwork or ceramics.

Dance activities may range from simple singing games and rhythmic exploration to more complicated folk and square dances and creative or modern dance. For older retardates, social dancing is a popular co-educational activity.

Dramatics may include puppetry and creative or informal dramatics. Since it may be difficult for many mentally retarded children and youth to memorize and deliver lines effectively, the emphasis may be on improvised dialogue in some dramatic ventures. However, it *is* possible to do much more elaborate dramatic productions with mentally retarded children. As an example, 65 children and young adults from Letchworth Village for the Mentally Retarded in Thiells, New York, a state institution, put on a full-scale performance of the musical "Oklahoma" before 3000 guests at the New York City Hilton Hotel. The individuals, aged 8 to 35, with an I.Q. range between 30 and 79, prepared the show as a climax to a fund-raising campaign for the school. The residents rehearsed steadily for the performance for six months and did an almost professional job of remembering their lines and cues.

Music may provide a release for tension and emotions, stimulate language and communication, improve group interaction and enhance self-image. Improving the musical abilities of the retarded promotes their sense of accomplishment and their ability to use their leisure constructively. At the Plymouth State School, music is presented as therapy and as education. The program for each of these forms includes the following:

Listening Behavior

1. Sitting quietly and attentively listening to music played on a phonograph, tape recorder or instrument.
2. Improving the attention span until the resident can participate in a classroom for 30 to 45 minutes.
3. Discussing what has been heard.
4. Improving comprehension of instructions.
5. Giving creative interpretations of what has been heard.

Gross Motor Activities, Coordination and Rhythm

1. Developing basic movements of walking, marching, running, jumping, tiptoeing, hopping, galloping, skipping and skating.
2. Clapping hands to strong rhythmic music.
3. Using rhythm instruments for marking simple and compound meters.
4. Participating in a rhythm band (playing when music begins, stopping when music stops, playing alternately and at different times).

Musical Games

1. Understanding the idea of the game by verbal or demonstrative instructions.
2. Taking turns.
3. Group participation.
4. Heading the group.

Singing

1. Humming.
2. Singing parts of songs.
3. Singing song in correct melody and rhythm.
4. Singing a song within the proper key.
5. Singing with the correct words.
6. Singing a complete song with a group.
7. Singing a complete song alone.
8. Leading others in song.

Ear Training

1. Recognizing various recorded sounds.
2. Differentiating stop and go.
3. Differentiating between high and low, fast and slow, loud and soft, musical and non-musical sounds.
4. Describing musical moods (happy, sad, funny, serious, etc.)

Instrumental Music

1. Playing simple musical instruments, (kazoos, hum-a-zoos, harmonicas, drums).
2. Learning the names of various instruments and recognizing them by sight.
3. Learning to play the more difficult instruments (tonettes, recorders, guitar, autoharp, piano).
4. Learning to play chords.
5. Playing by ear.
6. Reading music.

In some cases, different creative activities may be combined with each other. For example, German composer Carl Orff's "Orff-Schulwerk," involving music, movement and language, has been a successful form of creative dramatics with mentally retarded children at the San Francisco Center for the Handicapped.[26] Morgan describes an improvisational, open approach to acting out or moving to themes based on familiar surroundings in the "real" world, children's songs, fairy tales, adventure stories or simple exploration of concepts and ideas. Appropriate themes are selected according to participants' chronological ages and levels of comprehension, and children participate with considerable enthusiasm.

In another interesting experiment, approximately 125 college students conducted a week-long summer camp for 72 multi-handicapped mentally retarded individuals from the Lynchburg (Virginia) Training School and Hospital. With the assistance of faculty members from the fields of recreation, special education, psychology and nutrition at Virginia Polytechnic Institute and State University, the students emphasized music and movement activities.[27] Singing, creative movement,

---

[26]David Morgan: "Combining Orff-Schulwerk with Creative Dramatics for the Retarded." *Therapeutic Recreation Journal,* Second Quarter, 1975, pp. 54–56.
[27]Gene A. Hayes and Cynthia Crain: "Music and Movement Activities for the Multi-Handicapped Mentally Retarded in a Residential Camping Environment." *Therapeutic Recreation Journal,* Second Quarter, 1979, pp. 14–20.

musical games, sensory awareness and socialization activities, simple folk and square dancing and parachute play were all part of the camp's program.

Games

Games are extremely useful in recreational programs for retarded children, youth and adults. They may include quiet table games, more active equipment games, social games and mixers carried on in groups and active outdoor or gymnasium games.

Games provide an important environment for learning social skills, as well as the opportunity to have fun in simple ways. Many retardates who have never really learned to play can have this experience for the first time in a game. Games provide the opportunity both to compete against others and to cooperate closely with others in a team effort. Specific games may require participants to learn and obey rules, to work with number concepts, to develop alertness, to practice memory or to dramatize roles.

Obviously, games that involve complex rules or highly developed skills are not appropriate for the mentally retarded. It is important, in leading games, not to use those activities which depend on all participants functioning correctly. Even if one or two players do not understand the point of a game, or are not able to participate successfully, it should be possible for the overall group to continue to play it with enjoyment.

Some institutions, such as the Rainier State School in Buckley, Washington, have published pamphlets listing the needed equipment, teaching procedures and time required to play specific games. Richard Endres, Patient Program Supervisor of the Brainerd State Hospital, Brainerd, Minnesota, has compiled a collection of basic games (relays, tag games, simple ball games, follow-the-leader and elimination games) that he has used successfully with the retarded.[28]

Social Activities

One of the most important elements in a program serving mentally retarded teen-agers and adults is the social program. Most retardates find it extremely difficult to mingle and be accepted by nonretarded persons in their age range. Often, the retardate's social skills and confidence are extremely limited because of this exclusion.

It is essential to provide club activities, dances, parties, trips and similar activities to meet the important social needs of retarded youth and adults and to prevent isolation and withdrawal. These programs may vary according to the setting. In an institution, social activities should not only provide fun and social contact but also contribute to the overall social development of participants.

---

[28]Richard Endres: *Modified Game Activities: Improvisation Is the Key.* Brainerd, Minnesota, State School Manual, 1971.

At the Rainier School, for example, recreation is used to develop social skills and to help the retarded learn to use leisure independently and creatively. Hough writes that "exchange dinners" between halls and units of the school are a popular co-educational activity. Often these dinners are followed by games, dancing and informal conversation. Proper table manners and social behavior are encouraged by the supervising staff. She continues,

A social atmosphere is also provided through parties and entertainment planned and carried out by staff and/or volunteer groups. . . . The Residents' Canteen is another medium wherein skills learned . . . include: money handling, purchasing refreshments by name and cost, dancing, table games, social etiquette, group activity participation and interaction, and facility rules. Essentially, this is a place for the practice of skills. However, the recreation leader offers a reinforcing element by correcting inappropriate behavior, assisting each person who may have trouble with reading the name of an item he or she desires to purchase, and helping the person in recognizing the value of money. The program is primarily for use in one's leisure time and not structured as a class.[29]

Other social activities at the Rainier School also are geared to the personal growth of teen-age retardates. For example, one program designed for the Placement Unit (youth and adults who might be discharged but who lack the skills needed for community living) is the Holly and Cedar Leisure Time Activity Club. Hough describes this program as an extremely popular one that deals not only with activity but also with exploration and group discussion in the following areas:

Program content developed with the participants to include: grooming and care of clothing; personal hygiene; physical conditioning and posture; boy-girl relationships and dating procedures (with supervision); party and picnic planning; behavior problems discussions for correction and understanding of right and wrong; self-motivating hobbies; service projects; community based functions and other special items as brought up by the membership. . . . Special emphasis is made on the development of each individual's attitudes toward responsibility in work and play, as fellow men and women, and in general, life itself.[30]

Within this program, the development of potential leadership abilities receives special attention; members of the club are encouraged to act as activity leaders and planners.

In the community, as indicated earlier, many public recreation and park departments and voluntary agencies provide services for the retarded, such as the YMCA or YWCA. For example, since the mid-1960's, the San Bernardino, California, YWCA has cooperated with the San Bernardino County Council of Community Service to sponsor a recreation club for educable retarded men and women over 18. Known as the YW "Merri-Mixers," the club meets weekly, and its members take part in

---

[29]Barbara A. Hough: "Activities for Youth." *In* Larry L. Neal: *Recreation's Role in the Rehabilitation of the Mentally Retarded, op. cit.,* p. 65.
[30]*Ibid.,* p. 66.

social activities such as arts and crafts, games, refreshments or Ping-Pong, along with trips, parties and other special events. Programming is flexible and changes from year to year, according to the interests of the group members. The membership rotates as some young members take jobs or enter job training and new members are referred to the group.

Living Skills

Many recreation or activity therapy programs in state and private institutions include a strong component of special living skills. As indicated earlier, some of these—particularly those related to social behavior—are included in club and other social programs for teen-agers and adults. Not infrequently, special classes or workshops may be held in such activities as cooking, sewing or the repair of simple equipment.

LEARNING SHOPPING SKILLS

In a study of the needs of mentally retarded individuals living in the community, Williams and Ewing explored their shopping abilities. They found that mildly retarded persons could learn to use a mass transit system, identify the types of stores that sold different kinds of products, make a selection, pay for it and count their change. However, the complexities of balancing the quality of an item against its cost and making a logical choice from a large array of products were too difficult for the subjects of their study.[31] Clearly, activity programs should focus on such needs and develop training and guidance strategies that will help the mildly and moderately retarded to shop successfully.

Camping Programs for the Retarded

There is rapidly growing interest in camping for the retarded. One of the pioneer programs has been Camp Confidence, the Northern Minnesota Therapeutic Camp, an independent organization intended primarily to provide year-round camping and outdoor recreation facilities for mentally retarded residents at Brainerd State Hospital; it also serves groups sent by Daytime Activity Centers in the hospital's receiving area and families of the retarded.

Tent sites, picnic areas, cabins and a lodge have been constructed on a 140-acre wilderness site with over half a mile of lakeshore frontage. Activities include winter sports (ice-fishing, snowmobiling and tobogganing) archery, swimming, boating, nature study and other activities suited to the natural setting. Richard Endres has

---

[31]Randall D. Williams and Sheryl Ewing: "Consumer Roulette: The Shopping Patterns of Mentally Retarded Persons." *Journal of Mental Retardation*, August 1981, p. 145.

outlined a number of categories to show how camps of this type may serve different classifications of mentally retarded persons, both institutionalized and living in the community. On a year-round basis, a number of the following programs might well be conducted simultaneously:

1. One-week programs for individuals considered capable of *independent* or *semi-independent community living*. Emphasis on outdoor education curriculum, with participants coming to camp approximately every six weeks.
2. Two- or three-day *vacation camping*. Primarily intended for hospital residents working in industrial programs, who have little or no vacation opportunity. Less emphasis on outdoor education and more on recreational programs. Participation for such individuals suggested every three to four months.
3. *Day camping programs*. Primarily intended for children participating in special education classes at the parent facility (hospital). Instructors would serve as the major counselors for day camping experiences.
4. Two- or three-day *independent living skills camp*. Operated in separate units (away from the main camp complex), with six to eight individuals and one counselor living together with emphasis on home and camp living skills (cooking, clean-up, and so on).

In addition, as campers become proficient in various phases of the outdoor education curriculum, they might take part in two- or three-day *overnight tent camping* programs. Also, families of the retarded might enjoy meeting and camping together with similar families in a *family tent-and-trailer camping area*. Through the years of its existence, Camp Confidence has continued to be innovative in its programs and services; recently it developed an outstanding wildlife sanctuary.

Perhaps its most unique success, however, is in mobilizing support from local business people, parents' groups and other auxiliary organizations. Even a U.S. Army Reserve Engineer Battalion, located in Brainerd, assisted in constructing facilities. Relying heavily on major fund-raising efforts for its support, the camp sponsors an annual celebrity golf tournament at the Brainerd Golf and Country Club, with an art fair, Italian fiesta, boxing exhibition, painting demonstration, awarding of thousands of dollars in spectator prizes and numerous other events. Other tournaments, coffee days, "swap fairs," stage shows and programs are sponsored by businesses and community groups, senior citizens and teen organizations. With the assistance of such fund-raising efforts, Camp Confidence provides year-round camping and outdoor education programs to Minnesota's mentally retarded residents and their families—*free of charge*. That it is able to do so is a tribute both to its own leadership and advisory board and to the willingness of many citizens to support a program that meets an important community need.[32]

HABILITATIVE CAMPING

For retarded children and youth living in the community, such special camping programs might prepare them to move into camping programs with nondisabled peers. In writing about "habilitative camping," Marilyn Herb, Recreation Director

---

[32]*The Camp Confidant.* Newsletter of Camp Confidence, Brainerd, Minnesota, Third Quarter, 1981, pp. 1–4.

of the Fairview Hospital and Training Center in Salem, Oregon, stresses the need to give campers real responsibilities in planning and carrying out program activities. Only if this is done can camping produce the maximum social, emotional, physical and intellectual growth in retarded participants. The stress must be on the camper's abilities, not disabilities. She asks,

1. What responsibilities can be assumed by the camper?
2. How do these responsibilities affect the function of the camp?
3. Are duties and activities geared to camper abilities?
4. Who assigns these duties, you or campers?
5. Do your activities have carry-over values?
6. Are the activities new, or have campers been involved in like programs before?
7. What is the potential for camper planning, executing, and evaluating programs?
8. Do activities stress anticipation, participation, and reflection?
9. How can activities be broken down to meet the needs of varied levels of participants?
10. Is the program the result of direct or indirect professional involvement?[33]

Some camping programs may be eligible for federal funding. For example, the Porterville State Hospital in Porterville, California, operates an extensive on-grounds camping program for mentally retarded residents at Camp Vandalia, an 18-acre site on the hospital property, and other camping experiences made possible with the help of the District VII California Council for Retarded Children, Boy Scouts and Girl Scouts, YWCA and Easter Seals. The Camp Vandalia program is financed primarily by a federal Title I grant as an "Outdoor Education for the Handicapped" project, with assistance from a strong parents' association. The site itself is also made available to outside community groups, particularly those affiliated with the hospital, involved in service to special populations or assisting in its development and maintenance.

SCOPE OF THERAPEUTIC RECREATION FOR THE RETARDED

This chapter has given examples of recreation programs and activities designed to meet the needs of the mentally retarded. How widespread *are* such programs? No fully comprehensive information has been gathered about all institutions and community programs. It is obvious that practices vary widely around the United States and Canada, but that public concern about the needs of the mentally retarded has grown steadily.

A mid-1970's report by Thériault and Witt on the status of Canadian recreation services for the handicapped showed that a substantial number of special projects

---

[33]Marilyn Herb: "Habilitative Camping." *In* Larry L. Neal: *Recreation's Role in the Rehabilitation of the Mentally Retarded, op. cit.,* p. 53.

for the mentally retarded were provided under the national Local Initiatives Program. The 21 programs serving the retarded were third only to the 60 programs for the aging and the 22 for the physically handicapped.[34]

Despite some of the excellent programs described in this chapter, it must be recognized that in many cases, inadequate staffing and funds have limited the care for severely and profoundly retarded residents in many institutions. Often they are extremely overcrowded; it is all that staff can do to keep up with their minimal physical needs. Aroused public opinion has, in some cases, resulted in improved funding and program development in such institutions.

For the last several years, there has been a ground swell of evidence that large institutions represent neither economical nor humane approaches to the care and habilitation of the mentally retarded. The March 1976 report of the President's Committee on Mental Retardation actually took the position that institutional commitment, either voluntary or involuntary, should be prohibited except in extreme cases and through due process. More and more states are developing networks of group homes in the community. In 1977, Pennsylvania, which operates the largest group home program in the United States, was able to care for 2100 residents in homes and apartments at a cost of $15 million a year, or approximately $7300 per person. In contrast, in the same state, one institution's budget for the fiscal year 1976 to 1977 for 1430 residents was $34 million, a cost of almost $24,000 per person. Recognizing that those in institutions are probably more severely disabled than those in group homes, thus requiring more care, the disparity in cost is still striking.

In a number of cases, lawsuits by residents' families have resulted in the closing of residential facilities serving the mentally retarded. In other cases, parents' groups have resisted this action, feeling that their children were cared for more effectively in an institution than in a community facility.

Nonetheless, more and more cities and states are moving toward community-based services for the mentally retarded. In group homes, it is not possible to provide a full range of needed services (a typical residential unit might have only ten to 15 residents, making it difficult to have enough specialized staff to provide all needed programs). Such units are likely to depend more heavily upon recreation facilities and programs in the community itself and to "mainstream" their residents, whenever possible, in integrated leisure settings.

Public and voluntary agencies in the community will need to have more expertise in serving special populations and will, in many cases, need to design programs specifically for them. Much progress needs to be made in this area. Mitchell and Hillman have commented,

---

The overall picture of recreation services for the mentally retarded in municipal recreation agencies suggests that a wide gap exists between the services provided and the services needed. Studies reveal that far too many recreation departments are not engaged in providing programs for which they should be basically responsible.[35]

---

[34]Roland Thériault and Peter A. Witt: *Recreation Services in the Local Initiatives Program of Canada.* Ottawa, Recreation Canada, Department of National Health and Welfare, December 1973, p. 3.
[35]Helen Jo Mitchell and William A. Hillman, Jr.: "The Municipal Recreation Department and Recreation Services for the Mentally Retarded." *Therapeutic Recreation Journal,* Fourth Quarter, 1969, p. 35.

Hillman stresses the need for improved coordination and intra-agency cooperation in the provision of services, as well as for improved research programs to determine needs and effective programs, better information services, training for staff, parent education and involvement and evaluation of participants. He wrote in the late 1960's,

---

... the overall effort to provide information services related to recreation and mental retardation has been sporadic. The need to consolidate efforts and planning in this area is reflected along with other prevalent needs. . . . Vital to the delivery of any service is that of planning. The contributions to either comprehensive planning for mental retardation or planning for recreation services to the retarded have been scant. . . . The need to collect data on such topics as residential areas, transportation methods, building, commercial and public recreation areas, along with the demographic aspects of the population, is often completely overlooked.[36]

Within the community, a number of alternatives exist for serving the retarded. Programs may be sponsored by separate voluntary organizations or public recreation departments or by joint efforts of both. When no program exists and interested parents or community leaders seek to initiate one, a process of community education, identification of need and organization is required. Avedon and Arje have developed a handbook for sponsoring groups that presents useful guidelines for carrying on this process.

Guidelines for Developing Community-Based Programs

1. *Assess retarded population and existing programs.* First, it is necessary to determine the size and make-up of the retarded population and the existing facilities and services within the area concerned. Usually such information can be gathered through the local chapter of the National Association for Retarded Children, public agencies such as the board of education or private agencies or welfare organizations serving the disabled.

2. *Assemble "framework" committee.* After determining the extent of need within a community, Avedon and Arje suggest, it is essential to develop a steering committee or "framework" of sponsors to plan and initiate action. This may include active parents of retarded children, representatives of community agencies, specialists in recreation and related rehabilitative services and similar individuals.

3. *Mobilize community interest and support.* To arouse community concern and promote involvement, it is desirable to have an initial, well-attended community meeting to discuss the need for, and ways of sponsoring, an inter-agency program. Those to be invited might include representatives of the public school system, public recreation and park department, voluntary social and recreational agencies, civic

---

[36]William A. Hillman, Jr.: "Federal Support of Recreation Services Related to Mental Retardation." *Therapeutic Recreation Journal*, Third Quarter, 1969, p. 10.

clubs, government, churches and synagogues and the general public. If successful, this meeting should evoke concern, gain the support of community leaders and agencies in beginning a recreation program for the retarded and result in the formation of an advisory and programming committee to form the program and publicize and gather funds for it.

4. *Developing funding support.* Potential sources of financial support for such programs include federal and state grants, Community Chest or other charitable funds, civic and service clubs, the municipal recreation and park department or the local chapter of the Association for Retarded Children. Not infrequently, money may be gathered from several sources (including fees from the families of retarded participants, if they can afford to pay them); at the same time, one agency may provide facilities free of charge, while another provides trained leadership and another provides equipment or transportation. Special fund-raising efforts, such as rummage sales, carnivals, theater parties or charity balls, may be used to raise initial funds and thereafter be repeated yearly.

An effective public relations program is necessary from the outset, both to support fund-raising efforts and to stimulate public awareness of the needs of the mentally retarded.

5. *Developing staff resources.* This is one of the most important considerations in getting a new program under way. Ideally, it is desirable to have the program directed by a recreation leader who has had direct experience with the mentally retarded and professional training in the field of therapeutic services. Since such persons are not always available, it is a reasonable solution to have the program directed by a qualified recreation leader, assisted by consultants or representatives of community organizations who are expert in the field of mental retardation—although not in recreation.[37]

In addition, it is necessary to make considerable use of volunteers—since the ratio of staff to retarded participants necessarily must be high. Young college students and even high school students often provide an excellent resource. Other volunteers may be recruited from civic groups, women's auxiliaries, fraternal orders, religious groups or service clubs. A program of orientation, in-service training and on-the-job supervision should be established for all workers, professional and volunteer alike.

Programs should include not only a wide variety of activities but also counseling for participants which will serve them in the various areas of development described earlier. When possible, program activities should include the nondisabled. Integration is most feasible with educable retardates, who are capable of functioning on a higher social level.

This chapter has dealt with the nature of the mentally retarded and presented a number of guidelines for developing recreation program services for this group, both in institutions and the community. It should be stressed that in many cases—particularly among the more severely retarded institutional residents—mental and social disabilities are complicated by physical factors. A substantial percentage of such retarded persons have visual, auditory or other physical disabilities which hamper their overall development and their participation in such programs.

---

[37]This section has been adapted from Elliott M. Avedon and Frances B. Arje, *op. cit.*

PROGRAMS FOR THOSE WITH LEARNING DISABILITY

A final concern of this chapter is the kinds of leisure services that should be designed to meet the needs of the learning disabled. The term "children with specific learning disabilities" refers to

> ... those children who have a disorder in one or more of the basic psychological processes involved in understanding or in using language, spoken or written, which disorder may manifest itself in imperfect ability to listen, think, speak, read, write, spell, or do mathematical calculations. Such disorders include such conditions as perceptual handicaps, brain injury, minimal brain dysfunction, dyslexia and developmental aphasia.[38]

Learning disabilities stem primarily from neurological origins and not from a visual, hearing or motor handicap, mental retardation or emotional disturbance. It should be stressed that learning-disabled children are *not* mentally retarded; indeed, such children, despite their frequent inability to read, write, speak or move with appropriate control, often have intellectual potential that is normal or better than that of the general population. The list of famous world figures who had some form of learning disability includes General George Patton, President Woodrow Wilson, Thomas Alva Edison and Albert Einstein. Nonetheless, many individuals with learning disabilities are misdiagnosed as mentally retarded or emotionally disturbed, chiefly because their behavioral impairment bears a surface resemblance to these other broad categories of disability. It has been conservatively estimated by the U.S. Office of Education that there are slightly more than two million children with learning disability in the United States, about 3 per cent of the population in the age group from birth to age 19 years. In 1970, Congress designated learning disabilities as a separate category of the disabled, funding a variety of special educational programs to meet their needs.

Mangel writes, "Most of these boys and girls have the potential to lead fulfilling, productive lives. They are intellectually competent. With skilled and compassionate handling by parents and professionals, they can overcome much or all of their handicaps."[39]

Sherrill points out that children with learning disorders vary widely but, despite their heterogeneity, tend to have certain common characteristics. These include hyperkinetic (hyperactive) behavior, easy distractability, dissociation, lack of social awareness, immature body image, poor spatial orientation and general clumsiness in physical activities. Clearly, such youngsters would function best in

---

[38]U.S. Department of Health, Education and Welfare, 1970, cited in Rhona Shulman: "Recreational Programming for Children with Specific Learning Disabilities." *Journal of Leisurability*, Ontario, Canada, January 1976, p. 13.
[39]Charles Mangel: "The Puzzle of Learning Disabilities." *The New York Times*, April 25, 1976, p. E-S 21.

programs and environments designed to meet their needs. Specialists in this field suggest that those working with hyperkinetic children should (a) establish a highly structured program; (b) work within a limited space; (c) eliminate distracting auditory and visual stimuli; and (d) use instructional materials that stimulate the child's interest and participation.[40]

Nonetheless, great numbers of the learning-disabled are not provided such assistance. Often, their continuing failure in school and in social activities, as well as increasing criticism, scorn and rejection by teachers, families and peers, results in devastating damage to the child's basic self-image. Maturational lag within various spheres of activity means that the disabled child falls far behind others, becomes socially isolated and often develops significant emotional problems. Recreation's unique role within this area is that it can provide both a sheltered and encouraging environment in which the learning-disabled can experience success for the first time in their lives and can also undertake new kinds of directed learning, both conceptual and psychomotor, to help them function more effectively.

Recently, a number of voluntary agencies and public recreation and park departments have initiated programs designed either to meet the specific needs of the learning-disabled or to integrate them into general recreation and camping activities. In many cases, the sheltered experience is most desirable at the outset.

For example, in a summer camping program operated by the Westchester County, New York, Association for Children with Learning Disabilities, a high ratio of skilled staff to campers provides careful, individualized instruction in arts and crafts, music, swimming, sports, perceptual and motor training and a variety of other nature-oriented activities and special events.

In a study of recreation programs for children with specific learning disabilities in Toronto, Canada, Shulman found the following general rationale underlying the development of such programs: (a) children with specific learning disabilities require remedial attention outside the classroom, much of which can be provided in a recreational atmosphere; (b) these children cannot function adequately in a regular community recreation program because they lack the necessary physical, social and/or behavioral skills; and (c) special programs can help develop the skills needed for later integration into regular recreation programs.

Shulman's study showed considerable contrast, in both parents' and professionals' attitudes about whether learning-disabled children needed to be placed in special settings and in the extent to which many of these children had already taken part in some regular community recreation programs. She concluded,

> . . . a great deal of the ambivalence experienced by parents and recreational personnel regarding recreational programs for these children is a reflection of the present lack of knowledge, imprecision and lack of direction in the field of learning disabilities as a whole.[41]

---

[40]Claudine Sherrill: *Adapted Physical Education and Recreation: A Multi-Disciplinary Approach.* Dubuque, Iowa, Wm. C. Brown, 1981, p. 416.
[41]Shulman, *op. cit.,* p. 18.

Given the extent of this special problem, however, as well as the considerable difficulty that many learning-disabled children have in taking part successfully in community recreation activities (in part because those who attend special schools are, in effect, isolated from normal neighborhood associations and play friendships) it seems clear that recreational professionals must pay increased attention to serving those with specific learning disabilities.

It was pointed out earlier in this chapter that many mentally retarded children are multiply disabled, with more or less severe physical impairments. The following chapter deals specifically with the nature of recreation services for various categories of physically disabled children, youth and adults, including the multiply disabled. This population represents a major concern for therapeutic recreation service because the numbers of individuals with physical disabilities are so great and because they have tended to be so poorly served in the past by community recreation agencies.

Suggested Topics for Class Discussion, Examination Questions or Student Papers _____

1. What are the unique characteristics of the mentally retarded on three diagnostic levels that influence the planning of recreation programs for this special population?

2. What are some of the special problems of mentally retarded individuals living in the community, with respect to social integration and ability to care for themselves? How can recreation and activity therapy programs help to overcome these difficulties?

3. Select a specific area of program activity described in this text, such as sports or camping, and show how it may be modified and planned to meet the needs of the mentally retarded.

4. There is some uncertainty about whether the learning-disabled require special, separate recreation programs. What are the key elements to be considered in programming for this population?

8

Recreation for the
Physically Disabled

This chapter deals with the major forms of physical disability as they affect both children and adults in modern society. Each type of disability is described, together with its effects on the individual afflicted, the resultant needs for recreation service and suggested program activities.

PHYSICAL DISABILITY IN MODERN SOCIETY

As a previous chapter indicated, an estimated 68 million Americans have some form of significant disability that limits their participation in various experiences, including recreation. A substantial number of the disabled have a serious physical impairment or chronic condition. For example, it was reported in the mid-1970's by the National Center for Health Statistics in the United States that 409,000 Americans were in wheelchairs, 1.1 million used heavy leg braces, 2.1 million used canes, 404,000 used walkers, 443,000 used crutches and 172,000 had artificial limbs.[1] Millions of others are blind, deaf or have other forms of physically limiting illnesses. In Canada, similar statistics of physical disability exist in proportion to that nation's smaller population.

Such statistics do not give a fully accurate picture of disability and its effects. Both the degree of physical disability and the *extent* to which it has proven to be a major limitation to the individual suffering from it vary widely within *each* disability. The great majority of physically disabled persons live in the community, either with their families or independently. Many of them, even those with extremely serious physical limitations, are able to engage in a wide range of recreational and social interests. Unlike the mentally ill person, who tends to be withdrawn and to avoid social contact or challenges that may be psychologically threatening, the physically disabled person is often eager to test himself or herself among the nondisabled. Unlike the mentally retarded individual, who has great difficulty

---

[1]*Trends for the Handicapped.* Washington, D.C., National Park Services and National Society for Park Resources, 1974, p. 4.

in establishing a meaningful bond of friendship with nondisabled peers, those with physical limitations are often well-integrated members of other social groups.

However, to provide adequate program service for the physically disabled, it *is* necessary to plan specifically for them, to provide programs geared to their needs and abilities, to modify activities and facilities and to provide sympathetic and capable leadership.

GOALS OF RECREATION FOR THE PHYSICALLY DISABLED

These goals include the following:

1. To contribute to the disabled individual's morale and adjustment to the hospital if he or she is being actively treated, for example, for stroke, heart attack or serious accident.
2. To contribute directly to the process of rehabilitation within the treatment setting by providing physical exercise that restores or helps to maintain functions of affected parts.
3. To provide opportunities for the constructive, creative and pleasurable use of leisure for individuals who are not in active treatment and are either in a special residential setting or in the community.
4. To enhance the social independence of individuals and provide satisfying group experiences in socially integrated settings, when possible.
5. To relieve the families of the disabled, both psychologically and in terms of the time commitment, from the need for unremitting care for the physically disabled member of the family.
6. To help physically disabled persons compensate for their specific impairments by finding satisfaction in other activities unaffected by their disabilities.
7. To promote healthful physical activity and prevent further physical deterioration because of disuse.
8. To expand the disabled person's involvement in community life and complement other social, vocational, educational or civic involvements in a rounded schedule of activity, thus promoting his or her "normalization."

As earlier chapters have pointed out, efforts to improve the lives of the physically disabled became common in the twentieth century, especially after World Wars I and II, when public awareness of the needs of disabled war veterans led to a broad concern for the total rehabilitation of the physically disabled. Efforts were made to establish programs that would permit vocational and social reintegration into the mainstream of community life. In addition to programs established by the federal government, many municipal governments developed multi-service programs for the physically disabled. Among these programs have been a variety of recreation-oriented services.

A number of states have taken significant steps to provide needed recreation services for the disabled. In Massachusetts, for example, a state law was passed in 1958 to promote recreation for the physically disabled and mentally retarded. Although responsibility for this overall function was assigned to the Director of Special Education in the Massachusetts State Department of Education, it was specified that the responsibility for actually organizing programs would rest with recreation and park departments in municipalities throughout the state.

In addition, there are a variety of voluntary organizations that have recognized the need of the physically disabled for recreation and are concerned with meeting their overall needs. As an example, the Easter Seal Society for Crippled Children and Adults is a national organization that operates through local chapters in cities throughout the nation. It provides special clubs and recreational programs in community centers, and in some cities also sponsors programs for the homebound physically disabled person.

In some cases, disabled adults themselves have organized to meet their recreational and social needs. An excellent example is the Metropolitan Activities Club in Birmingham, Michigan. The members of this club range in age from 18 to 72 years, and all have serious physical disabilities; many are in wheelchairs or on crutches. Members of the Metropolitan Activities Club assume total responsibility for fund-raising and the organization of activities, including bowling, basketball, swimming, square dancing, singing, arts and crafts and such special activities as parties and outings. Members also publicize their activities through a newsletter and yearbook and through radio and television appearances.

On a national level, such organizations as the National Wheelchair Athletic Association promote specific forms of activity for the orthopedically disabled. Wheelchair basketball was among the first sports to be provided for those who had lost the use of their lower extremities. In recent years, the range of activities enjoyed by such individuals has expanded to include archery, field events, marathon racing, swimming, table tennis, weightlifting, kayaking and boating, hunting, scuba diving, table tennis and a host of other sports. Organizations like the National Wheelchair Softball Association and the National Wheelchair Marathon Committee have been established.

In addition to such groups, many other organizations designed primarily to serve the nondisabled, such as the Boy Scouts of America, also provide special programs for the physically disabled. Although in many programs individuals with various types of disability take part in mixed groups, it is helpful to understand each major category of disability so that needs may be met most effectively.

RECREATION FOR THOSE WITH ORTHOPEDIC IMPAIRMENT

Sherrill points out that individuals who use prostheses, wear braces, maneuver wheelchairs, or ambulate with the help of crutches, canes or walkers may be assigned many labels. Often they are referred to as "crippled," "handicapped" or "disabled." Based on a designation used by the U.S. Office of Special Education, Sherrill prefers to use the term *orthopedically impaired* to describe those individuals who have been deprived of the full use of one or more of their limbs and whose condition is more or less static and incurable—although their level of physical capability may be dramatically improved.[2]

---

[2]Claudine Sherrill: *Adapted Physical Education and Recreation: A Multi-Disciplinary Approach.* Dubuque, Iowa, Wm. C. Brown, 1981, p. 476.

Orthopedic impairments are those that prevent individuals from properly performing the motor and locomotor functions of their body and limbs. Such disabilities may be concerned with the functions of joints, tendons, bones, nerves or peripheral blood vessels and may be caused by traumas, congenital conditions or infection.

Traumatic causes consist most frequently of amputation or peripheral nerve injury. Amputations may result from accidents, illnesses such as diabetes, or surgery. Lack of development during the prenatal period, for a variety of causes, may result in a baby's being born without one or more limbs. Paralysis or motor loss in the muscles of the hips, lower trunk, legs, feet and arms may be caused by accidents affecting lesions in the nerves at the brain or attached to the spinal cord. A person who has lost the use of both legs is said to be *paraplegic;* if all four limbs are affected, the person is *quadriplegic.*

Congenital conditions causing physical disability include the following: *spina bifida,* a condition involving incomplete neurological development, which may cause loss of bowel and bladder control or paraplegia; *congenital hip dislocation,* a malpositioning of the hip that weakens the leg and hip muscles and occurs more commonly among girls than boys; and *talipes,* a congenital condition commonly known as club foot. Other orthopedic conditions that tend to affect boys in the pre-adolescent or early adolescent periods are *coxa plana* and *Osgood-Schlatter disease,* both of which cause limping and pain in the legs or hips and may affect locomotion.

Infectious diseases that affect limb function include *poliomyelitis,* which may result in paralysis of one or more parts of the body, *osteomyelitis,* and *tuberculosis of the bone.* The incidence of these diseases has been reduced considerably by vaccines and improved medical treatment, but they still affect many persons.

Despite greatly improved services for the physically disabled, severe orthopedic impairments have marked effects on the social, psychological and even economic lives of those with disabilities. Individuals who become disabled by accident or illness often must find new ways of earning a livelihood, adjust to the attitudes of family and friends and discover new social and recreational activities to replace those that may no longer be possible.

The orthopedically disabled still face widespread rejection. The high value placed on physical appearance means that persons with crippling disease or missing limbs are often ostracized—either openly or in subtle ways. Particularly when the impairment is sudden—from an accident or severe illness—the problems of adjustment are extreme. Neser and Tillock write,

---

A patient generally needs a period of time, which may range from nine to fifteen months, in order to translate his lack of physical improvement into the psychological acknowledgement that his disability is permanent. His attempt to integrate this knowledge often results in his entering a phase characterized by deep depression and mourning. . . .[3]

---

[3]William B. Neser and Eugene Tillock: "Special Problems Encountered in the Rehabilitation of Quadriplegic Patients." *Social Casework,* March 1962.

Problems of the orthopedically handicapped are often accentuated by family attitudes. Financial difficulties resulting from the need for special care or equipment, as well as the need to devote considerable attention to the disabled child or adult, may cause family strain. Often, parents or relatives of the disabled become overly cautious or overprotective; as a result the disabled person becomes excessively dependent. It is essential that the orthopedically disabled person come to grips with his or her disability and be encouraged to seek out activities that *can* be performed with success.

Recreation as an Avenue to Recovery

For patients in hospitals or rehabilitation centers who are recuperating from a serious accident or crippling illness, a recreation program may divert attention from grief and provide constructive and rewarding ways of using time. It may lead to improvement in function and the development of *new* skills and interests that compensate for the disappearance of past abilities. Recreation contributes to the physically disabled person's ability to accept an impairment and to his or her growing independence and acceptance of a new status in life.

With intelligent modification of activities and equipment, it is possible for the orthopedically disabled to participate in a variety of sports, such as archery, bowling, table tennis, horseshoes, fishing or even such team games—depending on the exact nature of disability—as soccer, baseball, softball, basketball or football.

It must be recognized that the orthopedically impaired have an extremely wide range of capabilities, as well as limitations. A growing number of one-legged individuals have taken up downhill skiing, for example, with considerable success. At the first disabled Olympiad Games in Toronto, a one-legged Canadian, Arnie Boldt, soared over the high-jump crossbar at 6 feet, 1¼ inches, far higher than many two-legged athletes can jump. Claude Stevens, who won the silver medal in the discus at the Montreal Disabled Athletes Olympics, is 57 years old and totally disabled from the chest down—the result of a fall while he was in the merchant marine. Stevens had been hospitalized for nine years and, in his own words, was almost a "basket case," when two other wheelchair athletes persuaded him to take up sport: "I was swathed in rugs. I couldn't hold my head up without a rest. I had no interest in life. . . . I was literally an old man dribbling. Then my whole life changed."[4]

Today, Stevens is fit and bronzed, youthful and strong in appearance. He maintains a vigorous daily training schedule, including 2 hours of weightlifting, an hour of push-ups, an hour of road work in his wheelchair and additional hours of warming up, throwing the discus and shot-put. He maintains that competitive sport and the training it entails have changed his whole life outlook: "It makes you mentally alert, aware of things in an almost psychedelic way. (It is) the greatest cure for depression."[5]

---

[4]Ulick O'Connor: "Athletics: One Man's Path to a New Life." *The New York Times*, January 2, 1977, p. 2-S.
[5]*Ibid.*

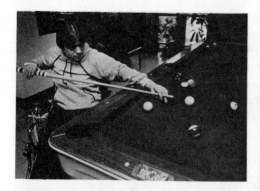

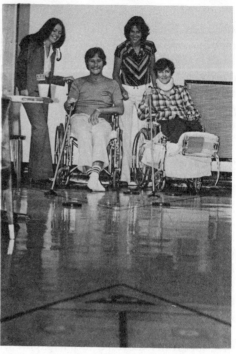

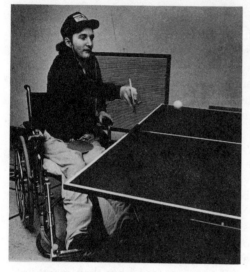

Physically disabled patients at the Williamsport, Pennsylvania, Hospital take part in pool, shuffleboard and Ping-Pong.

In another unusual example of individuals overcoming their physical disabilities, Carl Joseph, a one-legged New Jersey athlete, has high-jumped 5 feet, 11 inches, can dunk a basketball, has won 13 high school letters in football, basketball and track, and was named the year's most courageous athlete by the Philadelphia Sports Writers Association. He has played college football successfully and can cover a mile in under 6 minutes.[6]

Numerous other examples of unusual athletes who have serious physical disabilities may be cited. John Baker, a retired Air Force loadmaster, advertises himself as a one-legged parachutist and is a professional skydiving instructor and performer. He has recruited a team of eight amputee skydivers who call themselves "Pieces of Eight." Their exploits were featured on the television show *That's Incredible*. Wheelchair athletes have competed in major marathons, such as the New York, Boston and New Orleans marathons. They have been so successful that race officials have sought to bar them from competition and have listed them in separate cate-

[6]Bill Lyon: "A Real Wonder on Just One Leg." *The Philadelphia Inquirer*, February 2, 1982, p. D-1.

gories of racers. In the New Orleans Marathon, a wheelchair athlete finished first with a time of 2:07 and would have been declared the world record-holder for the event if he had been on foot.[7]

Obviously, not all orthopedically disabled individuals have the will or physical potential for such a degree of involvement in physical recreation. Quadriplegics, in particular, who have usually suffered almost total bodily paralysis as the result of a severe accident, find themselves in a condition of extreme helplessness, often to be followed by serious psychological problems, withdrawal and depression. The general goal in active treatment centers is to facilitate the return of the quadriplegic to his or her home by maximizing the patient's potential for self-management. Over a period of a year or more, many quadriplegics learn to accept their disability, pass through a period of mourning and develop certain physical capabilities, including bowel and bladder control, the ability to sit upright for a period of time and some degree of use of the upper extremities with the help of orthotic devices. Throughout this process, the recreation worker may work with patients at their bedsides or in small groups on the ward. Ultimately, as they begin to move out into the community, the recreation worker helps them to gain skills and competence that will help them to live independently in the community after discharge.

In addition to modified sports (described later in this chapter) the orthopedically disabled also may enjoy hunting, swimming and dancing. In the area of social activity, the orthopedically disabled are able to enjoy group games, parties, carnivals and similar activities and events. With sufficient motivation, *every* form of creative activity, such as art, crafts, music, drama or creative writing, may be enjoyed by the orthopedically disabled. Even when an individual is so severely disabled that he or she cannot grip a paint brush, it may be strapped to his or her arm, foot or chin.

RECREATION FOR THE CEREBRAL PALSIED

Cerebral palsy is a condition affecting the motor control centers of the body and is a result of lesions in various parts of the brain arising from injury, infection or faulty development. The condition is not regarded as an orthopedic disability but is a neurological impairment.

More than 600,000 children and adults are victims of this condition. It may occur before or at birth or at any time later in life, although 90 per cent of all cases stem from birth injuries or prenatal causes. These causes include maternal disease, severe maternal nutritional deficiencies, toxins, radiation therapy, incompatibility of Rh factors between the mother and the developing fetus or defective development of brain cells before birth and lack of oxygen to the developing brain (anoxia). Infectious diseases such as measles, mumps, whooping cough and encephalitis or accidents involving a severe head injury are responsible for most cases of cerebral palsy that develop after birth.

---

[7]As another example, three paraplegics climbed 8750-foot Guadalupe Peak, Texas' highest mountain, in five days of crawling and dragging their chairs across rocky ledges in torrid heat. *See* "Three Reach the Top in Wheelchairs," *The Philadelphia Inquirer*, July 18, 1982, p. 3-A.

The movement of the cerebral palsied is impaired, awkward and is often accompanied by postural malformations. Speech patterns are usually affected. The condition may cause a complete inability to control muscular functions or only a very slight lack of muscular coordination. Several types of dysfunction have been identified. These include (a) *spastic,* characterized by jerky and uncertain movements and tightly contracting muscles; (b) *athetotic,* typically showing uncontrolled, sprawling muscular functioning; (c) *rigid,* with extremely tight muscles and limited, resistant movement; and (d) *tremor,* characterized by uncontrollably shaking limbs. Eight-five per cent of all cases are either spastic or athetotic.

Cerebral palsy is classified as *mild, moderate* or *severe* in its impact. It may affect one or more parts of the body and often includes a degree of impairment in verbal ability, vision, hearing or intelligence, although the cerebral palsied person may be perfectly normal in these respects. Unless it is a mild case, the person with cerebral palsy has considerable difficulty being accepted by others. Drooling and jerky physical movements, constant facial grimacing and the overall physical appearance, as well as the hard-to-understand speech of many palsied individuals, tend to make normal social relationships extremely difficult. As a result, withdrawal and fear of social contact are common among many children, youth and adults with this impairment.

Although the condition cannot at present be cured, research has shown that intensive treatment, using a variety of approaches, can markedly improve the social, physical and intellectual capabilities of the cerebral palsied. The primary function of recreation services for the child with cerebral palsy is to promote normal growth and development by providing the kinds of experiences and activities other children receive.

The first step is to become familiar with the patient's total history, including the details of home life, attitudes of his or her family toward the impairment, medical history, present physical limitations, psychological make-up, present social involvement and interests and other accompanying symptoms or conditions he or she may have.

In planning programs for the cerebral palsied, it is necessary to select activities that do not produce tension and do not require quick response or performance. While programs should not be overstrenuous, and frequent rest should be provided, it is important to provide physical activities to counteract the obesity and poorly developed motor skills characteristic of many cerebral palsied persons. Simple games, easy rhythmic activities and swimming are particularly desirable.

The National Association of Sports for Cerebral Palsy, a program of United Cerebral Palsy Associations, Inc., provides competitive sports for individuals with cerebral palsy and similar conditions. A member of the United States Olympic Committee, this new organization, created in 1978, is one of the five recognized handicapped sports organizations in the United States. Events in which the cerebral palsied compete include, but are not limited to, archery, horseback riding, weightlifting, table tennis, wheelchair and ambulant soccer, bocce, bowling, riflery and track and field events. Athletes are grouped into eight classes, depending on their degree of disability and means of locomotion.[8]

---

[8]*National Association of Sports for Cerebral Palsy.* New York, United Cerebral Palsy Associations, 1982, pp. 1–2.

Facilities operated by United Cerebral Palsy in a typical center in New York City include two multi-purpose rooms, an arts and crafts shop, a music room, a library and apartments used for training the cerebral palsied in self-care and other life skills. Activities include arts and crafts, music, drama, table games, social events and trips, homemaking projects, physical programs and discussion groups. They consist of approximately 40 per cent active programs and 60 per cent quiet, varied according to age and the physical, mental and social levels of participants.

The heart of the adult recreation program consists of social clubs with 20 to 25 members of both sexes who meet weekly in all five boroughs of New York City. They emphasize social events, bowling, creative writing, discussion groups and other common club activities. United Cerebral Palsy also operates a camping program to serve the cerebral palsied and conducts research, promotes legislation and disseminates publications in this field. Strong emphasis is placed on self-help activities, playing a meaningful role in group decisions and program planning and especially on giving them the opportunity to mature and have meaningful relationships with members of the opposite sex. Nigro writes,

One element of programming that has not so far been mentioned is the pairing off of people into romantic alliances and love affairs and sexual activity at many levels. Obviously, if we are going to bring adults together, stimulate growth, bombard them with social experiences, and increase self-esteem and promote self-awareness, we must be prepared to deal with this very adult kind of behavior. Perhaps it is not so obvious, however, for frequently staff members in adult programs panic at the first sign of such goings on. It is essential that anyone involved in the conduct of programs for severely disabled adults expect and perhaps even encourage such activity. . . . the program design will have to include an element of sex education and sex counseling, for both the disabled themselves and for the staff who work with them. It cannot be stated emphatically enough that the people we are concerned with are adults and have to be thought of in that context, regardless of how they might behave or how retarded or dependent they might be.[9]

The concern with sex counseling has important implications for the entire field of therapeutic recreation service. Recent studies indicate that the majority of individuals with physical disabilities have some degree of difficulty with sexual relationships. National organizations that deal with various disabling conditions are often able to refer clients to sex counselors who specialize in working with the disabled. In the United States there are two such programs, the Human Sexuality Program at the University of California Medical Center, San Francisco, which provides sex counseling for the disabled, and the Physical Disability Program in Human Sexuality at the University of Minnesota Medical School.

Organizations like United Cerebral Palsy provide a wide range of such educational and habilitative programs—including therapeutic recreation service—to meet the need for the well-rounded development of their clients.

[9]Giovanna Nigro: *Sexuality in the Handicapped.* Lecture at Institute of Rehabilitation Medicine, New York, November 1973; and Giovanna Nigro: "Recreation and Adult Education." *Rehabilitation Literature,* September 1974, p. 270. *See also* Nadine Brozan: "Sexuality of the Disabled: A Growing Concern in Health Care." *The New York Times,* May 6, 1980, p. B-18.

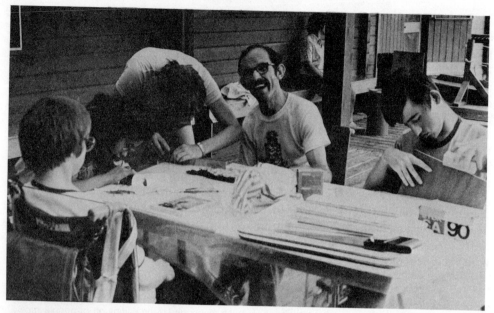

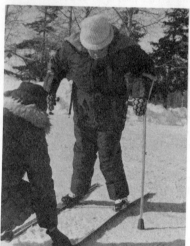
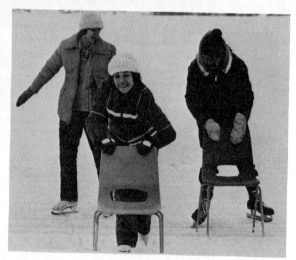

The Ontario, Canada, March of Dimes sponsors camping programs for physically disabled clients of all ages. Here they enjoy arts and crafts and adapted winter sports activities.

RECREATION AND MUSCULAR DYSTROPHY

Muscular dystrophy is the name given to a group of chronic diseases characterized by the progressive degeneration of the voluntary muscles. It is a noncontagious illness that weakens the victim, who is eventually confined to a wheelchair and ultimately to bed. Although its precise cause has not been determined, muscular dystrophy appears to result from an inborn metabolic defect—the lack of a specific enzyme essential for the conversion of food into tissues and energy.

There are four main types of muscular dystrophy: (a) *Duchenne*, which begins as a rule between the ages of 3 and 10, affects more males than females and is usually hereditary; (b) *juvenile*, which begins in adolescence and progresses slowly, sometimes not becoming severe until the victim reaches middle age; it is usually hereditary and affects both sexes equally; (c) *facioscapulohumeral*, which affects the facial muscles, shoulders and arms and makes very slow progress, rarely shortening the life of the person afflicted, although it may cause considerable disability; and (d) *limb-girdle*, which occurs from the first to the third decade of life and makes rapid progress, often causing death within five to ten years.

The disease is not usually fatal in itself, although in some instances it may cause heart failure. However, since muscular dystrophy patients cannot combat infections well, even the most trifling cold may result in suffocation. It is estimated that there are over 200,000 persons affected by muscular dystrophy in the United States. Almost two thirds of these are children, a high proportion of whom die before reaching adulthood.

Recreation is extremely important for those who have this disease. It helps to satisfy their basic human needs for recognition, creative expression, sense of accomplishment and group association. It may even retard the progression of the illness by strengthening those muscles still functioning well. Prolonged bed rest or confinement to a wheelchair can lead to limb atrophy and weaken patients unnecessarily.

Activities for those suffering from muscular dystrophy include arts and crafts, card playing, table games, informal music, modified sports and camping. Since the disease results in marked physical deterioration in its later stages, it is often necessary to modify activities and use ingenious devices to permit participation.

For example, a game like checkers may be played with the use of an instrument held in the mouth to move the pieces across the board. Electric shufflers are used for card games, and racks have been constructed to hold the cards while they are played. Harmonica playing is often recommended because it is a good exercise for the lung muscles; a device holds the instrument in front of the player's mouth so he need not use his hands. Arts and crafts may be simplified, and special devices may be used to hold tools or equipment. Sports are usually played with light, easily held equipment (whiffle bats and plastic balls) and with modified rules and court dimensions.

RECREATION AND MULTIPLE SCLEROSIS

Multiple sclerosis is an organic disease that affects the nervous system in a variety of ways. Most often it attacks the spinal cord, resulting in partial or complete paralysis of the legs and, at times, the trunk and arms. It is often mistaken for other illnesses, since its symptoms are unpredictable; sometimes there are periods of remission and even partial or complete recovery from the disease. Symptoms of multiple sclerosis include partial or complete paralysis of parts of the body, numbness, double or otherwise defective vision, noticeable dragging of the feet, loss of control of bowels and bladder, poor balance, speech difficulties, extreme weakness or fatigue, a pricking sensation in parts of the body, loss of coordination and tremors of the hands.

The disease is caused by a disintegration of the coating over the nerves and the formation of scar tissue that interferes with nerve impulses and causes malfunctioning. Multiple sclerosis usually occurs between the ages of 20 and 35 years, rarely appears after 45, and is slightly more frequent in women than men. Its effects differ markedly from patient to patient. Some individuals are able to maintain job and family responsibilities and make an excellent adjustment to their illness. Others have severely crippling conditions followed by symptom-free periods. Still others are completely paralyzed and permanently incapacitated.

The National Multiple Sclerosis Society is an organization that serves persons afflicted with this illness in a variety of ways. It conducts research, provides medical and other referral services and offers recreational and social programs through local chapters. Through clubs and organized social programs, it provides companionship (including home visiting for the severely afflicted) and organizes picnics, parties, theater programs and visits to sports and other entertainment events. There are comparatively few special recreation programs operated by voluntary or public recreation agencies for those with multiple sclerosis alone. Instead, they are normally served by programs geared to meet the needs of adults with a variety of physical disabilities.

RECREATION AND CARDIAC MALFUNCTION

More than 50 per cent of all deaths in the United States today are the result of heart disease, a statistic that may be attributed both to the larger number of people who reach middle age today (owing to the elimination of other illnesses that attacked younger people in the past) and to changed styles of living. A second major factor is the high incidence of rheumatic fever among children, which causes cardiac damage in over two thirds of those attacked.

Heart disease is generally classified under the following headings: (a) *rheumatic heart disease*, which usually occurs among children between the ages of 6 and 12 as a result of rheumatic fever that inflames and scars the heart valves; (b) *hypertensive heart disease*, which occurs as a result of high blood pressure or hypertension or in association with arteriosclerosis (hardening of the arteries); and (c) *coronary heart disease*, which occurs most often among middle-aged and older persons who have had one or a series of heart attacks. Other causative factors include congenital heart disease resulting from birth defects; anemia, which places a burden on the heart; and conditions brought on by such diseases or infections as diphtheria, myocarditis and endocarditis.

While the symptoms of heart disease vary, the most significant impact on their victims is that they impose an immense burden of fear. Heart disease carries the constant threat of death; although most individuals with cardiopathic conditions do not have the obvious impairments associated with other physical disabilities described in this chapter, they nonetheless are acutely aware of the danger of their condition. Thus, for both children and adults who are afflicted by heart disease, the normal urge to engage in physical recreation is frustrated.

Many children with heart conditions are excessively restricted and become socially immature because they are shielded from any form of play and isolated from involvement with their peers. Fait writes, "Such children need to be counseled into a better course of adjustment, one which recognizes the restrictions as essential but points up the effective and enjoyable life which is possible within the limitations."[10]

Similarly, it is important that adults with heart disease be helped to take part in a regimen of safe but enjoyable recreational and social activities in order to prevent inactivity and social withdrawal. If they do not, they tend to become so obsessed with their illness that they are isolated and lack normal outlets for energy, as well as other forms of release, which may result in a high degree of emotional tension and actually promote heart disease. However, certain safeguards should be kept in mind:

1. Competition in recreational activity should be avoided or kept to a minimum, since it may cause a high level of emotional stress that is dangerous to the cardiac condition.
2. Children should not be permitted to overexert themselves in physical play or in the duration of any sort of recreational activity and should therefore be carefully supervised.
3. Individuals with heart conditions should be given frequent rest periods to prevent strain or exhaustion.
4. Environmental conditions, such as bad weather, heat or cold, may have an effect on cardiac patients; attention must be given to such factors in planning recreation programs.

Associations serving persons with heart disease have classified them in three categories according to the degree of malfunction. Those in the *least serious class* are able to engage in active sports, such as swimming, softball, bowling, tetherball and similar pastimes, although care must be taken to avoid violent expenditures of energy or sustained periods of heavy activity. On the *middle levels of illness* more moderate activity is required, and for the *most seriously ill* only extremely quiet recreational activity, which can be carried on in bed or a sitting position, should be used. Since heart patients normally have full use of their vision, limbs and other body parts, they are readily capable of taking part in table games, cards, arts and crafts, music and similar sedentary activities. Recently, many individuals who have suffered serious heart attacks have taken up jogging as part of their physical rehabilitation program. It seems probable that active recreation under careful medical supervision for heart disease sufferers or those who have recovered from heart attacks will be expanded in the years ahead. In addition, regular exercise reduces the risk of cardiovascular disease, Sherrill points out, through a carefully monitored program of activity.[11]

---

[10]Hollis F. Fait: *Special Physical Education*. Philadelphia, Saunders College Publishing, 1978, p. 172.
[11]Sherrill, *op. cit.*, pp. 401–405.

RECREATION FOR THE BLIND

An estimated 90 million Americans have some degree of ocular malfunction; 3.5 million have a permanent noncorrectable eye defect. Approximately one million persons lack the ability to read ordinary-sized newsprint and are regarded as functionally blind. The legal definition of blindness is vision of 20/200 or worse, meaning that, at 20 feet, the legally blind person can see what a person with unimpaired vision can see at 200 feet. Based on this standard, there are an estimated 430,000 legally blind persons in the United States.

Thus blindness, commonly thought of as the total lack of vision, may include varying levels of sight. Statistics on blindness are often inconclusive owing to different legal and medical definitions of it. Nonetheless, it is obvious that it represents a major physical deficiency for persons of all ages in the United States. It is particularly important for those concerned with therapeutic recreation service because those affected by blindness do not usually have other limiting physical impairments and tend to live a normal life span; however, the effect of blindness is often to limit severely the individual's social integration and other life functions.

There are several causes of blindness: (a) *infectious diseases,* such as measles, scarlet fever, typhoid fever and so on; (b) *accidents* causing injury to the eyes; (c) *functional disorders,* such as diabetes or vascular disease; and (d) a number of miscellaneous causes, including cataracts, genetic defects and poisoning.

As indicated, most persons considered legally blind have some degree of residual vision and can distinguish light from darkness, see major forms or perceive movement. They are, however, extremely limited in mobility and in many aspects of daily living, since so many routine activities are heavily dependent on visual perception. Sometimes they develop motor disabilities, poor posture and other physical impairments. The degree to which blindness affects the individual depends to some extent on when it developed. Some studies have shown that a person who becomes blind during the course of his or her lifetime tends to have more difficulty in adjusting than those who are born without vision. Another study has shown that individuals with no useful vision at all are better adjusted, particularly in group situations, than those with *some* vision.

As a result of blindness, many persons tend to become withdrawn; they lack initiative and are deficient in social relationships, particularly when they are overprotected or when social opportunities are denied them. Some blind persons experience anxiety and depression, while others become hostile; a variety of neurotic problems may develop as a consequence. That these are not the inevitable effects of blindness is demonstrated by the fact that many blind persons lead full and happy lives, hold jobs, raise families and play meaningful roles in their communities.

Because services for the blind have frequently been inadequate, many blind persons are poorly developed physically. Often they are lacking in locomotion, kinesthetic awareness and coordination. Approximately two thirds of the visually impaired children in public schools are not given adequate physical education programs. Often, without appropriate physical release, they experience a high level of tension. Many blind persons develop "blindisms," which are habits such as rocking, rubbing their eyes or waving their hands back and forth, which appear to stem from the repressed urge for physical movement.

All these factors reinforce the strong need of the blind for varied and interesting recreational outlets. Basically, such programs have three major purposes for the blind:

1. As an end in themselves—to satisfy the normal human needs and drives that the blind share with all persons.
2. As a diagnostic and evaluative tool—to determine the capabilities, weaknesses and needs of the blind individual.
3. As a specific tool in rehabilitation—to develop physical, social or intellectual growth or to minimize overall disability.

Since many blind persons are not employed and possess great amounts of leisure time, it is important that they be provided with the means of using this time productively and enjoyably. Recreation can satisfy creative urges, release tensions, promote self-esteem and physical health and strengthen social ties. It is essential, in planning programs to meet the needs of the blind, that this not be done *for* them but *with* them. Ireland writes,

---

A thorough understanding of the blind person is the only reliable basis upon which a recreation worker can set both a realistic and idealistic goal. What might be an ideal and yet realistic goal for one person might be wholly inadequate for the next person. The most important task of the recreation person is to assist the blind person to fulfill his desires and to be aware of his needs as fully as possible.[12]

Under the sponsorship of the American Foundation for the Blind, Kelley has edited an excellent handbook on recreation programming for the visually impaired.[13] It stresses the need to distinguish between the *congenitally blind*, whose visual impairment occurred at birth or during the first five years of life, and the *adventitious blind*, whose visual impairment is due to later illness or accident. The adventitious blind can use visual memory to orient themselves to their environments and to visualize the tasks they are performing. The congenitally blind cannot do this and have difficulty in developing a realistic body image or sense of spatial organization. Recreation leaders must learn to work effectively with both groups and must adapt their instructional techniques so that the visually impaired can build confidence and enjoy recreational skills.

Blind persons today receive benefits in the form of education, rehabilitation services, Braille materials and income tax exemptions. Nearly all states have agencies that provide assistance with homemaking, counseling for parents of blind children, vocational counseling, training and placement, and information services. With respect to recreation, most blind individuals are served through special organizations concerned with this category of disability rather than through public or voluntary agencies for the general public.

---

[12]Ralph R. Ireland: "Recreation's Role in Rehabilitating Blind People." *Journal of Health, Physical Education and Recreation,* January 1958, p. 44.
[13]Jerry D. Kelley: *Recreation Programming for Visually Impaired Children and Youth.* New York, American Foundation for the Blind, 1981.

Programs Serving the Blind

An example of a special school for the blind is the Ontario, Canada, School for the Blind, a residential school that offers a three-phase curriculum: (a) academic; (b) social development; and (c) extracurricular. Out-of-school hours are supervised by residence counselors, who conduct Brownie, Guide, Cub and Scout groups. Such groups operate just as they would with sighted children and in some cases share programs with similar groups in the community. The goals in the Ontario School for the Blind are:

1. To provide healthy, vigorous, outdoor living activities related to the Canadian cultural milieu.
2. To give the children practical skills necessary to cope with independent living outside of the school.
3. To develop the child's personality to the fullest.
4. To integrate the visually handicapped with seeing children as much as possible and to guide them in handling themselves in such settings.

Trips and excursions are an important part of the program, and blind boys and girls in the school take part in track and field and wrestling meets, as well as in other clubs and associations in the community. Individuals are taught to travel, using the white cane for visibility, in order to facilitate independent mobility outside the school. Music in all forms, dramatics and other social and recreational activities are stressed for all residents.

A number of cities have organizations that serve the blind. The New York Association for the Blind, also known as the Lighthouse, is a private, nonprofit, multi-service agency, serving approximately 3300 blind persons each year. It is funded through donations, grants, special funds and endowments. The Lighthouse offers the following services: (a) a nursery-school-age play program, meeting twice a week; (b) a recreation program for rehabilitation clients, meeting four times a week; (c) a youth recreation program, meeting all day on Saturdays; (d) an adult education program in leisure activities, meeting two evenings a week; and (e) an older adult recreation program, meeting two evenings a week.

The facilities of the Lighthouse include bowling alleys, a swimming pool, social hall, kitchen and dining room, auditorium and stage, arts and crafts room, ceramics room, recreation hall and two residential camping areas. Since it is necessary to provide transportation for many of the participants in the program, it operates a fleet of four station wagons and private cars. The Lighthouse also offers residential accommodations for both men and women in its training program and has satellite programs elsewhere in the New York City area.

There are about 60 residential camps in the United States designed to serve the visually impaired. Some camps stress travel as an important vacation experience. For example, the Foundation for the Junior Blind takes 100 to 125 blind teen-agers travel camping each Easter vacation. Young blind campers have panned for gold in California's Gold Rush country, traveled widely elsewhere and attended a reception in their honor at the White House in Washington, D.C. Kaplan and Eskridge write,

... we have piloted an armada of 11 houseboats on the Sacramento River, and a flotilla of rubber rafts down white water rapids of the Colorado River through the Grand Canyon. And we have camped in the Santa Cruz Mountains, the thorn jungles of Mexico, and on an Arizona Indian Reservation.[14]

Such experiences are immensely valuable to the blind, not only for the pleasure they provide but also because of the horizons they open up for the participants and the confidence the teen-agers gain by encountering and mastering new challenges. A considerable amount of experimentation is being done today on new forms of technology such as computerized travel aids that are being developed by the American Foundation for the Blind that should help to make the visually handicapped more independent and capable of travel for business, personal and recreational reasons.[15]

In some cases, special community recreation programs are organized to serve the blind. These may involve the joint sponsorship of various private or government agencies; for example, in 1974, an innovative program for the blind was established by the National Park Service at Glen Echo Park in Maryland. It was begun at the request of the District of Columbia's school system to fill a strong need for programs in the creative arts for the blind. The Children's Experimental Workshop has featured high-quality instruction in dance, theater arts, pottery and design for hundreds of elementary and high school students with visual disability.

Specially designed parks, nature trails and other outdoor facilities marked by rope trails, Braille markers and sometimes taped interpretative messages also serve the blind today with varied forms of outdoor recreation and education. For example, the Roaring Fork Braille Trail in the White River National Forest near Aspen, Colorado, was developed as an experimental trail to provide environmental experiences for the blind.

Special Methods and Equipment

Some forms of recreational activity, such as listening to music or participating in discussion groups, require no special adaptations or methods for the blind. Others need to be presented with special care or modification. For example, in certain activities, such as playing a musical instrument or doing arts and crafts, it is helpful for the leader to perform the skill while allowing the hands of the blind to touch his throughout—thus "learning by feel." Similarly, the leader may move the hands or feet of the blind person through the skill. It is particularly important for the

---

[14]Norman Kaplan and Rob Eskridge: "Blind Teens 'Touch' Hawaii Via Travel Camp." *Camping Magazine,* March 1977, pp. 14–16.
[15]"AFB Developing Computerized Travel Aid." *American Foundation for the Blind Newsletter,* November 1981, pp. 1–2.

leader to give a full description of what is happening. In a game like bowling, for example, the leader must indicate not only the number of pins knocked down but also the placement of the remaining pins.

Since blind persons depend so heavily on auditory stimuli, special attention must be paid to sound and hearing. Whistles may be used to get attention or to give direction to runners in a race. Since sound is often lost or distorted outdoors, the leader should always face the participants and project his or her voice loudly when giving directions. In the play area, confusing noises in the background, such as a portable radio, may distract blind players.

Stability of the play environment is also important to the blind. They must be allowed to familiarize themselves fully with the room or outside space, and equipment or play materials should not be moved without warning. This stability will enhance their security and ease of learning new activities. Some specific kinds of equipment often used for the blind in sports and games include the following: (a) guide wires that enable blind individuals to run at top speed without fear, holding a short rope attached to a ring that slides along the rope without interference; (b) audible goal detectors (consisting of a motor-driven noisemaker that makes clicking sounds at a constant rate), which are used in basketball goal-shooting, to locate bases or to indicate orientations in other play situations, such as swimming pools; (c) audible balls for modified ball games, such as kickball, that have either a battery-operated beeper or bell placed inside; and (d) a portable aluminum rail for use in bowling that is movable from lane to lane and orients the blind bowler.[16]

In other sports, sighted or partially sighted companions may assist the blind athlete. Hundreds of blind children and adults are learning to ski today as part of a nonprofit, volunteer instructional program called Blind Outdoor Leisure Development (BOLD) begun in Aspen, Colorado, in 1969. The instructor and blind pupil are linked by a 12-foot long bamboo pole until the learner is ready to ski alone. At that point, the blind skier is accompanied on the downhill slopes by a sighted companion who calls out directions and warnings about the terrain ahead. In some cases, blind skiers have also worn wireless headsets through which nearby instructors broadcast turning directions. Given the speed and potential risk of skiing, the fact that many blind people are successful at it demonstrates that they, like other types of disabled persons, are capable of far more than they have been permitted to do in the past.

Today, several ski areas in Pennsylvania, including Spring Mountain in Montgomery County, Doe Mountain in Lehigh County and Chadds Peak in Chester County, provide regular skiing instruction for the blind, the mentally retarded and those with other physical disabilities. Here, too, the blind are accompanied by instructors who direct proper placement of the skis and give constant directions to the students. "The teacher becomes the eyes of the blind, watching out constantly for rocks, trees, poles and other skiers."[17]

---

[16]Linda Joseph: "Skiing . . . is Believing: Blind Skiers Reach New Heights." *WomenSports*, January 1976, pp. 28–29.

[17]Helene Moccia: "Blind Skiers Conquer a Mountain." *The Philadelphia Inquirer*, February 2, 1979, p. C-2.

RECREATION FOR THE DEAF

The most commonly accepted definition of the deaf regards them as those whose sense of hearing is nonfunctional for the ordinary purposes of life. Complete loss of hearing is much less common than partial loss, in which sounds are garbled and unclear or high or low sounds are lost. There are several ways of classifying deafness. It may be categorized according to the time the loss of function occurred: (a) *congenital deafness,* meaning that an individual was born deaf as a result of pre-natal or natal nerve destruction or injury, illness of the mother during pregnancy, incompatible Rh factors between mother and child or prolonged labor; or (b) *adven-titious deafness,* referring to later loss of hearing caused by injury, infection or disease (measles, mumps, scarlet fever, diphtheria and meningitis are common causes) or psychogenic factors.

Deafness may also be classified as (a) *nerve deafness,* usually congenital in origin but sometimes resulting from accidents, illness or senility and regarded as the more serious in its effects; and (b) *conduction deafness,* resulting from changes in the recep-tion and conduction ear mechanisms. In many cases, both types of impairment may occur in the same individual. Finally, deafness may be seen more broadly as part of a concept of "auditory disorder," which is concerned with the total reception and interpretation of sound.

The effects of deafness are profound, since language and verbal communication are so important in all aspects of daily life. Because it is not a visible disability, people frequently show little understanding or sympathy toward the deaf and tend to regard them with hostile attitudes, epitomized by the label "deaf and dumb," which is often attached to them. In fact, many deaf persons learn to speak quite effectively, and deafness does not imply any mental subnormality. In some cases, since spoken language is such an important factor in development, the deaf may be weak in the capacity for abstract thinking, and in some children who are born deaf, this may be a contributing factor in mental retardation.

Deaf persons generally have good motor skills, although poor balance and diz-ziness may exist when the impairment is related to semicircular canal injury or cere-bral palsy. In some cases, they may be slightly less skilled in touch perception; on the other hand, they frequently have faster reflexes than the person with normal hearing, probably because their level of tension is high, resulting from the under-standable effort to compensate for their lack of hearing ability.

A primary objective of recreation and social programs for the deaf should be to integrate them with nondisabled peers. As in other areas of life, this poses a difficult problem because of the importance of verbal communication in most recreational activities. In many cases, deaf young adults who have spent 16 or 17 years in special schools for the deaf, with little social contact with the hearing population, continue to isolate themselves after graduation. Highly independent and proud, they often organize their own social clubs, sports groups, churches and state and national orga-nizations. Although such groups provide valuable services for the deaf, they con-stitute a barrier of self-imposed isolation that must be overcome.

Teaching the deaf or leading them in recreational programs requires careful attention to the means of communication. Involving them in games, dancing or other group activities where directions must be heard should be done carefully. In special situations in which skilled leaders are working with the deaf exclusively, reliance may be placed on the manual method of spelling out words with "finger language." However, in mixed groups or with leaders not familiar with this method, lip reading is the more useful approach. The recreation leader should stand close to the persons he or she is working with, facing them directly, and should speak slowly and clearly, enunciating each word distinctly. The leader may also use hand gestures and other forms of direct demonstration, visual aids or diagrams or may rely on persons with normal hearing in the group to assist deaf participants.

In leading the deaf in sports and games, it is important to recognize that because of past exclusion from childhood play in neighborhood playgrounds or schools, they may not be familiar with the rules and strategies of games, as most normal children tend to be. In facilitating play, a variety of devices may improve understanding and help the deaf participants overcome the effects of their impairment. For example, when they play flag football, they quickly learn that the best way to signal to have the ball "hiked" is to clap their hands—an unmistakable visual signal. In basketball, the official must not only blow a whistle but also simultaneously wave his or her hands to get deaf players' attention. Numerous other methods are used to compensate for the inability to hear verbal directions, signals or explanations.

A unique adaptation has been made in dancing. Hearing-impaired teen-agers and adults have learned to disco as part of the popular dance craze—moving to music they cannot hear, but whose vibrations they can sense through the floor. Recently, a new device, known as an *audio transducer,* has been developed. This disc-like object can be used to turn most surfaces into speakers and to make music "sound" much more vivid and real to the deaf.[18]

Examples of Programs Serving the Deaf

Educational, vocational, social and recreational services for the deaf may be provided in a variety of settings, such as special schools or classes, voluntary organizations in the community or programs provided by public recreation departments. Special centers to serve deaf and blind children have been established in a number of cities with federal funding under Public Law 90–247. These centers assist local agencies with grants or contracts empowering them to provide diagnosis, evaluation, education, social services and consultants to parents and teachers.

An example of a school for the deaf in New York City is the Lexington School for the Deaf, operated under the auspices of a board of trustees and the New York State Board of Education, with funding by the New York City Board of Education and private sources. This school serves some 400 students, almost half of whom are residents; all have auditory disabilities and some have multiple handicaps. Facilities operated by the Lexington School include a gymnasium, library, activity and game

---

[18]"Deaf Disco: Device Allows Hearing-Impaired to Dance." Associated Press Dispatch, September 20, 1979.

rooms, lounges, swimming pool, ballfields, playground, billiards room and arts and crafts shop.

The after-school recreation program includes a high proportion of physically active pursuits—all voluntarily participated in by students. It has been found that once they have learned the basic rules, skills or strategy in a given activity, deaf children tend to participate extremely successfully. Particularly in sports in which hearing is not an important factor, such as wrestling or swimming, they are able to compete with others on an equal footing; occasionally, deaf competitors have won NCAA or AAU wrestling championships. However, the school has experienced continuing difficulty in integrating its students in programs with nondisabled peers, a problem facing other community recreation agencies that seek to accomplish this goal.

THERAPEUTIC RECREATION FOR THOSE WITH OTHER PHYSICAL DISABILITIES

In addition to the impairments described earlier, there are a number of other diseases or disabling conditions that may require specially designed therapeutic recreation service.

Tuberculosis

An infectious disease that affects the pulmonary system, tuberculosis may necessitate long hospitalization in a sanitarium or rest home, together with sustained bed care and a nutritious diet. Although it once was regarded as a major health problem and often resulted in progressive disability and death, today its incidence has declined markedly, particularly among children. It continues to appear in persons of all ages, however, and a substantial number of persons have arrested cases. For such individuals, activity must be limited and precautions taken to prevent reinfection.

Recreation plays a vital role in making the long period of hospitalization more bearable. It provides pleasure and interest, strengthens morale and helps the tubercular patient avoid depression as well as gain a sense of usefulness and involvement. Recreation can also introduce new skills and interests to supplant those that the patient must give up. It may also contribute to the patient's physical fitness level without unduly taxing his or her energies.

Diabetes Mellitus

Diabetes mellitus is a disease in which the body is unable to properly ingest starches and sugars owing to an inadequate supply of naturally produced insulin. The highest incidence of diabetes is among middle-aged persons, although approximately 10 per cent of its victims are children. For the most part, diabetics can engage in a normal range of activities (some have been successful as professional athletes), and most can engage in the normal occupational, family and other community involvements of the nondisabled without danger. Diabetics tend to fatigue more easily than others, however, and care must be taken with respect to diet and regular medication. Therefore, camping or other residential programs serving diabetic persons must be designed to meet their health needs. When the condition is severe, it may necessitate hospitalization and a sharply limited regimen of activity.

It has been estimated that there are approximately 4.5 million diabetics in the United States; about 350,000 new cases are discovered each year. It is extremely likely that recreation leaders, physical educators and coaches will come into contact with many individuals who have this disease and therefore should be familiar with its causes and effects. For example, diabetics having insulin reactions may exhibit a wide variety of symptoms:

> The classic symptoms are increased "nervousness" or "shakiness," hunger, weakness, sweating, vision changes, irrational behavior, mental confusion and loss of coordination. A normally quiet, easygoing individual may become argumentative, irritable, and aggressive, and may exhibit uncharacteristic outbursts of temper. Occasionally diabetics in insulin shock are accused of being intoxicated or high on drugs.[19]

Since the onset of hypoglycemia may be quite rapid, requiring only hours or minutes to develop, it is important that the leader or coach be able to recognize the symptoms quickly. The normal treatment for insulin reaction is to compensate for low blood sugar by having the diabetic quickly eat or drink something sweet. The participant should have a prearranged signal with the coach or adult leader so that if he or she needs to leave an activity for this purpose, he or she can do it promptly, rather than trying to "gut it out" by staying in the game. The leader should also be aware of the possible implications of diabetes for healing after an injury and the effects of exercise, although self-care is the diabetic's own responsibility. Particularly for recreation leaders who are with youngsters on a round-the-clock basis, such as camp counselors, it is important to understand that a proper diet helps control diabetes. The meal plans for campers with diabetes should be well balanced and low in sugar, and should include two or three regularly scheduled snacks in addition to meals.

> During periods of strenuous exercise, such as swimming, hiking, and dancing, when sugar is burned up rapidly, extra nourishment is usually needed to keep the blood sugar from falling. If a vigorous camp activity is scheduled just *before* a meal, the camper with diabetes should not participate, *unless* additional food is provided beforehand. Extra food should also be allowed before periods of sustained exercise, such as a long hike.[20]

[19]David L. Engebretson: "The Diabetic in Physical Education, Recreation and Athletics." *Journal of Physical Education and Recreation,* March 1977, p. 19.
[20]*The Camper with Diabetes: Guidelines for Counselors.* New York, American Diabetes Association, 1982.

It is extremely important to see this disability in perspective. Many top college and professional athletes, as well as individuals in all other spheres of life, have been diabetics who have learned to live with and control their disability successfully.

Other Disabilities

In addition to the disabilities already described in this chapter, therapeutic recreation can be of immense value to those with other types of physical impairments. Sherrill, for example, describes the use of adapted physical education and therapeutic recreation activities with such illnesses or disabilities as asthma, sickle-cell anemia, cystic fibrosis and epilepsy.[21] Sometimes recreation may be used to meet a special need of such groups. For example, individuals with kidney malfunction must be rigged up to a blood-cleansing mechanism—a dialysis machine—often three times a week for three to five hours at a time. In some dialysis centers, quiet activities like recreational art programs have been developed to counter the boredom and poor morale that might otherwise affect patients undergoing dialysis. Epileptics in particular are frequently found in many therapeutic recreation programs.

Finally, it should be recognized that substantial numbers of disabled individuals do not fit within any one category, but have multiple impairments. The San Francisco Recreation Center for the Handicapped serves 1300 children, youth and adults in its camping programs, most of whom are multiply handicapped:

Some are in wheelchairs, on crutches, or bedfast, have severe speech impairments, visual handicaps and hearing losses. Many are unable to feed themselves and require assistance with toileting. While the majority are primarily mentally retarded, some are in addition partially sighted, deaf, hard of hearing, neurologically handicapped, emotionally disturbed or a combination of these handicaps.[22]

MODIFICATION OF FACILITIES FOR THE PHYSICALLY DISABLED

It is important that architectural barriers be eliminated so that persons with impairments may use parks, playgrounds, community centers or a variety of other special recreation facilities. This problem, which does not affect the mentally ill or retarded, *does* affect hundreds of thousands of individuals, young and old, who are in wheelchairs or on crutches or who have limited powers of locomotion. A 1967 report by the Bureau of Outdoor Recreation emphasizes this need:

---

[21]Sherrill, *op. cit.*, pp. 361–397.
[22]*Annual Report.* San Francisco Recreation Center for the Handicapped, 1981.

> It is clearly evident . . . that great numbers of disabled persons are not receiving the benefits of our nation's recreation resources. The severity of their disabilities, architectural barriers, non-acceptance by society, and slowness of the recreation profession to adjust its programs and facilities to their needs all have contributed to a serious lack of opportunity.[23]

Similarly, in 1975, a lead editorial in *Parks and Recreation* identified "access" as the most important issue affecting the modern park and recreation facility. The problem of making park and recreation facilities accessible must be attacked vigorously and on all levels.

To promote this effort, a national hearing on the recreation needs of disabled persons was held in Boston, in October 1976, by the Architectural and Transportation Barriers Compliance Board, in cooperation with the National Recreational and Park Association and the U.S. Department of the Interior. The hearing brought together recreation professionals, state and federal park officials, private recreation developers and representatives of various types of disabled persons. In addition to gathering information about the needs of the disabled and current trends in this field, the conference members formulated recommendations to the President and Congress to promote compliance with existing laws and standards to ensure access to recreational facilities for the disabled.

The United States of America Standards Institute has published a pamphlet suggesting ways to adapt facilities so they can be used readily by the physically disabled. Specific design details have also been established in a number of states for park and recreation facilities. For example, the New York State Council of Parks and Outdoor Recreation published a handbook of design standards for various types of facilities in order to make them accessible to the physically disabled. These standards must be followed by all municipalities that wish to qualify for state or federal assistance. Examples of such standards follow:

1. Parking facilities should have special parking stalls designed for wheelchair users. The parking area should be close to the recreation site and paved with a nonslip surface. An opening of 30 inches should be maintained between guardrails to permit a wheelchair to pass.
2. Walking trails should have a minimum width of 48 inches in order to be accessible to disabled persons. They should be smoothly graded without steep inclines and with sufficient area to turn around at various places on the way. Ramps should be used where necessary. Doors of buildings should have a minimum clear opening of 32 inches, with the threshold close to the floor.
3. Food service areas should have special service areas in at least one concession where wheelchair users may be served and seated. Public telephones mounted on poles at appropriate heights make it possible for wheelchair users to make calls unaided.
4. For toilets to be made accessible, ramps with sufficient width should be installed to reach stations that are above-grade. Urinals should be floor-mounted, no higher than 19 inches above the floor and equipped with horizontal handrails. Hand-driers, soap dispensers and mirrors should be at levels accessible to wheelchair users.

---

[23]*Outdoor Recreation Planning for the Handicapped.* Washington. D.C., Bureau of Outdoor Recreation, April 1967, p. 1.

Many other specific guidelines indicate the ways in which recreation and park agencies should provide access for the disabled. Swimming facilities can be made more useful by providing a paved walk leading to the swimming area. Sloping handrails or ropes mounted on posts make it easier to get into the swimming facility. Bathhouses should have enlarged dressing room facilities with a bench, guardrails and outward-swinging doors for wheelchair users.

Spectator areas, picnicking, camping and boating sites should have similar modifications or design features. Fishing areas should have a paved surface at the water's edge, with a protective handrail to make the sport safe for the physically disabled. Auditoriums should have seats missing in some rows, with a level surface, so wheelchair users may sit there rather than in crowded aisles or at the back of the hall.

A number of playgrounds, parks and other facilities have been designed for use by the physically disabled. For example, a unique playground was developed for disabled preschool children at the New York University Medical Center's Institute of Rehabilitation Medicine. Planned by the well-known architect, Richard Dattner, it includes a ladder leading to a tree house (which may also be reached by ramps) a waterfall, tabletop sandboxes and similar features that contribute to children's play opportunities and overall development. A special playground with large animal forms and modified equipment has been developed by the Child Study Center in Fort Worth, Texas.

Ideally, such specially designed facilities should not be for disabled persons alone, since this tends to reinforce their isolation from the rest of society. Instead, the facilities should attract and serve their families, as well as other nondisabled individuals. Recently, the U.S. Department of Housing and Urban Development funded an architectural competition for the most innovative designs for special playgrounds that would integrate disabled and normal children. Each design incorporated various forms of experimental play equipment leading to individual and group play on various levels of difficulty or complexity.

Need to Strengthen Efforts

Despite these successes in making recreation and park facilities accessible to the physically disabled, there is a need to redouble such efforts in the years ahead. Many park systems and other facilities have not yet been remodeled to permit access, while others continue to be designed without adequate consideration for the guidelines that have been presented. For example, a study of five outdoor recreation projects that had been funded by the Bureau of Outdoor Recreation in the state of Georgia and developed during the early and mid-1970's found that fewer than 20 per cent of the minimum standards of accessibility for the physically disabled had been met.[24] Arrangements for adapting mass-transit vehicles and other public build-

---

[24]Charlene Drosselmeyer Farmer: "A Study of Five Land and Water Conservation Fund Projects in Regard to Accessibility and Usability for the Physically Handicapped." *Therapeutic Recreation Journal,* First Quarter, 1976, pp. 27–30.

ings to improve access for the physically disabled have been limited by high costs and the lack of adequate funding.[25]

In an analysis of Canadian guidelines for barrier-free swimming pools, Adair points out the need to remove physical obstacles in order to provide a more dignified and supportive environment in which disabled persons may mingle freely with the nondisabled. He stresses the need to provide facility managers, recreation professionals, social planners, architects, engineers and physically disabled persons themselves with appropriate guidelines and with the strong rationale for developing such facilities.[26] Finally, recreation and park administrators in communities throughout the United States and Canada should take the initiative in reviewing all facilities developed since the passage of relevant federal or state legislation, as well as all facilities receiving federal funding, to ensure that they are in compliance with the law. As an example, the city of Des Moines, Iowa, has assigned capital improvement funds to carry out a comprehensive study of the accessibility of leisure facilities to the handicapped, in cooperation with housing, engineering and other human services personnel in city government.[27] All communities should take such initiatives on a regular basis.

Policies to Facilitate Travel

Travel has always imposed special problems for the physically disabled; strong efforts have been made generally to improve recreational travel opportunities for the disabled (see p. 177). Such states as Oregon, New Jersey and Michigan have constructed new rest areas along the highways with special aids for disabled persons, or have stipulated that restaurant chains or lodging chains with concessions along major thruways must provide facilities to meet the needs of disabled persons. In addition, both voluntary agencies and commercial travel agencies are now making increased efforts to provide travel facilities and arrangements for the disabled. Carr writes,

---

... thousands of severely handicapped persons are today making the tourist rounds, including those afflicted with muscular dystrophy, multiple sclerosis, myasthenia and polio. Paraplegics, even quadriplegics, as well as the blind, the deaf and the retarded are also taken on major trips by agents.[28]

Some travel firms are specializing in foreign travel for the physically disabled. With a highly competitive market today, instead of discouraging tourists in wheel-

---

[25]"Access for the Handicapped: One Barrier Is Money." *The Philadelphia Inquirer,* July 5, 1981, p. 5-C.

[26]Bill Adair: "Barrier-Free Swimming Pools." *Recreation Canada,* April 1979, pp. 10–13.

[27]*Study of Handicapped Accessibility.* Des Moines, Iowa, Department of Parks and Recreation, William Foley, Director, 1982.

[28]Stanley Carr: "The World From a Wheelchair: Travel for the Handicapped." *The New York Times,* February 23, 1975, p. 10-1.

chairs who require special aisles and mechanical lifts in buses or ramps and large elevators, airlines and hotels are going out of their way to make necessary adjustments to serve such travelers.

In various ways, facilities and equipment are being modified to serve the disabled in many public and commercial settings. The construction of all major federal and state buildings, including university structures and office buildings, is increasingly being geared to serve the physically disabled. Elevators are being designed with slow closing speeds and with controls and alarm boxes set at appropriate heights on their walls. Nature trails have been developed in many national and state parks for the blind, with special guide ropes and Braille signs pointing out natural features.

In many other ways, attention is being given to meet the needs of the physically handicapped for recreational opportunities. Much progress needs to be made, however, particularly in improving public acceptance of the physically disabled in recreation areas. A larger number of recreation and park administrators must accept the needs of the disabled as a high-priority program concern.

In summary, efforts to provide more opportunities for enriching and creative recreational involvement for the physically disabled are relatively recent. The extent to which many seriously impaired individuals have been able to overcome their disabilities and take part in a wide range of challenging activities would not have been believed a few decades ago. Their courage and determination have been truly impressive. At the same time, it is essential to recognize that the problem has *not* been fully addressed and that many millions of physically disabled persons continue to lead tragically limited lives for lack of leisure opportunities, counseling and instruction. Meeting their needs must be a high-priority concern of all professional recreation personnel, including both community and therapeutic recreation specialists.

Suggested Topics for Class Discussion, Examination Questions or Student Papers

1. How does the problem of providing recreation for the physically disabled person differ sharply from that of planning for the mentally ill or retarded individual?

2. Select a specific type of physical disability, and then select a major category of recreational involvement, such as sport. Based on the specific needs of the population chosen, outline a set of goals and then show how the activity would be designed to fulfill these goals.

3. We frequently underestimate the capability of such groups as the blind or orthopedically disabled. Discuss this point, using information from this chapter or from your personal observation. In your reply, deal with the psychological aspects of physical disability.

4. Discuss the need for specially designed or modified facilities to serve the physically disabled, showing how present facilities often limit or bar their participation. How can fuller support for such efforts be developed among administrators, planners and designers, and the public? Related to this, what are some recent trends in travel for the disabled?

9

Recreation and the Aged

This chapter deals with the aged population in modern society. It discusses the aging process and the special problems that face older persons in the world today, including leisure, its uses and values. It analyzes various types of settings in which recreation and related services are provided for older persons. The bulk of statistics and illustrations provided are drawn from the United States; however, the pattern of service to the aged is quite similar in Canada.

THE AGED IN AMERICAN SOCIETY

Who are the aged in American society? The 1980 U.S. Census indicated that there were 25.5 million persons 65 years old or older, 28 per cent more than in 1970. They constituted over 10 per cent of the entire population.[1] The percentage of Americans in the older age bracket is growing rapidly:

When the first census was taken in 1790, half the people in the country were 16 years old or younger, and as recently as 1970 the median age was under 28. But as the nation moves into its third century, its people too, are getting older. The median age will . . . reach 35 by the year 2000 and approach 40 by 2030. Over the same span, the number of people over 65 will more than double to 52 million—one out of every six Americans.[2]

It is predicted that within about 50 years, one of every five Americans will be 65 or older, and there will be one retired person for every two of working age, compared with one retired person for every five workers at present.[3] Within the over-65 population, the ratio of women to men is about four to three; there are six million more females than males in the population, largely because women live

---

[1]John Herbers: "Sharp Rise of Elderly Population in 70's Portends Future Increases." *The New York Times*, May 23, 1981, p. 1.
[2]"The Graying of America." *Newsweek*, February 28, 1977, p. 50.
[3]Patricia O'Brien: "The Elderly: As Population Ages, Economic Planning Must Change Radically." *The Philadelphia Inquirer*, January 29, 1980, p. 10–A.

290

longer. This disparity increases with age. About 70 per cent of older Americans live in their homes or with relatives, whereas about 25 per cent live alone or with a nonrelative and about 5 per cent live in institutions.

Why is the aged population a matter of special concern for those involved with health and welfare services in the United States and Canada? This population's role in society has been shifting rapidly as a result of increased life span, changes in family structure and social attitudes, population shifts in our cities and other economic and psychological factors. Many older people today lead isolated, unhappy lives. They are often relegated to a position of inferiority within a youth-oriented culture. They are stereotyped and misunderstood and often shunted aside following retirement from business or family responsibility; they reach a point at which their lives become empty and meaningless, and they deteriorate both physically and psychologically.

This is not an inevitable part of aging. It happens only because society permits it to happen. In order to understand the phenomenon, it is necessary to examine the following: (a) the process of human aging; (b) the social and psychological implications of aging; (c) the economics of retirement and aging; (d) the needs and problems of older persons; and (e) the role of recreation and related services in programs for the aged.

THE PROCESS OF HUMAN AGING

First, it must be understood that aging is a universal process, although it varies greatly from person to person. It is generally regarded primarily as a physiological development, although it obviously has social and psychological components as well. *Gerontology* (study of the aging process and of aged persons in society) and *geriatrics* (the branch of medicine dealing with medical problems of the aged) have both contributed greatly to our understanding of this stage of life.

Although age 65 is considered the beginning of old age, the process is not strictly age-correlated and can vary tremendously among individuals. Some persons begin to show signs of aging in their 40's or 50's, and others remain extremely vital and alert well into their 80's. In general, the process of aging includes the following physiological changes:

1. Slowing of biological functions
2. Breakdown in functioning of body systems
3. Reduction in physiological reserve
4. Altered structure of cells, tissues and organs

These changes decrease the efficiency of the functioning of body systems and begin to bring about progressive disabilities of the heart and nervous system, the five senses (especially vision and hearing) and the motor abilities of older persons. Geriatrists have concluded that such changes are due to both internal and environmental causes. One of the obvious factors influencing the process of aging is the availability of competent medical care. Yet, a National Health Survey found that one in four persons aged 65 and over had not been to see a physician for two years or more—a reflection of the inadequacy of our social concern and practical provision of services for the aged in society.

It is necessary to recognize that many persons have misconceptions about the older people in American society that are usually detrimental to this segment of our population. In an effort to correct such stereotypes, the National Council on Aging formulated ten basic concepts of aging that may be summarized as follows:

Aging is a universal and normal process, which varies uniquely from person to person. Aging is not necessarily accompanied by illness, and one's life-style may greatly enhance one's chances for a healthy old age. Older people represent a span of three generations, each with its own characteristics. Despite stereotypes about them, older people can and do learn and change; old age is not inflexible. Older people wish to remain self-directing; they are vital human beings, who need only develop or maintain existing capacities to lead productive, rewarding lives.[4]

It should also be clearly understood that aging has two major aspects: *biological* and *sociogenic*. Biological aging refers to physical changes that occur in an individual as he or she grows older. In contrast, sociogenic aging refers to the role in which society places people when they reach a given chronological age. Schrock comments that a holistic definition of aging would communicate the idea that the changes associated with aging are normal and continuous, resulting in both losses and gains. Aging occurs on a continuum; there are no precise demarcations between the various stages of life. Older people often experience change so gradually that they develop successful coping skills and accept changes that occur as a normal part of life.[5]

It is a misconception that great numbers of aged persons necessarily become *senile*. Hickey points out that this over-used term has become something of a catchall for symptoms stemming from, or resembling, chronic brain syndrome. However, "senility" tends to cover a host of behavioral or chronic health problems typical of old age, often inaccurately and inadequately diagnosed. Hickey stresses that only a small proportion of older persons who appear to be forgetful and confused have actual brain damage resulting from a hardening of the arteries. The majority are suffering from other problems, such as nutritional deficiencies, heart disease, drug problems or depression, which are clearly treatable. Hickey concludes, "Thus, the representation of old people as 'typically senile' and generally suffering from the cognitive deteriorations of old age is simply an inaccurate generalization."[6]

Finally, it has been predicted that medical science will soon be able to extend the average human life span to 85 years and that these additional years of life will be healthy, for the most part. Two leading medical researchers reported to the American Association for the Advancement of Science that we are on the verge "of

---

[4]Adapted from statement of National Council on Aging. Reprinted in *Recreation*, February 1963, p. 67.
[5]For a useful discussion of the aging process, see Miriam Martin Schrock: *Holistic Assessment of the Healthy Aged*. New York, John Wiley, 1980.
[6]Tom Hickey: *Health and Aging*. Monterey, California, Brooks/Cole Publishing Co., 1980.

becoming a society in which nearly all individuals survive in a healthier state to advanced age, and then succumb . . . over a narrow age range."[7]

Despite such statements, however, it must be recognized that many aged persons in modern society have been seriously affected by a variety of social changes entirely apart from the biological process of aging: enforced retirement, exclusion from meaningful roles in community life and shifting patterns of family involvement.

PROBLEMS FACING OLDER PERSONS

Compulsory Retirement

Early retirement, which has become widespread in American life as a result of pension and Social Security plans and Civil Service or personnel regulations in most businesses, has enormous implications for older persons. For many, retirement from work brings a loss of prestige and status. In a society that places great emphasis on work and productivity, being cut off from a job commitment means a drastic change in lifestyle. Coupled with the general tendency in our society to value youth and denigrate age, it means that older persons who no longer play a meaningful role in society tend to feel useless and to lack a sense of self-worth and dignity.

Added to this is the problem of economic insecurity. The major sources of income for the elderly retired person are Social Security, employment pensions, welfare programs, savings and assistance from family members. Retirement almost always decreases income, however, and Social Security or pension benefits have no cost-of-living clauses to compensate for inflation. Certain expenses, such as medical costs, frequently increase sharply for older persons. As a result, many face an economic nightmare; their meager incomes barely stretch to meet their basic needs. In 1975, *Time* pointed out that

---

About a third of all aged Americans are plagued by poverty. Despite pensions, savings and Social Security, which will disburse $72 billion to 33.5 million recipients this year, fully 4.75 million of the nation's aged exist on less than $2,999 a year — well below the Federal Government's poverty line.[8]

In May 1977, the U.S. Senate Special Committee on Aging issued an annual report showing that poverty among the elderly was rising steadily, particularly among older blacks. Over half of this population group was living in poverty or near-poverty. Obviously, a large part of this problem is derived from the fact that older persons are customarily forced to retire from work and accept a sharply

---

[7]Victor Cohn: "Average Human Life Span Said Soon to Be 85 Years." *The Philadelphia Inquirer*, January 10, 1982, p. 7-F.
[8]"New Outlook for the Aged." *Time*, June 2, 1975, p. 45.

reduced standard of living, whether or not they are capable of continuing to do the job effectively. It has been pointed out that a substantial proportion of those over age 65 or 70 *would* be capable of continuing to do a full day's work; indeed, lawsuits have been initiated, with the support of the American Medical Association, challenging the federal government's retirement policies (see p. 328 for examples of other resistance to compulsory retirement).

During the first years of the Reagan administration, government officials sought to rebut the prevailing stereotypical view of older Americans as destitute, enfeebled, neglected and unfed. Reagan officials argued that most retired Americans live in houses they own, have adequate incomes, are in good health and do not need major new benefits.

On the other hand, Dr. Alex Comfort, in his popular work on aging, *A Good Age*, argues vigorously against retirement on both economic and psychological grounds. He describes "oldness" as a political institution and a social convention, based on a system "which expels people from useful work after a set number of years," bolstered by a large body of ignorant folklore that depicts the elderly as weak-minded and incompetent. He writes,

Retirement is another name for dismissal and unemployment. It must be prepared for exactly as you would prepare for dismissal and unemployment. You are about to join an underprivileged minority . . . (and) at a set age you will be deprived of half your income . . . [9]

In a study comparing the morale of employed and retired men over the age of 65, it was found that the retired individuals had distinctly poorer morale. Thompson considers four factors to be responsible for the morale problem: the retired had more negative evaluations of their health and were more functionally disabled, poorer and older. These factors, rather than retirement alone, accounted for the poor psychological adjustment of retired persons.[10] He concluded from the study that, while work undoubtedly was important, other pursuits could compensate for it; life in retirement could be as pleasant and fulfilling as continued employment.

In a review of research on attitudes toward retirement, MacNeil and Teague comment that much current writing on the subject is based on the idea that retirement is "forced." They argue, however, that a number of research studies do not support this view. Instead,

Most people look forward to retirement and most people like retirement when they get there. . . . (one authority) argues that the work ethic is overestimated and that, given adequate resources, most people "show no reluctance to embrace leisure roles."[11]

---

[9]Alex Comfort: *A Good Age.* New York, Simon and Schuster, 1976, p. 29.
[10]Gayle B. Thompson: "Work vs. Leisure Roles: An Investigation of Morale Among Employees and Retired Men." *Journal of Gerontology,* Third Quarter, 1973, pp. 339–344.
[11]Richard D. MacNeil and Michael L. Teague: *Therapeutic Recreation Journal,* Second Quarter, 1980, p. 7.

Shifting Family Roles

Traditionally in American society, several generations lived together. Older persons continued not only to receive the affection and support of their children or grandchildren but also to play meaningful roles in family life. With the shift toward urban and suburban living in apartments or one-family houses, increasing numbers of older persons are living alone in small apartments or single-room units. This is particularly true of women who have lost their husbands; the life expectancy of women at birth is 74 years, 13 years greater than that of men.

Many aged persons are faced with the problem of living alone, without family and with few friends. Often they are unable to take care of themselves properly. Particularly in run-down areas of larger cities, where they are often victims of thieves or muggers, old people tend to be afraid to leave their homes, and thus they are deprived of the opportunity for social contacts. The need for companionship does not diminish for older persons; with the breaking of other ties and an increased amount of leisure time, their loneliness becomes all the more difficult to bear. In some cities, it is not uncommon to see older persons sitting on benches along malls in the middle of crowded traffic or spending their entire days in bus or train terminals—just to be near people.

In a Canadian report on changing roles in retirement, Sissons and Vigoda point out that while we tend to think of older persons as married or recently widowed, the reality is that great numbers of senior citizens are single and have been so for a substantial period of time. Either they have never married or they were divorced at a much earlier age and did not remarry. In either case, their needs are distinctly different from those of their married counterparts; in many cases they have learned to be much more self-sufficient and happy with a single lifestyle. Another interesting phenomenon today is the growth of families that have two generations over age 65 as a result of greater longevity. Sissons and Vigoda comment that newly retired couples may find themselves in the unusual situation of being caught "between independent adult children and strong-willed elderly parents."[12] The point is that today's aged live in a wide variety of family structures and have changing roles. They should not be stereotyped by those who plan leisure services for the elderly.

Other Stereotypes of Aging

Frequently, older people behave in ways that younger people find childish. For example, many older people seem to live in the past and refuse to change or even be concerned with what is happening in the present. Although this is sometimes considered evidence of senility, it is quite understandable. For many aged persons, the present is bleak and unpleasant; they would *rather* live in the past. Childish behavior is also frequently considered a symptom of aging. However, in many cases

---

[12]Annabel Sissons and Debby Vigoda: *Leisure Can Be Pleasure: Changing Roles in Retirement.* Ministry of Culture and Recreation, Province of Ontario, 1981, p. 27.

it is the result of a self-fulfilling prophecy: when older people are expected to be childish and when they are treated like children, they naturally become helpless or petulant.

Complaints about being ill, often verging on hypochondria, also may be readily understood. Dr. Ewald Busse comments that when someone keeps criticizing the older person unjustly and

> . . . makes him feel unwanted, uncomfortable, he may retreat into an imaginary illness as a way of saying, "Don't make things harder for me. I'm sick and you should respect and take care of me." It is clear from our studies that if the older hypochondriac's environment changes for the better, he will too. He will again become a reasonable, normal person.[13]

It is also important for the older person or those around him to recognize that certain forms of behavior, such as forgetfulness, typically increase with aging but are not necessarily signs of senility. Altman points out that many conditions can produce symptoms that mimic senility, with the result that many older people are falsely labeled senile when their symptoms are due to depression, thyroid gland malfunction, pernicious anemia, effects of routine medication or other conditions that can be effectively treated or cured by psychotherapy or drugs.[14] Dr. Eric Pfeiffer, a Duke University psychiatrist, sums up the point,

> The most important stereotype regarding the elderly is that a certain amount of emotional instability, forgetfulness, depression and withdrawal is normal and therefore does not warrant medical intervention. On the contrary, early treatment might prevent deterioration or institutionalization, or both.[15]

It is also clear, however, that many older persons *do* find difficulty in adjusting to their changed status in life. One common problem is alcoholism. Although this is not commonly thought of as a disease of the aged, it was reported in the late 1960's that in the previous decade the death rate for alcohol-connected disorders had risen by more than 52 per cent for white males between the ages of 60 and 69 and by 114 per cent for white females in the same age group. Similarly, suicide appears to be a special problem of aged persons. Studies of elderly persons have shown that an unusually high proportion of persons over the age of 60 commit suicide; in fact, almost 30 per cent of suicides in the United States are in this age group. The rate of self-inflicted death among white American males over age 65 is three times that at the ages of 20 to 24, and research suggests that many of the fatal "accidents" among the elderly are actually suicides in disguise.

Researchers have concluded that many older persons, rather than directly

---

[13]Ewald Busse, in "The Old in the Country of the Young." *Time,* August 3, 1970, p. 51.
[14]Lawrence K. Altman: "Senility Is Not Always What It Seems To Be." *The New York Times,* May 8, 1977.
[15]Eric Pfeiffer, cited in "Can Aging Be Cured?" *Newsweek,* April 16, 1973, p. 57.

injure themselves, place themselves in life-threatening situations which tend to increase the possibility of their demise. A significant segment of the older population apparently no longer *wishes* to live and withdraws from active roles.

This point of view has been expressed in a theory of adjustment formulated in the early 1960's, known as "disengagement" theory.

DISENGAGEMENT THEORY

Cumming and Henry, who developed this theory, perceived aging as an inevitable mutual withdrawal or disengagement by older persons from others in the society. Withdrawal may be initiated on either side; the aged person may withdraw dramatically from some groups of people while remaining relatively close to others. Disengagement

---

. . . may be accompanied from the outset by an increased preoccupation with himself; certain institutions in society may make this withdrawal easy for him. When the aging process is complete, the equilibrium which existed in middle life between the individual and his society has given way to a new equilibrium characterized by a greater distance and an altered type of relationship.[16]

In essence, the theory suggests that society should accept the needs of older persons for a "dramatically reduced social life-space" and permit them, in effect, to disengage themselves from meaningful life relationships and move into roles of greater isolation. However, a number of leading sociologists and gerontologists have not been willing to accept this point of view. A Harvard sociologist, Chad Gordon, writes, "Disengagement theory is a rationalization for the fact that old people haven't a damn thing to do, and nothing to do it with."[17]

THE ACTIVITY APPROACH

In contrast, many authorities on aging favor an approach that sees successful adjustment as dependent on the aged person's ability either to find substitutes for activities carried on in previous years or to maintain such activities for as long as possible.

Both the "disengagement" and the "activity" approaches to adjustment have been criticized because they fail to take into account the wide individual differences in modes of adjustment; the two approaches deal with only one aspect of this process.

Obviously, people respond differently to the challenge of aging, depending on their family and marital status, their physical health, their economic status and their

---

[16]Elaine Cumming and William E. Henry: *Growing Old: The Process of Disengagement.* New York, Basic Books, 1961.
[17]Chad Gordon, in "The Old in the Country of the Young," *op. cit.*, p. 54.

psychological well-being. Reichard carried out a study of how retirement affected five different groups of men according to their personality types—the "mature," the "rocking chair," the "armored," the "angry" and the "self-haters."[18] In each category, there was a different response to retirement; several of the groups adjusted to it with relative ease. Reichard concluded that an understanding of personality types is essential for those who work with the aged, since the method of successful adaptation and role alignment of one group is not necessarily appropriate for another.

As one example of the falsity of certain stereotypes regarding the aged, one might point to the widely held belief that older persons normally no longer engage in sexual intercourse—and the dependent view that any older person who does is therefore "different." Research carried out at the Center for the Study of Aging and Human Development at Duke University indicated that between 40 and 60 per cent of different groups of subjects between the ages of 60 and 71 years reported that they still engaged in sexual intercourse with some frequency. Additional research has revealed that considerably older persons continue to have sexual relations successfully; such behavior seems to involve a continuation in modified form of earlier life patterns. Indeed, in some regions where large numbers of older retired persons settle, such as southern Florida, observers have noted that growing numbers of elderly people are having emotionally close, long-term affairs—often to the dismay of their children and grandchildren:

Rather than marry, many elderly men and women pair off in what one geriatric counselor calls "unmarriages of convenience"—relationships established for companionship and sex but never formalized because, as married couples, they would receive less income from Social Security and other retirement benefits than they do by remaining single.[19]

The point is that life does not *stop* at 65 or 75 years of age. The same needs and interests tend to continue; many of the weaknesses or problems demonstrated by older persons stem from their difficulty in adjusting to social, psychological, economic or physiological change.

According to Duke University researchers, the key factor in long and successful aging is remaining active on all three major levels—psychological, physical and social. Much depends on the attitudes the individual forms about the prospect of aging during his or her early years:

Those who lived longest were the ones who refused to give in. If widowed, they usually remarried. If retired, they took up hobbies. They took long walks and watched what they ate. And they took old age in stride. "The decision to have an active mental, physical and social life is really the important decision," says Dr. Eric Pfeiffer. "It's a yea-saying to life."[20]

---

[18]Suzanne Reichard, et al.: Cited in *Retirement Roles and Activities*. Washington, D.C., Report of 1971 White House Conference on Aging, 1971, pp. 20–21.
[19]"Romance and the Aged." *Time*, June 4, 1973, p. 48.
[20]Eric Pfeiffer, in "Can Aging Be Cured?", *op. cit.*, p. 66.

RECREATION'S ROLE WITH AGED
PERSONS

It is obviously important for older people to have a range of interesting recreational opportunities available to them, both to fill their long leisure hours and to meet, in a positive way, some of their important needs. What exactly are these needs, and what contribution does recreation make to them?

Improves Physical Health

A number of studies have established that physical recreation makes a significant contribution to the health of the aged, particularly in terms of cardiac function. Moderate and enjoyable exercise frequently means that individuals need not take certain drugs to relax. Exercise also helps to prevent progressive breakdown of the body systems. There is evidence that the satisfaction derived from continued physical activity is linked to human longevity.

Raymond Harris, a leading cardiologist, suggests that physical activity for older persons should include four basic elements: (1) relaxation; (2) endurance exercise to condition the heart, lungs and circulation; (3) muscle-strengthening exercise; and (4) stretching exercise to improve joint mobility and reduce the aches and pains accompanying the aging process. He writes,

---

Proper exercise can delay or at least retard changes associated with age in the musculoskeletal, respiratory, cardiovascular and central nervous systems. Even when these systems have already deteriorated due to lack of physical conditioning or to disease, partial improvement of fitness and other functions may be obtained when properly prescribed and adequately supervised exercise is followed for an extended period of time.[21]

Recognizing this need, a growing number of public recreation and park departments have initiated physical fitness programs for elderly residents. For example, the Chicago Park District operates 16 such programs in neighborhood gymnasiums throughout the city, including warm-up exercises, gymnastics, floor hockey and similar activities. Recently, C. Carson Conrad, Executive Director of the President's Council on Physical Fitness and Sports, conducted fitness workshops for thousands of elderly persons in 32 cities.

Leslie points out that the trend toward more exercise for the elderly is in sharp contrast to the prevailing opinion in the past. Exercise was customarily thought to be inappropriate and perhaps harmful for older persons. While it is still essential

---

[21]Raymond Harris, M.D.: "Leisure Time and Exercise Activities for the Elderly." *In* Timothy Craig, ed.: *The Humanistic and Mental Health Aspects of Sports, Exercise and Recreation.* Chicago, American Medical Association, 1975, p. 100.

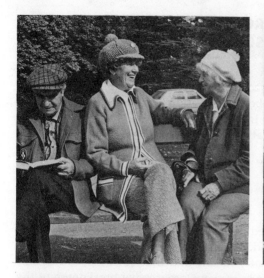
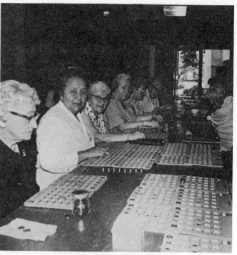
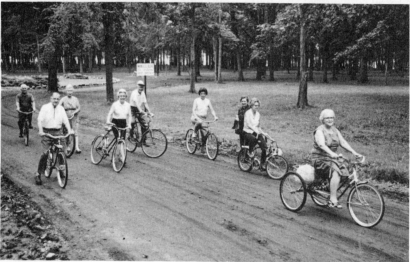

Elderly residents of Vancouver, Canada, enjoy a park and play bingo in a community center, while Flint, Michigan, senior citizens belong to a city-sponsored bicycling club.

to plan stress exercise programs under medical supervision (a policy that should be applied for all adult participants), Leslie reports that

> . . . current medical opinion is highly supportive of regular physical exercise both for the "healthy" person as one of the variables in staying healthy and as a means of rehabilitation for (older) persons recovering from certain illnesses or surgeries.[22]

[22]David K. Leslie: "Prescriptive Exercise for the Aged." *Therapeutic Recreation Journal*, Second Quarter, 1980, p. 39.

In addition to calisthenics or other therapeutic exercise programs, there is considerable value in older persons taking part in such recreational activities as horseshoes, croquet, pool, bowling, hiking, canoeing, fishing and gardening—all of which provide both pleasure and diversion as well as muscle toning, stretching and healthful relaxation and breathing benefits. Today, a growing number of older persons are taking part in more vigorous and active sports. In France, for example, elderly persons in *clubs d'animation* (vitality clubs) are encouraged to take part in a wide variety of physical activities, including exercise classes, hiking, swimming and cross-country skiing. Bowling, bike riding, tennis and jogging are becoming increasingly popular with the elderly. Despite the stereotype that generally assumes that people give up active sports once they reach their 30's, many people in their 60's, 70's and 80's today are playing strenuous games, competing in track and field events and even running the marathon!

In Florida, St. Petersburg's Three-Quarter Century Softball Club is composed of two teams, the Kids and the Kubs, who play each other in three seven-inning games a week from November through March. All players are at least 75 years old, with a number of star outfielders and catchers ranging up into the high 80's and 90's. Another unusual program that has been of special interest to the University of Southern California's Andrus Gerontology Center is the Senior Olympics, in which elderly athletes compete under medical supervision in such sports as basketball, boxing, canoeing, the decathlon, diving, fencing, handball, karate, power-lifting, racquetball, rugby, squash, tennis, track and field, water polo and wrestling. Yasgur writes,

---

Men in their 60's who throw a discus well over 100 feet, 55 year old sprinters who crack the 24 second mark for 200 meters, 75 year old men who compete in 16 events over two weekends or win two tennis titles (in 100° heat), and women aged 60 and older who set records in swimming, sprinting, and field events can shame many persons 30 years their junior. Obviously, they must be doing something right.[23]

Of course, not all elderly people are capable of such strenuous activity. Such examples, however, demonstrate that we are far too limited in our vision of what older people can accomplish—and of the benefits to be derived from regular exercise.

Improves Emotional Well-Being

Meaningful involvement in social, physical and creative recreational activities tends to improve the morale of most aged participants. It takes their minds off themselves, their illnesses and their problems and provides a sense of accomplishment. Generally, recreational activities contribute to a positive outlook toward life.

---

[23]Stevan S. Yasgur: "The Senior Olympics: Games for Adults Who Won't Quit." *Geriatrics*, January 1975, pp. 120–125.

Research has shown that for many elderly persons, feelings of depression and helplessness, as well as accelerated physical decline, may be attributable, in part, to their lack of autonomy and control over their environment. Increasing the degree of choice and control in residential care settings has been shown to have a measurable positive effect on the morale and well-being of residents.[24] Clearly, recreation provides an area in which older people can make choices, exercise initiative and gain important satisfactions.

The type of activity is not as important as the extent to which it meets an individual's important emotional needs. For example, recent studies have shown that keeping pets tends to counteract feelings of loneliness, depression, helplessness, boredom and low self-esteem among older persons. Pets provide a feeling of being needed and respected; they offer love and gratitude. Researchers have concluded that

---

. . . pets help to satisfy dependency needs, produce pride of ownership, serve as child substitutes, link people to the natural world, give unconditional love, provide companionship and build confidence in their owners. . . . People who have pets not only live longer, they are healthier and better adjusted. . . . Dogs (for example) are catalysts in human relationships. They encourage owners to get out and around, which is particularly important for the lonely, isolated elderly.[25]

Many other kinds of leisure involvements provide comparable emotional benefits for the elderly.

Reawakens Creative Impulses

For many older persons, the recreation programs found in a home for the aged or a community-based senior center offer opportunities in the arts, music, theater or literature that awaken or revive creative impulses not felt for many years. Again, these stimulate intellectual functioning and emotional well-being and encourage a sense of vitality and energy.

Vintage, Inc., a multi-service senior center in Pittsburgh that is described later in this chapter, offers classes in ceramics, sewing, music, drama, dance, photography, creative writing and poetry. Three performing groups—in music, drama and chorus—have developed from these classes at Vintage. In many cases, elderly persons who had never engaged in such activities before discover they have an unusual degree of talent. The activities provide a new, important interest in life.

---

[24]Rudolf H. Moos: "Environmental Choice and Control in Community Care Settings for Older People." *Journal of Applied Social Psychology*, First Quarter, 1981, pp. 23–42.
[25]Deborah Lawson: "Pets Can Be Vital Psychological Aid to the Elderly." *The Philadelphia Inquirer*, May 31, 1981, p. 14-F.

Encourages Social Involvement

Obviously, recreation can provide an atmosphere conducive to developing friendships and to overcoming isolation and loneliness. For many older persons who have been widowed or divorced, such programs may even result in friendships between the sexes that develop into marriage. There is a surprisingly large number of such marriages among elderly persons who meet in recreational settings, although match-making is not, of course, the program's primary purpose.

In institutions as well as in community programs, recreation has been shown to have a positive effect on socialization. In Pennsylvania state hospitals and nursing homes a series of studies demonstrated that swimming, arts and crafts, games and other social pastimes measurably increased the positive social interaction patterns of aged mental patients or residents.[26]

Another significant social value of recreation is its potential for breaking down patterns of age segregation. In a growing number of cases, community recreation programs that serve people of all ages, or that deliberately blend senior citizens and young people in shared programs and events, have been successful in bridging the "generation gap" that too often separates the elderly from other age groups.[27]

Provides Meaningful Roles

As described earlier, an important need of many older persons is for significant roles in society to supplant job or family responsibilities that have disappeared. For many aged persons, projects undertaken in recreation programs include giving assistance to the homebound or hospitalized, to children needing adult guidance or similar ventures. Sometimes projects involve political campaigning, working in ecology or providing advice to minority-group members who are beginning a business and need help from experienced, retired business persons. The opportunity to contribute to society and to feel of real value to other human beings is of great importance to the aged.

There are numerous examples of such programs being initiated by public and voluntary agencies, often with federal or state financial assistance. For example, three such programs that have been highly successful in the United States are (a) the Foster Grandparent Program, which pays older people for working with dependent and neglected youngsters; (b) the Retired Senior Volunteer Program (RSVP), which pays expenses to a large number of retired individuals who provide volunteer services in such settings as libraries and hospitals; and (c) the Senior Corps of Retired Executives (SCORE), which reimburses thousands of retired business people who assist individuals and community groups in business management.

---

[26]See Herberta M. Lundegren, ed.: *Penn State Studies on Recreation and the Aging.* State College, Pennsylvania State University, 1974, pp. 61–66, 75–79.
[27]Pam Emory: "A Program That Mixes Older with Younger." *Parks and Recreation,* February 1979, pp. 17–19, 51.

Davis and Teaff point out that recreation can provide a useful way of maintaining role continuity among older persons. They describe a program implemented at the Byer Activity Center of the Dallas Home for Jewish Aged in Dallas, which sought to determine the past roles of residents and to encourage them to maintain and continue these through the Center's activity program. For example, residents might have taken pride and pleasure in the past in being a hostess, salesperson, organizer, entertainer, mother, family man, visitor, musician, artist, receptionist or signmaker. Through recreation, they may continue these past roles in satisfying ways. For example, an elderly resident who had been a successful businessman, and who had become increasingly lonely and depressed in the home, was given the following responsibilities in the center:

. . . counting money from the soft drink machine, collecting fees for luncheons and trips, serving as the treasurer of the organization's council, helping on the membership committee, reporting on business and stock market changes at the men's discussion group, and operating the center's "post office". . . . By providing the opportunity . . . to continue his past preferences and experience, he is able to gain status and recognition while participating in a leisure program that is meaningful to him.[28]

Offers Threshold to Other Services

Obviously, recreation itself can be an extremely important experience for older persons, simply because it fills their greatly increased amount of leisure time in a satisfying way. Without fulfilling involvement, life could become extremely boring and empty.

However, recreation is also valuable in paving the way for elderly persons to become aware of other vital social services. Frequently, aged persons come to a center for the first time because of its recreational and social programs. However, once there, they learn to avail themselves of other services or opportunities, either within the center itself or through a referral process.

Concrete evidence of the increasing importance given to recreation for the elderly is found in a summary of the use of federal funds under the Administration on Aging grants program for states and municipalities. Of the many millions of dollars spent to assist local programs in a recent year, 34 per cent was used to support recreation and leisure-time activities, including hundreds of senior center programs—a higher percentage than that granted to any other form of service for older people living in communities.

---

[28]Natalie Beers Davis and Joseph D. Teaff: "Facilitating Role Continuity of the Elderly Through Leisure Programming." *Therapeutic Recreation Journal,* Second Quarter, 1980, pp. 32–35.

PROGRAMS PROVIDED FOR AGED
PERSONS

Recreation services are provided for aged persons in a variety of institutions and community programs, including the following:

1. Senior citizen's centers and Golden Age clubs.
2. Special residential centers, such as "leisure villages" or "retirement communities," or special housing projects of residences for the "well aged."
3. Day-care programs to serve aged persons who live at home but have serious disabilities that require special supportive services.
4. Programs for the homebound aged person.
5. Geriatric units in hospitals or nursing homes or skilled nursing care facilities that serve the dependent aged person.

The following section includes a description of programs offered in each of these categories. Since only 5 per cent of aged persons in the United States live in institutions or nursing homes, the greatest number of those who are to be served are in the community. Typically, such individuals are likely to find a range of leisure opportunities and social contacts in senior citizen's centers, Golden Age clubs or similar social programs designed for the elderly.

Senior Centers

These are described by Anderson, who carried out the first nationwide study of such programs, as

> ... places where older persons come together for a variety of activities and programs, ranging from sitting and talking or playing cards to professionally directed hobby and group activities. Some centers also provide counseling services to help the individual make better use of personal and community resources; some assume responsibility for encouraging community agencies to provide more help to senior citizens.[29]

Senior centers are considered to be agencies that meet for substantial periods of time several days a week, have professional staff direction and offer more than one form of service. Usually, they operate in their own facilities and may be sponsored by a variety of agencies, such as municipal recreation and park departments, housing or welfare agencies or religious federations. In contrast, Golden Age clubs

---

[29]Nancy N. Anderson: *Senior Centers: Information from a National Survey*. Minneapolis, Institute for Interdisciplinary Studies, American Rehabilitation Foundation, 1969.

are usually social or recreational clubs for older persons operating under volunteer or nonprofessional leadership and meeting once or twice a week or even less frequently.

In her study of 1002 senior centers, Anderson found that all agencies provided *recreational programs*, 73 per cent offered other *community services* and 60 per cent offered *counseling services* as well. Slightly over one third of all responding senior centers offered all three types of services.

A later study sampled 25 per cent of over 4800 community agencies selected on the basis of three factors: the center or club had to serve older adults, meet at least once a week on a regular basis and provide some form of educational, social or recreational program. The National Institute of Senior Centers, a component of the National Council on Aging, determined the following results from the study:

1. Older persons in our society are increasingly recognizing senior centers as appropriate and accessible resources for meeting their needs.
2. A growing number of such centers today provide multi-service programs for a broad spectrum of older persons.
3. Many centers, however, are limited by inadequate facilities and lack of full public recognition and support.

On the last point, the report stated that

Area agencies on aging, local councils on aging and boards of voluntary agencies in many communities have not fully exploited the potentiality of Senior Centers as a place where persons needing or wanting services or activities find them available without any stigma attached. They also have not recognized the potential of Senior Centers and clubs to expand their function and to become multi-service facilities and multipurpose Senior Centers.[30]

Despite such reservations, the National Institute of Senior Centers report found that program activities offered in the centers that were surveyed could be broken down as shown in Table 9-1.

Kaplan summarizes the characteristics of users of senior centers as described in the National Institute of Senior Centers study report:

About half of all Center participants were in the 65 to 74 age bracket; nearly one quarter were between 75 and 84 years of age; 85 percent were whites and 10 percent blacks; three of every four Center participants were women; relatively few Center users came from professional and managerial work backgrounds (16 percent), while former blue-collar workers made up 47 percent; one third of Senior Center participants were so poor that they had difficulty with dues; almost 60 percent of those who came to Centers lived alone . . . ; about 10 percent in Centers were physically disabled; and about the same proportion were deaf.[31]

[30]*Report of National Institute of Senior Centers.* In Max Kaplan: *Leisure: Lifestyle and Lifespan, Perspectives for Gerontology.* Philadelphia, W. B. Saunders Co., 1979, p. 103.
[31]*Ibid.*, p. 104.

Table 9-1 Average Hours Per Month Each Activity Offered[32]

	Hours Per Month	Per Cent of Total
Active recreation	22	.05
Creative activities	58	.14
Sedentary recreation	61	.15
Nutrition counseling	15	.038
Education	22	.05
Counseling	34	.08
Information and referral	50	.12
Other services (employment, health)	40	.10
Meals on premises	64	.16
Governing activities	10	.02
Leadership development	11	.02

STANDARDS FOR SENIOR CENTERS

Based on such research and on three years of intensive information-gathering from many individuals and agencies, the National Institute of Senior Centers published a detailed set of guidelines for senior centers in 1978. It was intended to promote a meaningful philosophy of service and to upgrade the quality of senior center programs. The document was based on nine principles:

1. **Purpose.**   A senior center shall have a written statement of its purpose consistent with the Senior Center Philosophy and a written statement of its goals based on its purposes and on the needs and interests of older people in its service area. These statements shall be used to govern the character and direction of its operation and program.

2. **Organization.**   A senior center shall be organized to create effective relationships among the participants, staff, governing body and the community in order to achieve its purposes and goals.

3. **Community Relations.**   A senior center shall form cooperative arrangements with community agencies and organizations in order to serve as a focal point for older people to obtain access to comprehensive services. A center shall be a source of public information, community education, advocacy and opportunities for community involvement of older people.

4. **Program.**   A senior center shall provide a broad range of group and individual activities and services designed to respond to the interrelated needs and interests of older people in its service area.

5. **Administration and Personnel.**   A senior center shall have clear administrative and personnel policies and procedures that contribute to the effective management of its operation. It shall be staffed by qualified, paid and volunteer personnel capable of implementing its program.

6. **Fiscal Management.**   A senior center shall practice sound fiscal planning, management, record keeping and reporting.

7. **Records and Reports.**   A senior center shall keep complete records required to operate, plan and review its program. It shall regularly prepare and circulate reports to inform its board, its participants, staff, sponsors, funders and the general public about its operation and program.

---

[32]*Ibid.*

8. **Facility.**   A senior center shall make use of appropriate facilities for its program. Such facilities shall be designed, located, constructed or renovated and equipped to promote effective access to and conduct of its program, and to provide for the health, safety and comfort of participants, staff and public.

9. **Evaluation.**   A senior center shall have adequate arrangements to monitor, evaluate, and report on its operation and program.[33]

Each of these principles is in turn spelled out with detailed standards of recommended practices and guidelines for implementing them according to high professional standards. To illustrate the trend in senior center programming today, the following section includes descriptions of several centers throughout the United States.

FRANKLIN H. PIERCE CENTER

One example of a senior center may be found in Flint, Michigan, where the Franklin H. Pierce Center provides several hundred older persons with a wide variety of social activities, games, classes, musical activities, physical conditioning, weight-watching programs and trips. This center was built with funds from the city of Flint and is assisted by the city in its operation. It offers scheduled programs five days a week and also has special activities on weekends. The Flint municipal recreation department operates a Senior Citizens Services Division, which uses the Pierce Center as a headquarters. The department operates other programs throughout the city, including the publication of a newspaper for senior citizens.

Among the program activities offered in the Pierce Center for Senior Citizens are the following: card games and instruction, craft classes, men's and women's choruses, dancing, golf, shuffleboard, lectures, library services, supper club, bingo, a "Married 50 Years and Over" Club and a special program of recreation for stroke victims that seeks to rehabilitate these individuals physically and socially. City-wide, the Flint Recreation and Park Board provides the following services to aged persons:

1. Publication of the *Senior Citizens News*.
2. Sponsorship of the Genesee County Senior Citizen Orchestra.
3. Publication of news releases for all news media regarding aging and senior citizens' programs.
4. Development of a discount card program, giving reduced rates and prices to older persons.
5. Sponsorship of a bicycle club, ecology club and over-80 club.
6. Planning of one-day bus trips and more extended vacation trips for older persons.
7. Sponsorship of other special events, including city-wide dances, parties, luncheons, tournaments and similar programs for senior citizens.

---

[33]National Institute of Senior Centers: *Senior Center Standards: Guidelines for Practice.* Washington, D.C., National Council on Aging, 1978, p. 17.

VINTAGE, INC.

Vintage is a multi-purpose center for senior adults living in Allegheny County, Pennsylvania. It was founded in a Pittsburgh church in 1973 by several religious organizations, the Junior League of Pittsburgh and other community residents. In 1979 it expanded to a large remodeled mansion with a program ten times more extensive than the original. Its program elements include the following:

1. **Education.**   Project DARE (Developing Adult Resources through Education) includes classes and enrichment groups in several curriculum areas.
2. **Recreation and Social Activities.**   Includes cards, table games, bingo, bowling, parties, trips and special events.
3. **Nutrition.**   A lunch program, supported by voluntary contributions, including satellite programs at other sites in the community funded by the Area Agency on Aging.
4. **Information and Referral.**   General assistance on a wide range of problems, using other community resources.
5. **Clubs.**   Several special-interest groups that develop out of the class offerings at Vintage.
6. **Outreach.**   A continuing effort to contact isolated persons in the community and to mobilize improved community services for the aging; includes speaking engagements, slide presentations, a regular radio program and door-to-door community canvassing.
7. **Counseling.**   Individual or small-group assistance in problems of adjusting to retirement or daily living and personal growth and values clarification. Includes financial, legal, health, tax, Social Security, rent and other problem areas.
8. **Health Services.**   Health evaluation and education programs, including gynecological and rectal screening examinations in cooperation with the American Cancer Society, and other tests for diabetes and vision or hearing problems. Group seminars on other health and safety problems and needs of the aging.
9. **In-Home Services.**   In addition to other Vintage services made available to the homebound, the following are offered: (a) Meals on Wheels, two meals a day, five days a week, delivered to those unable to shop or prepare food; (b) Friendly Caller and Visitation service, an on-going weekly call or visit to shut-ins; (c) Homemaker or Home Health Aide visits, to assist with light housekeeping and tasks of daily living; and (d) Chore Services, for heavier housekeeping tasks.
10. **Service Management or Protective Service.**   A fuller level of service for clients receiving in-home care, who have severe mental or physical disabilities, and need a high degree of supportive service or other specialized assistance.
11. **Small Businesses.**   Elderly persons are involved in planning and operating several small businesses through the center, including a craft shop, a shoe repair shop, a resale outlet and a beauty/barber shop.
12. **Transportation.**   As a subcontractor to the Area Agency on Aging, Vintage coordinates transportation for eligible aged persons in the district, for varied critical needs, primarily medical appointments and hospital visits.

As a United Way member, Vintage makes use of various funding sources to meet the social, psychological and physical needs of the center's clientele. During its unique Christmas festival, for example, which brings together people of many races and nationalities, Vintage helps to create an atmosphere of mutual respect and good will that is essential to its success in an inner-city area with many ethnic groups and social problems.

LONG BEACH, CALIFORNIA, SENIOR CENTER

A similar but larger multi-service senior center is provided by several public agencies in cooperation with other private groups in the city of Long Beach, California. Several years ago, the senior citizens of Long Beach approached the city with the need to establish and manage a multi-service senior center. Based on information from many groups and a large advisory council, three city departments—Health, Human Resources and Recreation—remodeled an old telephone company building with the help of $1.6 million in federal and state grants.

Described as a "one-step shopping center" for senior citizens' needs, the 50,000 square-foot Long Beach Senior Center offers health and dental services, cancer screening, food service, employment counseling, referral services, social clubs, recreation, entertainment, classes, lectures, dances and even chartered trips.

The City of Long Beach Health Department runs the health clinic on the premises. Geriatric care of all types is available in the clinic, including cancer screening, blood pressure checks and more. . . . the Harbor Dental Association sponsors a dental care unit in the Center that specializes in denture care, fitting and repair. . . . a local community college, Long Beach City College (offers courses at the Center including) foreign language, composition, sociology, gerontology, and more.[34]

SEMINARS AND SERVICES

Obviously, few senior centers throughout the United States and Canada are likely to have as wide a range of services as those in Long Beach and Pittsburgh. However, most senior center administrators realize they must provide far more than bingo or birthday parties to meet the needs of the elderly in their communities.

Programs should help to support and improve the lives of older persons, particularly those in large cities who are isolated or dependent. For example, the Los Angeles Park and Recreation Department sponsors a series of seminars directly related to the needs of older persons on such topics as "consumer protection," "dental care," "fraud schemes" and "housing." These are scheduled at ten centers specifically designed to meet the needs of older residents and at more than 75 other facilities where programs for senior citizens are part of the overall departmental programs. In addition, Los Angeles sponsors a Senior Citizens' Federation that unites all older people in the metropolitan area in joint efforts to meet their needs in such areas as recreation, health and housing services, legal aid, Social Security, legislation and similar concerns. It sponsors major city-wide events for older persons, many of which attract thousands of aged participants.

Operating in cooperation with the Mayor's Departmental Council on Aging, the Detroit, Michigan, Department of Parks and Recreation provides extensive services for senior citizens. In addition to its own centers, it sponsors several in cooperation with the United Auto Workers, a labor union that has traditionally taken a

---

[34]Terri S. Langhans: "Multi-Service Senior Centers—A New Role for Recreation." *California Parks and Recreation*, February/March 1979, pp. 22–23.

strong interest both in recreation and in the needs of its retired members. The Detroit Senior Citizens program strongly emphasizes leadership among older persons, having them serve as volunteers or paid leaders in programs and encouraging their involvement in public service.

Like Los Angeles, Detroit provides information to older persons on reduced rates for transportation, food, housing, library service, resident camping for senior citizens, golf, fishing and other programs available at limited cost.

In numerous other cities throughout the country, recreation and park departments are providing services for elderly and retired persons, operating chiefly through senior centers and Golden Age clubs. In many cases club members themselves assume a great deal of responsibility for planning and carrying on programs and for providing volunteer leadership to help homebound elderly persons.

An important element of program services provided by senior centers was added in the mid-1970's when the federal government began to provide more than $125 million a year for nutrition programs. Administered according to federal and state guidelines and under the direct supervision of county or city agencies, this plan permitted centers of all types to provide low-cost or free meals daily to older persons who otherwise might have been unable to meet their nutritional needs adequately.

Residential Centers

Another important aspect of recreation service for the elderly may be found in residential centers that serve older people in our society. They are of several different types: (a) "retirement communities" or "leisure villages"; (b) special apartments or units in housing projects that are set aside for the elderly; (c) adult homes or residential facilities that provide full care, including meals and activities for the well aged; and (d) new communal arrangements of older persons living in groups independently, with some supportive services.

RETIREMENT COMMUNITIES

Many elderly persons are in relatively good health and are financially capable of independent living. Large numbers of such individuals have chosen in recent years to live in retirement villages or communities established specifically to attract older persons.

This concept, which began on the West Coast, has since gained popularity throughout the United States. Generally, it consists of houses or garden apartments designed for maximum convenience and safety. Normally, only persons beyond a certain age are eligible to enter such communities. They may do so by purchase of property, on a rental basis, through a condominium or cooperative arrangement or a variety of other financial procedures. Since the units may be extremely expensive, they tend to appeal chiefly to elderly couples who are financially independent.

Although services vary considerably, in many leisure villages, medical care is available as part of group plans. In some, meals are served in dining buildings as part of the overall plan; properties are maintained by central services, and house-keeping services may also be provided. Because of the convenience they offer, as well as the safety (most villages have elaborate security, and some are actually walled villages), retirement communities have become extremely attractive to many retired persons.

Some of the best known retirement communities include Rossmoor–Walnut Creek in California, Heritage Village in Connecticut and Sun City, Arizona, probably the largest of its kind with over 28,000 residents in the late 1970's, and expected to expand to 50,000 homeowners within several years. Sun City has six shopping centers, nine golf courses and five recreation centers (one containing Arizona's largest indoor swimming pool), as well as an amphitheater, a stadium, two lakes and the country's first synthetic-surface lawn bowling green. Typically, all retirement communities stress recreational facilities, hobbies, clubs and programs—both to attract new residents and to meet the interests and capability levels of residents. Rossmoor, for example, has over 160 different clubs, as well as philanthropic groups and professional associations of former teachers or engineers:

These clubs help to integrate newcomers into the community. They also help structure people's time, giving them someplace to be or something to do at fixed hours and days. This can be particularly useful for men accustomed to going to an office, but it is also a boon for their wives. . . . Not only does it get the men out of their way, but it also helps preserve the distinction between male and female roles, which often gets blurred with retirement. A surprisingly large number of Rossmoor's clubs are designated as being for men only or for women only.[35]

Increasingly, retirement communities are employing social or recreation directors to conduct these programs, and usually a members' council makes policy and helps to schedule activities.

SPECIAL HOUSING UNITS FOR THE ELDERLY

A somewhat different form of residential development for older persons is found in apartment buildings or other housing units for the elderly. Unlike retirement villages, which are usually in suburban or rural areas with many separate housing units over a large tract of land, these developments may involve a single high-rise apartment building or converted hotel or possibly garden apartments that are specially designated for older persons. In some cases, the housing units may involve a proportion of small apartments within a publicly assisted low-income or middle-income housing development that are set aside by prearrangement for senior citizens only. In such developments, usually there are also clubs and hobbies and in some cases a senior center as part of the entire structure—although the recreation facilities are much less impressive than in retirement communities.

---

[35]Sheila K. Johnson: "Growing Old Alone Together." *The New York Times Magazine*, November 11, 1973, p. 40.

RESIDENTIAL FACILITIES FOR THE SEMI-DEPENDENT AGED

In some cases, three or four different kinds of living arrangements may be provided within a large complex, including nursing home facilities for the ill and dependent aged, assisted but separate housing for the semi-dependent and relatively independent units for the well aged. In each case, recreation programs are likely to be provided at an appropriate skill level. As a later section will show, recreation in facilities serving residents with a serious degree of disability is necessarily more limited and more therapeutically designed than programs serving independent individuals.

In some cases, housing units for the elderly have been set up in which they live in a congregate, or "commune," environment and share skills and abilities to help maintain each other. Based on similar programs in England and Sweden, such living units require strong assistance from an outside agency. Typically, the Weinfeld Group Living Residence, a renovated townhouse complex in Evanston, Illinois, has 11 women residents, some of whom were formerly in nursing homes or psychiatric hospitals. With each others' help and with services from a cook, caseworker, activities therapist and other aides provided by the Council for Jewish Elderly, these elderly women are able to carry on successfully in the community. Such arrangements provide a sensible and humane living environment for older people who would otherwise have to be institutionalized.

In some cases, "total life care" facilities have been built to provide convenient and safe living for aged persons with a degree of disability. The responsibility for housekeeping, repairs, meals and grounds care is assumed by the community administration. There are emergency call buttons to an adjoining health care center that provides preventive, emergency and long-term medical or nursing care on both an inpatient and outpatient basis. A typical fee for admission to such a housing facility in the late 1970's ranged from $25,000 upward, with an additional monthly service charge for utilities, transportation, repairs, security, cleaning, linen and recreation facilities.[36]

Day-Care Services for Disabled Aged in the Community

A number of community centers or health complexes throughout the United States have established center programs providing vital medical, nutritional, social and activity programs that permit elderly disabled persons to live at home rather than be forced into nursing homes or hospitals. For example, one such program, held at the Mosholu-Montefiore Community Center in New York, serves approximately 85 patients with a mixture of medical and social services, including transportation, meals, art, music and occupational therapy, physical examinations and health counseling, escorting patients to medical appointments and nursing care.

---

[36]"Retirement Living: Total Life Care." *The Philadelphia Inquirer*, November 4, 1979, p. 10.

Recreation is a significant part of the overall program, with a full-time recreation therapist serving as part of the interdisciplinary team. Beckerman describes the role of the recreational program:

It consists of movies, current events discussion, trips, art, music and other activities. Participation in recreation is voluntary, with greatest involvement in arts and crafts. The overall purpose of the recreation therapy program is the opportunity for self-expression, physical exercise, and socializing. Through recreation, patients learn and sometimes relearn skills which they can utilize in their own home. Activities permit functioning at various levels of concentration, intensity and skill. Interaction between patients and group experiences create a familiar, safe environment. Over time, groups of patients begin to form their own communication network, encouraging dyad and triad involvement for formally isolated patients.[37]

Like other programs described, such programs permit individuals to continue to live in the community at considerably less cost and with much greater satisfaction than if they had to be placed in nursing homes or hospital geriatric units. In some cases, supplementary services such as podiatry, dentistry and ophthalmology may be provided, along with social services and more intensive counseling.

Such programs have grown rapidly in recent years. With Massachusetts, California and Georgia leading the way, *Time* magazine reports that some 800 day-care centers have been established in 44 states and Puerto Rico. For an increasing number of Americans, *Time* reports, day-care provides a happy solution to the problems posed by infirmity and old age:

For people . . . who are disabled but not in need of full-time nursing care, they fill the vital gap between neighborhood senior citizen centers, which are generally not equipped for the handicapped, and . . . institutionalization. For families of the infirm elderly they offer welcome relief from the strain of providing full-time care for an ailing relative at home and from the guilt that often comes from banishing that person to a nursing home, perhaps prematurely.[38]

Services for Homebound Elderly

A growing number of agencies have outreach services to assist elderly persons who have severe impairments and cannot readily leave their homes. These include health-aide or nursing care, friendly visiting, shopping and cooking help, telephone reassurance and similar services. In many cases, elderly persons who are mobile themselves assist by visiting the homebound regularly, either on a volunteer

---

[37]Sheba Beckerman: "Geriatric Day Care Center." Graduate paper at Herbert Lehman College, New York, 1975.
[38]Claudia Wallis: "Day Care Centers for the Old." *Time,* January 18, 1982, p. 60.

basis or as part of a program funded under the Older Americans Act. Such assistance does much to overcome the physical and psychological isolation of homebound elderly persons and to make their lives more comfortable and happy. Recreation may be provided on a one-to-one basis, with outside visitors bringing in hobby activities, teaching skills or helping the homebound persons use their leisure more creatively and enjoyably than before.

In an article on alternative kinds of community living arrangements for the elderly, *Newsweek* reported in 1977 that

One of the most impressive community-service programs is the Older American Resources and Services program (OARS) at the Duke University Center. Aside from providing legal, medical and at-home nursing care, OARS arranges for "chore workers" who cook and do odd jobs in the house, "meals on wheels" to provide shut-ins with home-delivered meals, and a volunteer corps of drivers who take the disabled on trips. "We try to come up with a service package to allow each person to stay in the community," says director Dan G. Blazer. In Massachusetts, officials of the Department of Elderly Affairs are experimenting with a variety of alternative-living arrangements. Instead of purely social Golden Age Centers, they have established eight day-care centers and are experimenting with boarding houses and communes, where small groups of residents can care for each other, and an "adoption center," through which old people can live with young families.[39]

Although the number of such experimental arrangements is small, they offer much hope for avoiding the institutionalization of hundreds of thousands of elderly persons. Today, however, the most widespread method of caring for elderly, disabled individuals who cannot, for physical or psychological reasons, care for themselves in the community is admission to nursing homes or geriatric units in hospitals.

Institutional Programs for the Elderly

Today, there are approximately 23,000 nursing homes in the United States, in addition to thousands of geriatric or chronic-care units in hospitals—some of them in state psychiatric hospitals for the disoriented or senile patient. Nursing homes are of all types, operated by public authorities, voluntary organizations and proprietary owners, many of whom rushed into this field when the federal government began to pay for nursing home care through Medicaid; by the mid-1970's, $4.4 billion of Medicaid's overall $12.7-billion budget was spent on the elderly. Monthly charges for elderly and chronically infirm patients ranged from $1200 to $1800 a month by the mid-1970's, with many unscrupulous operators providing seriously substandard services and facilities. Mary Adelaide Mendelson of Cleveland, a community-planning consultant who spent ten years studying institutions for the aged, concluded that nursing homes in the United States were a national scandal and

[39]"The Graying of America," *op. cit.*, p. 57.

wrote a book titled *Tender Loving Greed*. "There is a widespread neglect of patients in nursing homes across the country and evidence that owners are making excessive profits at the expenses of patients."[40]

To prevent such exploitation, a number of states have developed strong nursing home codes as well as accreditation and inspection procedures. It is within such codes that the strongest support of recreation as a vital service for the institutionalized aged is found. For example, Connecticut's State Department of Health has established the following code for approval of nursing homes:

Standards for Certification of Therapeutic Recreation Program by Connecticut State Department of Health

I. Physical Requirements
   A. There shall be adequate space to accommodate recreation program in the form of recreation rooms and/or day spaces.
   B. There shall be separate facilities for administration of program, and for storage of supplies and equipment.

II. Administration
   A. There shall be a professional recreation director or a person having equivalent experience and training, who shall direct and supervise the recreation program in the institution. This program director shall be approved by the State Department of Health. Upon approval, two weeks' in-service training is required, and will be arranged by the State Department of Health.
   B. The program director will be other than a regular employee of the institutional staff, and will wear street dress.
   C. The program director will be required to work the number of hours per week as determined by the licensed capacity of the institution as follows:

5–14 beds	10 hours per week (at least 3 days)
15–29 beds	20 hours per week (5 days)
30–59 beds	30 hours per week (5 days)
60–120 beds	40 hours per week (5 days)

   For *each* additional 60 beds or fraction thereof, 40 hours per week is required.
   D. The program director shall generally work Monday through Friday, except for special program events on holidays and weekends or evenings. Work schedule shall be filed with the State Department of Health.
   E. The State Department of Health shall be notified immediately when any change in program director occurs.

III. Records
   A. Monthly reports shall be submitted *by the 10th of each month* to the State Department of Health and shall include:
      1. Advanced Monthly Program Calendar
      2. Current month's Patient Participation Record
      3. Budget breakdown on program costs
   B. Four additional records shall be kept on file at the facility:
      1. Patient Interest and Progress Record
      2. Volunteer Interview Record
      3. Volunteer Sign In Record
      4. Clergy Sign In Record

---

[40]Mary Adelaide Mendelson, in "New Outlook for the Aged," *op. cit.*, p. 46.

IV. Program Requirement
   A. The program shall be planned from *individual patient/resident needs and interests.*
   B. Activities shall be regularly scheduled and planned monthly in advance.
   C. There shall be diversified group and individual activities to include *per week:*
      1. *Art or Craft Program*
         a. Individual art or crafts for patient/resident at bedside where indicated.
      2. *Games* such as bingo, horse racing, bowling, and shuffleboard.
         a. Participation should be encouraged in special interest or small group games such as cards, checkers, chess and dominoes.
      3. *Cultural Activity* —music, literature, drama, adult education.
         a. Individual interest to be pursued and encouraged.
      4. *Religious Assembly* —conducted by clergy and/or volunteers.
         a. Individual pastoral and lay visits should be encouraged.
      5. *Personal Services* —to include letter writing, reading to, library service and patient/resident visitation.
   D. At least two of the following activities shall be scheduled per month:
      1. Film
      2. Birthday party
      3. Entertainment program
      4. Special event such as holiday party, picnic, bus trip, or carnival.
   E. Special Interest or small hobby group activities shall be provided.
   F. The program shall be evaluated and revitalized periodically with new ideas and/or adaptation of standard activities.
   G. Work activity, community service, out trips, group discussions, current events, story telling, puppets, marionettes, skits, variety shows, and fashions, as well as hobbies should be incorporated in general programming when interest and capabilities so indicate.
   H. Effort should be focused to secure volunteer assistance for all programs and especially for personal patient/resident contact as friend to friend.
      1. Interviewing, screening and orientation of volunteers is necessary.
      2. Supervision, evaluation, and coordination of volunteer efforts is required, with staff as well as with general program.
      3. Recognition of volunteer assistance should be encouraged by administrator and staff of facility.

V. General Information
   A. Renewal of certification will occur yearly from date of initial accreditation.
   B. Approval may be withdrawn by the State Department of Health at any time should the institution fail to meet the requirements outlined in the above specifications.
   C. Approval will be automatically revoked within 30 days after the resignation of a program director. Re-certification must be made in the name of program director replacement.
   D. Special seminars for program directors will be offered periodically by the State Department of Health, which program directors shall attend.
   E. Program Directors should avail themselves of continuing training and educational opportunities through professional organizations and educational institutions.

Many other states have similar requirements. For example, New York state law requires that for each resident in a nursing home there must be at least a half hour of planned leisure activities each week. Activities must be available seven days a week and should include both individual and group programs at various levels. Typically, a nursing home housing 200 residents should have a recreation staff consisting of one full-time director and volunteers, two full-time recreation therapists, one part-time specialist and one full-time clerical worker.

The responsibilities of the program director would be to (a) prepare weekly, monthly, biannual and yearly schedules of programs; (b) designate work assignments for therapists and volunteers; (c) attend staff and resident council meetings; (d) seek out community resources and arrange cooperative programs with interested groups; (e) interview new residents and determine their recreational needs and interests; (f) design individual and group activities as needed; and (g) maintain records of each resident's progress and evaluate both residents and the overall activity program.

GUIDELINES FOR RECREATION IN NURSING HOMES

Despite the negative publicity about nursing homes, there are many excellent ones throughout the United States and Canada that live up to such guidelines and go far beyond them. What *are* the elements of effective recreation in such settings?

Hisek suggests the qualities required for effective leadership in nursing homes.[41] Recreation therapists should have a positive outlook, be able to work independently and be creative, outgoing and willing to learn new skills and accept new ideas. It is essential for the leader to be able to relate to residents, to respect their dignity and gain *their* respect, and to understand their likes, dislikes and needs.

Suitable Activities

Since many residents are bedridden, confined to wheelchairs or otherwise limited physically, it is necessary to avoid physical activity of a strenuous nature. However, it certainly is possible to provide games that require a moderate amount of activity for those residents who are able to take part. Although many older persons in extended-care facilities have limited mental capabilities, others are perfectly capable of enjoying activities that require verbal or intellectual participation.

In general, activities fall into the following classifications:

1. *Arts and crafts*—particularly activities such as knitting, needlepoint, crocheting or similar crafts that do not require elaborate shops or complicated equipment.
2. *Music*—both as a participatory activity (group singing, rhythm instruments or small ensembles) and as a form of entertainment.
3. *Dramatics*—in the form of skits, recitations, pantomimes or creative dramatic programs.
4. *Dance*—with social, folk and square dancing involving those residents who are physically able to take part, and with simple rhythmic movement involving even patients in beds or wheelchairs.
5. *Religious services*—including Bible readings, hymm singing, meditation or rosary programs or more formal worship services. Volunteer groups frequently come from the community to assist in such activities and then extend their involvement to include personal visiting and other recreational activities.

---

[41]D. Hisek: "Recreation Planning for a Nursing Home." *Therapeutic Recreation Journal*, Second Quarter, 1978, pp. 26–27.

6. *Films*—may include travelogues or popular movies shown to all residents or home movies or slides of residents' families, which may be viewed individually in their bedrooms or dayrooms.
7. *Other activities*—include special interest groups such as *hobbies* (gardening, cooking, scrapbook collections or photography), *social programs* (such as parties, bingo, birthday events or discussion groups), *games* (adapted bowling, golf, shuffleboard, horse racing and toss games) and *trips and outings*.

Programs should be geared to residents who are bedridden or have limited mobility as well as to those who can get around easily. Beauty parlor and other self-care activities must be brought to residents who are confined to their rooms. Even if a resident can benefit from no other activities than visits and conversation, it is important that they be provided. Often, patients who have few interests and who at first resist involvement gradually begin to participate more fully.

Whenever possble, programs should give elderly residents the opportunity to take on meaningful responsibilities or provide needed services themselves. Residents of the A. Holly Patterson Home for the Aged in Uniondale, New York, for example, spend many hours stuffing envelopes for UNICEF, the March of Dimes and similar charities. Patients serve on a residents' council and on committees to greet new residents and counsel them when they are having difficulty making the transition. In many other ways, they assume meaningful responsibilities in the institution.

In the nursing home or skilled nursing care facility, recreation is more than an amenity or frill. Just as in the outside world, if stimulating and interesting activities are not provided for the patient who is confined to a bed, wheelchair or dayroom, boredom, lethargy and low morale will inevitably result. Vital and absorbing recreation is essential to maintain alertness and interest and, indeed, to reverse a patient's isolation and withdrawal. In a study titled "Effects of an Individualized Activity Program on Elderly Patients," Salter and Salter point out that elderly patients suffering from psychological disorders and long-term physical illness are often considered to be in an irreversible state of decline. On the other hand, they describe an individualized program of activity applied to 21 such patients that included reality orientation, activities of daily living and recreational activities, such as games, arts and crafts, singing, social programs and outdoor activity. The researchers reported that

---

Those with the motivation to participate in the available activities increased from 14 per cent to 76 per cent in just four months. Many who had not cared for their daily necessities, walked, or talked in years came to do so once more, some to the extent that they could leave the hospital.[42]

They concluded that individualized approaches should be used much more widely in geriatric institutions. Dulcy Miller, a leading nursing home administrator,

---

[42]Carlotta de Lerma Salter and Charles A. Salter: "Effects of an Individualized Activity Program on Elderly Patients." *The Gerontologist*, October 1975.

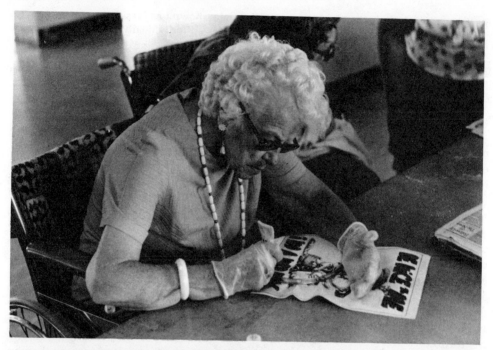

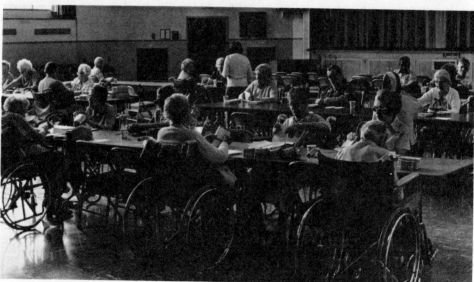

Elderly residents of the A. Holly Patterson Home in Nassau County, New York, take part in arts and crafts and community-service activities, such as volunteer mailing projects.

has agreed that recreation in a nursing home implies far more than just spending leisure time enjoyably; instead, it is part of a total concept of patient care:

Social rehabilitation of patients in a nursing home setting is effected through a treatment program that includes medicine, nursing, physical therapy, religion, occupational therapy, social work services and recreation. With optimal patient function the goal of the long-term care facility, recreation plays a particularly important part in the totality of professional disciplines. Consequently, the administration of a progressive nursing home is committed to the encouragement and development of the imaginative recreation service.[43]

Miller points out that therapeutic and diversional programs must be planned in terms of various levels of patient capability. Such activities as music, reading, gardening, crafts or games may be used individually or on a group basis to help integrate individual patients into the community of patients. In addition, programs for the entire patient population, such as religious services or celebrations, music or dance performances or other entertainment may provide colorful highlights.

Patients with organic brain damage may enjoy simple, rhythmical musical activities, simple crafts or repetitious exercise, parties or similar events. On the other hand, those patients who may have suffered physical impairment but whose brain function is sound will enjoy more sophisticated programming, including discussion groups, art and music appreciation, more complicated games and entertainment on a higher level.

Recreation personnel in nursing homes frequently complain that the service they provide is not understood, or supported, by other members of the staff. Therefore, Miller suggests that the administrator should assist recreation personnel in maintaining satisfactory intra-staff relationships:

. . . by interpreting the recreation program to other departments, seeking cooperation of the nursing and housekeeping departments as to scheduling to provide ample time for activity programs and by lending the weight of her position to experimental projects. The administrator also assists the staff in organization of written material of an administrative nature, e.g., development of manual and resources file.[44]

Activities must be scheduled at hours of greatest leisure and must avoid conflict with nursing care or medical treatment. It is usually possible to provide some individualized programs in the morning, but afternoons usually offer the largest segment of completely free time; therefore, most group activities are scheduled after lunch. In some homes, with supper over early, individual activities or special events may also be planned for the early evening hours. As much as possible, patients

---

[43]Dulcy B. Miller: "Nursing Home Setting." *Parks and Recreation*, January 1967, p. 38.
[44]*Ibid.*, p. 54.

should be involved in planning, both in choosing desirable activities for the program and in actually running parties and other special events. Many of the special techniques described in Chapter 4, such as sensory training and remotivation, may also be provided as part of the activity program. In some nursing homes, libraries operated by residents meet the leisure needs of more alert patients and provide an area in which they can offer volunteer help. Daily newspapers and current magazines, including publications in large-print editions, help residents keep in touch with the outside world. Speakers, films, slide showings, visits by outside groups and trips to places of interest in the outside community, including shopping by residents who are able to travel independently, all help to maintain contact with the outside.

As with persons with other types of disability, aged persons in institutions have traditionally been given little voice in deciding issues afecting their own lives and have often been treated as children. Today, there is a fuller effort to involve them meaningfully in policy-making and to give them a greater degree of freedom in determining their own behavior.

It was pointed out earlier in this chapter that aged persons often are capable of maintaining sexual relationships, contrary to widespread stereotypes. This has led to a serious policy question regarding the right of older persons in nursing homes to maintain sexual relationships. A federally funded workshop for nursing home operators in Arkansas, conducted by the National Association of Social Workers and funded by the Department of Health, Education and Welfare, considered a proposal for providing "privacy rooms" in which aged persons could hold hands, pet or engage in sexual relations. The proposal was presented by a sociology professor at Henderson State University, who contended that segregation of the sexes and lack of privacy in institutions for older persons afford almost no opportunity for physical or emotional contact:

I am not advocating copies of *Hustler* magazine and a water bed, but these people are human beings. They enjoy petting, holding hands, kissing. All those things that make us feel good make them feel good, too. Age has nothing to do with the fact that you need nurture and comfort.[45]

The proposal was almost universally opposed by the nursing home operators, arguing that patients might "abuse" privacy rooms. In the brochure of at least one home for the elderly, however, the policy is established that roommates of the opposite sex are not "frowned upon"; one's choice of a companion is the individual's decision, not the home's. Clearly, this is part of a larger trend toward treating the disabled as normal people, with normal desires and rights. As an earlier chapter showed, groups with physical disability today are also being given fuller rights and assistance in establishing appropriate sex roles and living patterns for themselves.

Given the tremendous variety in services for the aged in nursing homes, health-related facilities, proprietary homes and community-based services or cen-

---

[45]"Sex for Aged Issue in Arkansas." *The New York Times*, March 13, 1977, p. 26.

ters, it would appear that there is a growing need for government to expand its role on all levels if the needs of aged persons in modern society are to be met more adequately. What *are* the major functions of government with respect to aged persons, at present?

ROLE OF THE FEDERAL GOVERNMENT

The federal government has provided varied forms of help for older persons in the United States for several decades. Since 1935, when Social Security was established, it has provided retirement income for a large number of elderly persons.The Medicare and Medicaid programs greatly relieve the burden of medical costs for the aged by helping to pay hospital bills, bills for stays in extended-care facilities and medical bills for those who live at home. In addition, it has set standards for the care received in various types of facilities licensed to serve the aged.

A second major contribution was the passage of the Older Americans Act of 1965. Many of the programs initiated by this law have had recreational elements. In some cases, programs have supported community services for aged persons, particularly senior centers and multi-service programs. In others, such as the Foster Grandparents Program initiated by the Administration on Aging and supported at the outset by the Office of Economic Opportunity, older persons have been paid to work full- or part-time with disadvantaged children. In other programs, such as employment projects funded by the U.S. Department of Labor, older persons have been placed in jobs as community aides—many with recreation responsibilities.

Under Title IV of the Older Americans Act, many research programs and demonstration projects have been funded. These have tended to focus heavily on the process of successful aging and the kinds of community services required to promote healthy adjustment in later life. The goals of such projects have been described by the Social Rehabilitation Service of the Administration on Aging in the following terms:

Each project focuses on the older American and a specific factor which contributes to his living a wholesome, meaningful and satisfying life—as free as possible from fear, loneliness, and undue disappointment. The need for differentiating the problems of various sub-groups of older persons and of tailoring solutions to the needs and resources of the community and of the particular persons to be served are also recognized in the projects funded under Title IV.[46]

It must be recognized, however, that the federal government in the United States has been less active in helping the elderly than many European countries. In the Scandinavian countries, for example, city governments, with assistance from the national government, run housing developments where the aged can live close to

---

[46]*Aging*. Washington, D.C., Social Rehabilitation Service of Administration on Aging. U.S. Department of Health, Education and Welfare, January 1969, p. 6.

transportation and recreational activities. These governments provide a much wider range of subsidized housing, transportation and day-help service.

STATE PROGRAMS FOR THE ELDERLY

An important section of the Older Americans Act was Title III, which funds state programs for the elderly. In order to receive grants, states are required to organize state-wide agencies and develop plans for serving the aged, subject to the approval of the Secretary of Health and Human Services.

Although this overall program has met the needs of only a small fraction of aged persons, it has obviously been a step in the right direction. With its assistance, a number of states have moved ahead aggressively to provide recreation programs and services for the elderly. Among these have been Michigan and Connecticut.

Michigan

The state government of Michigan has organized a Commission on Aging to coordinate the issuance of funds from Title III. The state's attitude is reflected in the statement of Governor William Milliken, made to the 1971 Conference on Aging: "In this youth-oriented culture of ours, we have sent too many of our older citizens to a kind of early death—a quiet limbo where they will live out their remaining years without becoming a burden to our pocketbooks or our consciences."[47]

Michigan aids communities in establishing low-cost housing and developing community centers for the aged. Such centers customarily provide a wide range of services, including free community education at local schools (several Michigan school districts are leaders in the field of school-sponsored adult education and recreation); telephone calls, visitations and similar services for elderly shut-ins; counseling; trips; and other social activities. The state provides funding to the Institute of Gerontology at the University of Michigan and to Wayne State University to conduct research or hold workshops on problems of the aged.

Connecticut

For a number of years, Connecticut has been a leader in recognizing the importance of recreation in programs for the aged. In 1960, with the support of funds from the U.S. Public Health Service, the Connecticut State Department of Health employed a recreational consultant to supervise the organization of recreation programs in institutions, hospitals and nursing homes. This consultant, Dorothy Mullen, reached a number of major objectives, among them having the State Depart-

---

[47]"Report of 1971 Michigan Conference on Aging."

ment of Health establish standards for programs and staff at institutions serving the chronically ill and aged.

Under Mullen's leadership, the state also provided a variety of consultative services to improve patients' activities programs. Connecticut also has emphasized the use of skilled volunteers. A yearly conference recognizes the important contribution made by volunteers and also provides them with needed skills training.

Such efforts on the part of the states are generally reflected in programs in large cities. For example, the New Haven Department of Parks and Recreation has assumed a major responsibility for providing programs for the elderly. Its programs include a number of senior centers and a "Mobile Workers Outreach Program" (which assists elderly persons in a number of low-income housing units), a "Meals on Wheels" program, a "friendly visiting" program, an Annual Senior Clubs Council Hobby Show, fairs and many similar activities. New Haven is the site of many state-wide meetings on the aged and of conferences of the Connecticut Council of Senior Citizens. Overall, it has tackled many aspects of the aging problem and has used a number of approaches, ranging from direct service to legislation and research in retirement preparation to improve programs for the aged.

ROLE OF UNIVERSITIES

Closely associated with the work of the federal and state governments have been university programs that address problems of the aging. For example, a number of universities have established Multidisciplinary Centers of Gerontology with funding under the 1978 Amendments to the Older Americans Act. Under Title IV-E, dealing with National Aging Policy Study Centers, these centers carry out multidisciplinary activities that focus on major problems and concerns of the aged. The centers' functions range from training professionals in the field of aging to carrying out basic and applied research and disseminating new information about professional services for older people.

Research on Aging and Recreation

Research on aging and recreation has taken a number of different directions. A number of studies have sought to determine how older people spend their time and the nature of their leisure preferences. Moss and Lawton, for example, examined the day-to-day activities of older persons in four "life style" categories: independent community residents, independent public housing tenants, recipients of social and/or health-related in-home services and those on waiting lists for admission to long-term care facilities.[48]

Other studies have examined the leisure preferences, problems and needs of

---

[48]Miriam S. Moss and M. Powell Lawton: "Time Budgets of Older People: A Window on Four Life-styles." *Journal of Gerontology*, First Quarter, 1982, pp. 115–123.

the general population of elderly persons. McAvoy, for example, studied the leisure involvement of several hundred individuals over age 65 in the state of Minnesota.[49] Still other studies have addressed themselves to subgroups within the aging population, such as the rural elderly with visual impairment.[50] In general, such research has supported the importance of recreation and leisure in the lives of the elderly, and has established a substantial relationship between various dimensions of well-being and psychological health and satisfaction with the use of leisure time. McAvoy writes,

---

Individual studies . . . have concentrated on different aspects of successful aging and activities. These studies found that participation in social activities, and in leisure activities in general, is related to life satisfaction and the process of successfully aging. In a specific look at the motivations which prompted a sample of 540 elderly persons to engage in recreation activities, one study found that socializing was the most important motivation. This was followed by self-fulfillment, feeling close to nature, physical exercise, and learning, in that order.[51]

Much of the research on aging has dealt with the problems of geriatric patients in institutions—in part because hospitals and extended-care facilities provide subjects and controlled environments for scientific investigation and in part because funding has been made available for research in institutions. Most research has shown that much of the deterioration of older persons is not organic but results from their circumstances.

It has been found in a number of experimental projects that "confused, deteriorated and withdrawn" geriatric patients have made dramatic improvements as a result of recreation programs geared to promoting social interaction. As simple a remedy as "beer and tender loving care," applied in a conscientious program of recreation and social activity, has made remarkable changes in the lives of badly deteriorated patients. Their self-awareness, general ability to function and cooperation with hospital staff have all been improved markedly. In many cases, the development of such programs has made it no longer necessary to prescribe drugs to geriatric patients. Obviously, such research findings have important implications for the administrators of extended care facilities.

PREPARATION FOR RETIREMENT

For the overall aged population, some researchers have pointed out, learning to use free time productively poses a major challenge. Pfeiffer and Davis, of Duke

---

[49]Leo H. McAvoy: "The Leisure Preferences, Problems and Needs of the Elderly." *Journal of Leisure Research*, First Quarter, 1979, pp. 40–47.
[50]Vira R. Kivett and Dennis Orthner: "Activity Patterns and Leisure Preferences of Rural Elderly with Visual Impairment." *Therapeutic Recreation Journal*, Second Quarter, 1980, pp. 49–57.
[51]Leo A. McAvoy: "Needs of the Elderly: An Overview of the Research." *Parks and Recreation*, March 1977, p. 33.

University, have concluded that because of the strong work orientation in American society, a great number of older persons find extreme difficulty in accustoming themselves to the constructive, creative and guiltless use of leisure. They conclude, "In order to avoid serious dissatisfaction, our society must provide either more training for leisure in middle age, or more opportunity for continued employment in old age."[52]

Major business concerns, including utility companies, banks and oil companies, as well as industrial unions and government agencies are preparing their older employees for retirement. In April 1977, for example, IBM announced a program designed to prepare employees for an active and stimulating retirement. IBM grants up to $2500 for courses that might equip employees who are within five years of retirement to go into a new career or simply to gain new interests and skills.

Weiner comments that in many preretirement education programs, the subject of leisure has been relegated to "second-class status." Often it is the last topic to be covered, given the shortest time allotment and approached simply as a collection of activities. Yet, he writes,

> ... the research ... on retirement and retirement planning clearly indicates that retirement represents a transition from a work to a leisure role and that leisure orientation, attitudes and participation patterns are notable predictors of retirement planning and life satisfaction in retirement.[53]

Other universities and study centers are examining the probable effects of an increasingly older society. New forms of medical care could extend the life span markedly. If and when this occurs, scientists agree that it will be necessary for us to develop entirely new approaches to our social structure and economy as well as new personal and family attitudes toward the elderly.

Even if the government designs better programs to serve the aged the programs will solve only part of the problem. *Time* magazine comments,

> The ranker injustices of age-ism can be alleviated by governmental actions and familial concern, but the basic problem can be solved only by a fundamental and unlikely reordering of the values of society. Social obsolescence will probably be the chronic condition of the aged, like the other deficits and disabilities they learn to live with. But even in a society that has no role for them, aging individuals can try to carve out their own various niches. The noblest role of course, is an affirmative one — quite simply to demonstrate how to live and how to die.[54]

This comment suggests a unique role that has begun to face more and more recreation workers in chronic-care and nursing home facilities—helping terminally

[52]Eric Pfeiffer and Glenn C. Davis: "Free Time Poses Problems to Elderly in Our Society." *Geriatric Focus*, February 1971, p. 1.
[53]Andrew Weiner: "Pre-Retirement Education, Accent on Leisure." *Therapeutic Recreation Journal*, Second Quarter, 1980, pp. 18–19.
[54]"The Old in the Country of the Young," *op. cit.*, p. 54.

ill patients accept the reality of dying and live to the fullest during their remaining months or years. In her pioneering work, *On Death and Dying*, Elisabeth Kubler-Ross suggests that the psychological process of dying has five stages: *denial and isolation, anger, bargaining, depression and acceptance.*[55] The recreation therapist is in a unique position to counsel the dying patient informally and to help him or her in the terminal phase of life. In at least one American hospital serving primarily terminal patients, Calvary Hospital in New York, the therapeutic recreation staff has played a major role in this effort.

THE MILITANT ELDERLY: GRAY PANTHERS

Aged persons themselves are beginning to fight for improved benefits for the retired. Some six million elderly have joined the National Council of Senior Citizens and the American Association of Retired Persons to lobby for improved legislation and better social services. As an estimated 17 per cent of all registered voters, the elderly have the potential to exert considerable influence on government.

The American Association of Retired Persons has been active in fighting for increased Social Security and Supplemental Security checks. In an April 1977 referendum in Los Angeles, the association was successful in prohibiting mandatory retirement for the city's 45,000 municipal employees. Consciousness-raising has now reached the elderly in full force, resulting in the establishment of a unique organization called the Gray Panthers. Their leader, Maggie Kuhn, a retired Philadelphia social worker in her 70's, says, "Most organizations tried to adjust old people to the system, and we want none of that. The system is what needs changing." To do this, the Gray Panthers have agitated for better housing and medical care, along with improved employment opportunities for the elderly.

By the early 1980's, the Gray Panthers had expanded to a strong grassroots organization with 110 networks in over 30 states. In addition to promoting new work concepts such as job-sharing and phased retirement, the Gray Panthers have exposed abuses of the elderly in nursing homes and elsewhere and have strengthened rent control and condominium conversion laws. The Gray Panthers have been particularly vigorous defenders of the Social Security system and have opposed federal funding cuts affecting the elderly.

It seems clear that within an increasingly mechanized society and with more and more stringent union and Civil Service regulations, the amount of available work is not going to expand and the work life of a great number of people will not be lengthened. Retirement is a reality that must be faced. Clearly, the task of providing creative and rewarding involvements for older persons is going to be the responsibility of those who care for the elderly. Recreation will continue to be a major element in such programs—not "thumb-twiddling" or bingo alone, but a full range of cultural, social and creative activities—including structured opportunities for older persons to provide meaningful volunteer services to society.

---

[55]Elisabeth Kubler-Ross: *On Death and Dying.* New York, Macmillan, 1969.

LEISURE AS A "CON"

In his popular book, *A Good Age*, Alex Comfort comments that "leisure is a con." What he means is that older people are deprived of meaningful occupations and are "brainwashed" into "buying" trivial, commercialized forms of amusement—part of what he describes as a "phony aging package."[56] Realistically, although some older persons are able to continue in their jobs well into the 70's or 80's, most cannot. The challenge is to make *their* leisure as meaningful, challenging, educational and purposeful as possible—so that it is not just a matter of "killing" time but of using it fruitfully.

An excellent example of the type of activity attracting growing numbers of elderly persons is the ELDERHOSTEL program. Over 300 colleges and universities throughout the United States and Canada offer low-cost one-week residential academic programs for older adults. The great majority of such ELDERHOSTEL programs are offered during summer months. They combine the opportunity for serious academic study with extracurricular and recreational activities, often in attractive or unusual environments. The 1980 ELDERHOSTEL brochure included a number of programs at Hawaiian colleges which dealt with the history of the Hawaiian Islands, their legends and culture, oceanography and the reef habitat, and exploration of volcanoes, verdant jungles and coastal areas. Numerous other equally attractive offerings are provided each year for participants who are often in their 70's and 80's.

CHALLENGE FOR RECREATORS

In conclusion, it should be stressed that if recreation professionals are to play an increasingly meaningful role with the aging, they must establish their expertise, and they must do so by *action* rather than words. The recreation and park profession must develop a fuller sense of responsibility toward this group and must greatly expand its programs for the aging in the years ahead. Many millions of older persons are still unserved. Clearly, they need leisure programs and allied social services.

We have tended to be pessimistic in our appraisal of the effects of aging in modern life. An extensive study by Louis Harris and Associates, *The Myth and Reality of Aging in America*, indicates that the problems of older people are very much like those of younger people—except for health and fear of crime, which affect them inordinately. Substantial numbers of older people see themselves as useful to the community or are already involved in community service. Despite the real hardships they face, older persons tend to be only slightly less satisfied with their lives than those under 65 years old; the stereotype of aged people as a totally deprived population, economically and socially, is not justified.[57]

---

[56]Alex Comfort, *op. cit.*, p. 124.
[57]Louis Harris and Associates: *The Myth and Reality of Aging.* Washington, D.C., National Council on the Aging, 1975.

David Gray points out that the final issue of old age is that of integrity and courage against despair. Integrity, he says, is acceptance of one's life and a sense of comradeship with others—a determination to make the best of one's circumstances. Gray urges us to discard the damaging stereotype of elderly people and to embrace the concept of a life cycle with a rising curve of growth throughout most of life. For therapeutic recreation specialists, the challenge is clear—we must help the elderly make the most of their human potential. He concludes,

Our nation is in need of the awareness, intellect, perspective, time and power of our senior citizens. . . . The role of the social agency is to work with them to release the enormous reservoir of energy and competence our elderly citizens represent. In the end we will all benefit and not the least among the beneficiaries will be the senior citizen himself.[58]

The message is clear. For the aged, as for the other kinds of individuals discussed in this text, it is essential that we think of them not as handicapped or even disabled but rather as special populations with unique potentials and resources. The task of the therapeutic recreation specialist is to use the unique medium of recreation and leisure, along with certain allied forms of service, to help release these human resources, so that the aged, as well as other special populations, can maximize their own lives.

Suggested Topics for Class Discussion, Examination Questions or Student Papers

1. What are the unique problems of the aged in modern society that differ from those of the past? In your reply, deal with questions of retirement and changing family structures in our communities. How can recreation and related services play a significant role in meeting the needs of older persons?

2. To what extent *are* the needs of aged persons being met today, with respect to recreation and leisure? How must we change our thinking about older people and recreation, if leisure is not to be a "con," as Dr. Alex Comfort puts it?

3. Outline a model program of recreation or activity therapy for a specific type of setting, such as a nursing home or senior center.

4. How may education for leisure and leisure counseling help older persons use their retirement in more dynamic and satisfying ways?

---

[58]David E. Gray: "To Illuminate the Way." *Parks and Recreation*, October 1976, p. 33.

10

Programs and the
Socially Deviant

This chapter is concerned with the role of recreation in programs designed to serve socially deviant children, youth and adults. It deals with homes and special schools for children who have come from families unable to care for them, or who cannot function adequately in the community or in regular schools. It also considers correctional institutions and special programs designed for drug-addicted or alcohol-dependent youth and adults. It concludes with a description of community-based programs intended to prevent delinquency and other forms of antisocial behavior.

The problem of antisocial and deviant behavior is an important one for the entire recreation and park field. Westover, Flickinger and Chubb point out that crime and vandalism reduce the quantity of available recreation resources, deter participation and diminish the quality of recreation opportunities. A substantial percentage of residents avoid urban parks because of their fear of crime.[1] If for no other reason than this, it is essential that recreation and park professionals be concerned with the growing rate of juvenile and adult crime.

However, within the field of therapeutic recreation, there is a sharply increased awareness of the need for improved services in correctional facilities and community delinquency-prevention programs to cope with socially deviant behavior.

The concept of social deviance includes such problems as juvenile delinquency, drug addiction, alcoholism, aggressive and hostile behavior, truancy and sexual promiscuity. Recognizing that deviation may take a variety of such forms, this chapter deals primarily with those groups requiring special care or rehabilitation because they are socially maladjusted and unable or unwilling to conform to the demands of society.

Delinquency is the most common reason why young persons are committed to institutions. One state police manual describes the juvenile delinquent as " . . . a child of more than seven and less than sixteen years of age, who does any act which would be a crime if done by an adult. . . ."[2] Other codes list a variety of minor offenses as the basis for a charge of delinquency. Commonly, children below the

---

[1]Theresa N. Westover, Theodore B. Flickinger and Michael Chubb: "Crime and Law Enforcement." *Parks and Recreation*, August 1980, pp. 29–33.
[2]*New York State Police Manual*, 1971, p. 109.

age of 16 or 18 who are "incorrigible, ungovernable, or habitually disobedient and beyond the lawful control of parents or other authorities" are subject to juvenile court action and may be committed to institutions for care of deviant youth.

The problem of juvenile delinquency was described by the President's Commission on Law Enforcement and Administration of Justice in 1967 as the "single most pressing and threatening aspect of the crime problem in the United States." It found that one out of every nine children is referred to juvenile courts for an act of delinquency before his or her 18th birthday. To illustrate the seriousness of this problem, 52 per cent of those charged with burglary, 45 per cent of those charged with larceny and 61 per cent of those charged with auto theft are juveniles.

Over the past two decades, crime has increased steadily. Between 1963 and 1973, while the population increased by 8 per cent, the crime rate increased by more than 100 per cent. It was reported in 1977 that the prison population had risen by 13 per cent in the previous year, to a new high of more than 283,000 persons in federal and state prisons. In addition, there are about 160,000 inmates in local jails at any given time; up to four million persons are held in such institutions during the course of a year. Total government expenditures in the criminal justice system almost tripled between 1970 and 1978, from $8.5 billion to $24 billion.[3]

Clearly, criminal behavior represents a major concern for modern society. Since it is in childhood and youth that socially deviant behavior and delinquency are established, it is in this early period of life that strong prevention programs must be established.

THE CAUSES OF SOCIAL DEVIANCE

The causes of delinquency have been widely debated. There are basically two schools of thought—one that sees delinquency as a psychological or psychogenic problem and another that sees it primarily from a sociological or cultural viewpoint.

The psychological view regards habitual antisocial or criminal activity as an outcome of defective personality structure, stemming from feelings of inferiority, poorly developed control mechanisms or inadequate or disturbed family relationships. The typical delinquent has a relatively weak ego, is highly insecure and has a strong tendency toward aggressive and hostile behavior.

The sociological view of delinquency sees it primarily as the result of cultural and environmental factors. This view is supported by evidence that there is a much higher percentage of delinquent behavior in low-income areas—marked by slum housing, poor schools, broken or unstable families and the lack of desirable adult models—than in middle- or upper-class neighborhoods. The sociological view rejects the notion that juvenile delinquency indicates a disturbed or disorganized personality and suggests instead that the youthful lawbreaker may be a member of a cultural group that deliberately rejects "establishment" values and regulations and determines its own code of peer behavior.

---

[3]"Criminal Justice System: Public Expenditures and Employment." In *Statistical Abstract of the United States*, U.S. Bureau of the Census, 1980, p. 192.

Talcott Parsons suggests that the problem is chiefly one of masculine identification. In this view, delinquents are protesting female domination and affirming their own masculine self-image through antisocial behavior.[4] Block and Neiderhoffer regard delinquency as the result of inadequate societal processes for helping adolescents become adults; in their view, gangs engage in criminal activity as a way of stating their independence and adult identity.[5]

Merton explains socially deviant behavior as a form of protest by disadvantaged and racial minority youth. He writes,

---

When a system of cultural values extols . . . certain *common* success goals *for the population at large,* while the social structure rigorously restricts or closes access to . . . these goals for a *considerable part of the population* . . . deviant behavior then results on a large scale.[6]

The theory that the frustrated aspirations of lower-class youth are responsible for delinquent gang behavior was most fully developed by Cloward and Ohlin. They established a set of categories of urban youth gangs, including *fighting* gangs who derived their status chiefly from making war on the community and on other gangs, *criminal* gangs concerned mainly with financial gain through theft, racketeering and similar activities and *retreatist* gangs, who are involved chiefly with drugs, sex and alcohol as forms of escape.[7]

This view seems strongly supported by the preponderant number of black, Hispanic and other minority-group youth in prisons and correctional facilities today. Muth pointed out that during the 1960's prisons became even more "ghettoized" than they had been in the past. Poor persons and members of racial minority groups provided almost 75 per cent of the incarcerated population.[8]

RELATIONSHIP BETWEEN RECREATION AND DELINQUENCY

Recently, writers on juvenile delinquency have tended to minimize the role of play and recreation in the prevention of antisocial behavior. There has been considerable evidence, however, that there is a meaningful relationship between the leisure and recreational patterns of many youth gang members and their criminal activities. This relationship takes two forms.

---

[4]Talcott Parsons: *Essays in Sociological Theory.* Glencoe, Illinois, Free Press, 1954, pp. 304–306.
[5]Herbert Bloch and Arthur Neiderhoffer: *The Gang: A Study in Adolescent Behavior.* New York, Philosophical Library, 1958, p. 17.
[6]Robert K. Merton: *Social Theory and Social Structure.* Glencoe, Illinois, Free Press, 1957, p. 105.
[7]Richard A. Cloward and Lloyd E. Ohlin: *Delinquency and Opportunity: A Theory of Delinquent Gangs.* New York, Free Press, 1960, pp. 20–30, 161–186.
[8]Edmund H. Muth: "Prison Recreation in 1990." *Parks and Recreation,* September 1974, p. 28.

1. Play itself frequently is used in antisocial ways; leisure becomes the time in which early delinquent patterns are established. Tannenbaum writes,

---

In the beginning, the definition of the situation by the delinquent may be in the form of play, adventure, excitement, interest, mischief, fun. Breaking windows, annoying people . . . playing truant — all are forms of play. . . . To the community, however, these activities may and often do take on the form of nuisance, evil, delinquency, with the demand for control . . . punishment, police court.[9]

It seems probable that the relationship between the play impulse and delinquent activity is particularly high among middle-class and wealthy youth:

In the case of the low-income teen-age thief, often the drive represents a craving for possessions that the parents can't afford or simply won't consider buying. . . . But for the youth from a better and even high-income background, the stimulus is curiosity, a desire for "kicks," and escape from boredom . . . they want a thrill.[10]

Often, what begins as random or occasional behavior related to minor theft, gang fighting, drug experimentation or sexual exploitation gradually becomes more consistent and serious. When a child is arrested and brought before a juvenile court, and particularly when he or she is sent to a youth house, the pattern of behavior becomes fixed. Ultimately, what began as casual, impulsive play becomes serious criminal behavior.

Based on this understanding of the roots of juvenile delinquency, thousands of communities throughout the years have initiated recreation programs for youth. These programs have been seen as a valuable means of preventing juvenile delinquency for the following reasons: (a) successful youth recreation programs take teen-agers "off the streets" and involve them in positive and attractive leisure programs; (b) they help youth burn up their exuberant energy and express hostile, aggressive or competitive drives in constructive and useful ways; (c) the programs meet many of their needs for group affiliation and approval by others, which might otherwise be the basis for gang activity; (d) they expose them to the influence of helpful adults who provide desirable models and help to promote favorable social values; and (e) they help to attract young people into organized programs where they may then become involved in other needed tutorial, vocational or counseling programs.

Many civic leaders, police officials, judges and probational authorities have attested to the value of recreation in minimizing youth crime. In a study of the effects of a Boys' Club in Louisville, Kentucky, it was concluded that this youth

---

[9]Frank Tannenbaum: *Crime and the Community.* New York, Columbia University Press, 1938, pp. 17–20.
[10]*The New York Times,* December 1, 1968, p. F-1.

organization had helped to reduce juvenile delinquency. In 1976, after the program had been in operation for over two decades, the chief of police of Louisville stated,

---

Reported crimes in the areas served by this agency in 1975 were below the total in other parts of Louisville. When young people are actively involved in constructively supervised activities, their opportunity to participate in crime is greatly reduced.

Boys' Clubs in Louisville not only prevent juvenile delinquency, but also are a prime positive influence on the lives of many boys in underprivileged areas. The care and concern offered by effective youth workers helps develop a strong character and values which are carried by the young into adult life.[11]

---

2. A second important element of the relationship between recreation and juvenile delinquency is that youthful offenders typically have not learned to use their leisure in constructive and creative ways. It has been found that their family lives usually lack shared recreational pastimes and that they usually avoid taking part in organized community recreation programs.

As a consequence, many socially deviant youth have extremely narrow recreational interests. A former reformatory warden has written,

---

Among the inmates of correctional institutions there are many who have no knowledge or skills which will enable them to make acceptable use of their leisure. Most of them lack the avocational interests of the well adjusted. They cannot play, they do not read, they have no hobbies. In many instances, improper use of leisure is a factor in their criminality. Others lack the ability to engage in any cooperative activity with their fellows; teamwork is something foreign to their experience. Still others lack self-control or a sense of fair play; they cannot engage in competitive activity without losing their heads. If these men are to leave the institutions as stable, well-adjusted individuals, these needs must be filled; the missing interests, knowledge, and skills must be provided.[12]

Beyond this, Flynn emphasizes once again that most youthful and young adult offenders commit crimes during leisure hours. After they have been in a correctional institution or prison, the majority of inmates do not return to environments that provide for wholesome leisure activities. She writes,

---

More often than not, these offenders return to areas where the street is their principal recreation area and the neighborhood poolroom or bar is their social center. The incarcerative environment, coupled with long hours of nothing to do, leads, not infrequently, to the pursuit of criminal activities.[13]

---

[11]John H. Nevin, cited in "Officials Still Claim It's 'Critically Valid' . . . Boys' Clubs Reduce Delinquency Rates." Brochure of National Boys' Clubs of America, 1976.
[12]Garrett Heyns: "Penal Institutions." In *Annals of the American Academy of Political Science*, September 1951, pp. 71–75.
[13]Edith E. Flynn: "Recreation—A Privilege or a Necessity?" *Parks and Recreation*, September 1974, p. 57.

TYPES OF INSTITUTIONS

There are many different types of institutions serving socially deviant or dependent children and youth. These include the following:

1. State youth camps, frequently set in rural surroundings, emphasizing conservation work and outdoor living.
2. Cottage schools or homes operated by public, religious or voluntary agencies that tend to serve youth from broken homes or with a degree of emotional disturbance or problems of social adjustment who may or may not have been involved in delinquent activity.
3. Youth houses or "remand" centers that hold young people until their cases are brought before the courts.
4. Other penal institutions, ranging from jails to state and federal prisons, for older individuals who have been convicted of crimes.
5. Narcotics addiction treatment centers or rehabilitation centers for alcoholics.

Although statistics vary, it is estimated that the national recidivism rate is 65 per cent for adults and 75 per cent for youths—meaning that about two thirds of those who are committed to correctional facilities, jails and penitentiaries return to these institutions under new charges and convictions.[14] Senator Charles Percy of Illinois points out that about 80 per cent of all crimes are committed by persons who have previously been through the criminal justice system—and that for many inmates, prisons serve as little more than "graduate schools of crime."[15]

What this suggests is that in many cases treatment centers for the socially deviant are defeating their own purpose. Many young people who enter such institutions leave after a year or two far more hardened to society and knowledgeable in crime techniques than when they entered. Amos writes,

The ineffectiveness of our institutional programs is partly to blame . . . because many of the youngsters who return to their neighborhoods carry with them the added sophistication of a one-year course in delinquency, manipulation, conning, utilization of the sub-cultural codes, and assume roles of leadership and influence among other youngsters in their areas.[16]

Young people who enter such institutions often have immature expectations of authority figures stemming from earlier parent-child conflicts. They have confused self-images regarding their own worth, vocational goals, personal skills and sexual identification. Usually, they are listless and tend toward the passive use of free time;

---

[14]*Ibid.,* p. 34.
[15]Charles H. Percy: "Rehabilitating a Captive Audience." *Parks and Recreation,* September 1974, p. 25.
[16]William E. Amos: "The Future of Juvenile Institutions." *In* Ruth Cavan, ed.: *Juvenile Delinquency.* Philadelphia, J. B. Lippincott, 1969, p. 26.

yet they have a great deal of pent-up energy and hostility. They tend to have a low tolerance for failure or frustration and desperately need to acquire skills, training and a sense of accomplishment. A graduate student at Lehman College in New York wrote of the girls he worked with at Girls' Youth House (known as Manida), a short-term detention center for adolescent females:

The girls range in age from eight to seventeen, but generally the majority are between fourteen and fifteen. They are almost entirely from lower socio-economic backgrounds and it is the exceptional girl whose family is intact. Reflecting the racial patterns of poverty in New York City, the girls are mainly black and Spanish-speaking, although there are a few whites. The girls are referred to Manida by the courts for a variety of offenses, ranging from petty thievery to prostitution, drug abuse and even homicide. Many are referred because their families have no control over them. . . . Many of the girls have had sexual relations (a significant number of them are pregnant) and almost all have had experience with drugs (from just experimentation to hard-core addiction).

. . . many of the girls share similar emotions when they come to Manida. Many are close to hysteria, a reaction both to society's estimate of their offense as being immoral (especially sexual offenses) and also to parental rejection (half the girls are there because of parental petitions of incorrigibility). The girls are scared and have tremendous feelings of guilt. They are also often bitter, hurt from previous experience (particularly with men) and court experiences. They have little faith in adults.[17]

Although such youngsters are sent to correctional facilities to be rehabilitated, most of their time is often spent in learning—particularly in the case of male juveniles—about better ways to commit crimes and establish peer relationships on the basis of their own toughness and resistance to societal values. Barker and Adams write, "They often react against the dominant value structure and develop the feeling that anything that is valuable and acceptable for the dominant culture is wrong for them and vice-versa."[18]

This sense of alienation and resistance is understandable. The mere fact of the institutional setting militates against the resident's responding to even the most intelligent and constructive treatment. MacIver writes, "Technically, the institution is a place where the youth is sent for friendly guidance and training, but for the youth himself, it is a prison, a punishment. He is cut off from all familiar associations. He is under restraints that he bitterly resents."[19]

Within this context, then, it is essential that the program be one that provides a variety of needed kinds of experiences and human relationships, including counseling services, group discussions and therapy, academic education, vocational classes, work experience and recreation.

---

[17]Steven Berman: "Recreation at the Girls' Youth House." Graduate paper at Herbert Lehman College, New York, 1971.
[18]Gordon Barker and W. Thomas Adams: *In* Ruth Cavan, ed., *op. cit.,* p. 435.
[19]Robert M. MacIver: *The Prevention and Control of Delinquency.* New York, Atherton Press, 1966, p. 163.

GOALS OF RECREATION IN TREATMENT
CENTERS FOR THE SOCIALLY DEVIANT

The goals of recreation in youth camps and other correctional facilities include certain unique elements:

1. Recognizing that institutional life represents an unnatural and limiting kind of living arrangement, a primary purpose of recreation is to improve morale and to help make the setting more bearable and enjoyable. The lack of freedom and a high level of anxiety, tension and boredom can all be alleviated by a well-organized program of enjoyable activities.
2. A second purpose of recreation in the institutional setting is to help individuals learn new recreational skills; discover talents and interests and generally learn to use their leisure in socially acceptable and constructive ways.
3. Recreation provides a means of improving the social adjustment of participants; through it, they are helped to develop constructive social relationships with adults or with their peers, to learn to become cooperative group members and to accept social rules and values of sportsmanship and responsibility.
4. Generally, recreation may help the individual participant gain a more favorable self-concept and a sense of accomplishment and personal worth, as well as the knowledge that he is using his free time in a productive and acceptable way.
5. By providing a release for energies and drives that are pent up in prison, recreation may help to reduce the danger of friction and hostility; sports and creative and social activities are particularly useful in this respect.

McCall writes that the delivery of leisure services in correctional institutions should have two major purposes: to relieve the daily tensions that are created by incarceration, and to develop both existing and new leisure skills that benefit the inmate and may be pursued after his or her release.[20] In the relatively small number of correctional centers and prisons that have well-staffed and well-equipped recreation programs and facilities, inmates are likely to experience leisure opportunities, challenges and satisfactions that they never knew before incarceration.

But it should be clearly understood that while recreation is an important element in the rehabilitative process, it can accomplish little by itself. Decker writes,

---

Recreation is not a cure-all. It does not prevent, control or cure unacceptable behavior. But it does have an important role in the total rehabilitation process.... If a program is well-planned and adapted to the participants, they can be guided and assisted in learning self-control and self-discipline, engaging in cooperative enterprises, building more constructive social relationships, and acquiring interests that replace undesirable past interests.[21]

A former prisoner, Ray Speckman, agrees:

---

[20]Gail E. McCall: "Leisure Restructuring." *Journal of Physical Education and Recreation*, April 1981, p. 38.
[21]Larry E. Decker: "Recreation in Correctional Institutions." *Parks and Recreation*, April 1969, p. 32.

Recreation is an aid to the rehabilitative process, not a rehabilitative panacea. To treat it as such does not do justice to prison recreation programs or the people charged to administer and facilitate them.[22]

Nonetheless, there is growing agreement among many authorities, including the National Advisory Commission on Criminal Justice Standards and Goals, that prison administrators need to give much more attention to leisure and recreation opportunities. In some cases, the value of recreation has been documented. For example, Garibaldi and Moore describe an Indiana court where it had been determined that 92 per cent of the prisoners placed on one-year probation were arrested again for subsequent criminal acts. To reduce the recidivism rate in that court

. . . a condition of probation was added that required each man to learn new leisure skills. This new condition, along with the other conditions of probation, were strictly adhered to, and 24 months later the recidivism rate was 14 percent for those men placed on one-year probation.[23]

RECREATION IN CORRECTIONAL INSTITUTIONS

Despite the growing awareness of the need for recreation in correctional settings, in many youth camps, training schools, jails or prisons, the provisions for recreation services are extremely limited. In part, this lack stems from a traditional and still widely held concept of such institutions as places meant for the *punishment* rather than the *rehabilitation* of inmates. Although this viewpoint is gradually being replaced by more constructive views, the fact is that a brutal and harsh attitude toward offenders has characterized American penal institutions until comparatively recently.

Among the more brutal measures employed in the recent past were the following:

In North Carolina, a decade or so ago, men were thrown naked into solitary confinement cells, where guards used high-pressure water hoses from time to time to ''knock them up against the wall.''

In Maryland, inmates were disciplined until recently by receiving a meal only once every 72 hours.

---

[22]Ray Speckman: "Recreation in Prisons—A Panacea?" *Journal of Physical Education and Recreation,* April 1981, p. 47.
[23]Michele Garibaldi and Mary Moore: "The Treatment Team Approach." *Journal of Physical Education and Recreation,* April 1981, p. 28.

In Pennsylvania, until the mid-1950s, recalcitrant prisoners were placed for long periods in dark, damp underground holes.

In Arkansas, until the late 1960s, men were whipped on the bare buttocks with rawhide straps (flogging was practiced in 26 prisons as recently as 1963), and some were tortured by having needles pushed under their fingernails.[24]

Given this record of extreme harshness, it is understandable that meaningful educational, vocational, counseling and recreational services have been slow to enter many youth correctional institutions or adult prisons. Even where there is a desire to provide such services, staff limitations and overcrowded facilities have made it difficult to do so. The former U.S. Attorney General, Ramsey Clark, pointed out that 95 cents of every dollar spent in the early 1970's was for custodial care, and only 5 cents was for rehabilitation.

Even when a more positive philosophy of rehabilitation prevails, many youth houses and prisons are so overcrowded and lacking in well-trained staff and adequate budgets, that meaningful rehabilitation goals simply cannot be met. Numerous examples might be cited. In one such case, a children's shelter in New Jersey, the superintendent described what the institution had been like when she took over a few years earlier:

There was a lot of fear, uncertainty about who was in control. Staff people were paid less than garbage collectors. . . . it was difficult to attract talented people who would work at this as their main job. Their primary loyalties were elsewhere.

People were kicked, punched, beaten — children as well as staff members. We had riots and police intervention. Mace (a chemical spray) was used arbitrarily. Children have told me that staff members would walk down the hall and say, "Good morning, Henry" — and squirt Mace. It was hell. The staff hated to come to work because riots were so frequent.[25]

Other examples may be drawn from institutions in New York City—probably little better or worse than those in other large cities. Typically, a world of "fear, violence, filth and degradation" was described by prisoners who answered an uncensored questionnaire about conditions in the Tombs, a municipal house of detention for men. The use of force by guards and the lack of adequate medical care, schooling or other services, plus extreme overcrowding, made this facility a "dungeon of fear," in the words of one prisoner. In other centers, the shortage of caseworkers, teachers and recreation personnel limits programs markedly. Rikers Island, a reformatory jammed with almost twice the number of inmates originally planned for it, is marked by beatings, sexual abuse and suicides; observers have described it as an "island of idleness." There, writes one reporter,

---

[24]"Prisons Curb Brutal Discipline; Find Relaxed Controls Effective." *The New York Times,* May 15, 1971, p. 14.

[25]Darrell Sifford: "The 'Nice Lady' and the Snakepit." *The Philadelphia Inquirer,* March 28, 1978, p. D-1.

... teenagers can associate with accused felons and spend the day talking about the best kind of drugs to take, the most lucrative crimes, their real or imagined sexual experiences and the people they've beaten up. There is time, lots of time, for them to plan great crimes because their days are not disrupted by such unpleasantries as education, work, or sports. They get three meals a day and a place to sleep.[26]

Unfortunately, the national pattern is much the same. Flynn pointed out in the mid-1970's that a study of all jails and penitentiaries built in the United States during the preceding decade revealed that the majority of institutions seemed to have been built to perform but one function—"to warehouse men at the lowest possible per capita cost." Some buildings were constructed with no day-rooms, no auditorium, no gymnasiums and almost no facilities for outside recreation. This study concluded, based on the much higher level of inmate morale in the institutions that did provide adequate recreation, that such facilities and programs should no longer be viewed as luxuries but rather as essential elements in correctional programs, critical to the physical and mental health of all inmates.[27]

Other reports show that a high percentage of state maximum-security prisons in operation today were built during the nineteenth century. A national survey conducted in 1970 by the Law Enforcement Assistance Administration showed that 550 of 4021 jails counted were constructed during the 1800's, and six in the eighteenth century! Of 3300 jails located in cities and counties of more than 25,000 population, 83 per cent have no recreation or educational facilities of any kind.[28]

Such conditions undoubtedly have been largely responsible for a number of the bloody and destructive uprisings which have taken place in prisons in recent years—at Attica, New York, in 1971, at the Kansas State Prison in 1973, at Washington State Penitentiary in 1979 and at New Mexico State Prison in 1980.

Even when adequate facilities are provided (and a growing number of newer penitentiaries and prisons are being built with striking new architectural designs, making them resemble college campuses more than maximum security prisons), the lack of skilled staff members with training in recreation and appropriate attitudes often makes it difficult to provide adequate programs.

Despite this generally negative picture, there are a number of good programs of recreation in youth institutions throughout the United States. One evidence of improvement in this area has been based on lawsuits and court decisions which have guaranteed prisoners the right to out-of-cell exercise and recreation. Barbee and Calloway report that 33 states are currently under federal order to improve prisoners' living conditions and to provide recreational services to all inmates.[29]

Among the states to have moved vigorously into the improvement and reform of their correctional institutions are Ohio, Illinois, Georgia, Nebraska and California.

---

[26]Joseph Feurey: "Idle Rikers Teens Get Crime 'Tutoring'." *New York Post*, February 20, 1970, p. 22.
[27]Flynn, *op. cit.*, p. 35.
[28]*Ibid.* For a fuller discussion of recreation in local jails, *see* Carroll R. Hormachea: "Recreation Programs for Local Jails." *Journal of Physical Education and Recreation*, April 1981, pp. 44–45.
[29]Jim T. Barbee and Jim Calloway: "The Courts and Correctional Recreation." *Journal of Physical Education and Recreation*, April 1981, p. 40.

EFFECTIVE STATE PROGRAMS

Probably the leading example of a state that has reformed its correctional program is Illinois. There, in 1968, Governor Richard Ogilvie moved to merge separate state departments and boards dealing with youth offenders, adult correction facilities and penal institutions into a single state department with cabinet-level representation.

As part of this effort, Illinois took the following actions: (a) it raised its correctional budget sharply; (b) it established a strong central administrative staff to provide research, long-range planning, program analysis, policy evaluation, public information and medical and professional services; (c) it established a larger, full-time Parole and Pardon Board; (d) it developed a variety of new community-based programs, including four halfway-house community centers for parolees, six new work-release centers, ten group homes for youth parolees, a special services unit in Chicago to provide counseling and job placement for youth parolees and a new pre-release program to aid adults about to be discharged; (e) it developed several new minimum security facilities with emphasis on vocational and educational treatment programs; and (f) it expanded professional counseling and vocational and educational services in all facilities. Within two years, the recidivism rate dropped sharply for youth and adults who had access to the new programs and procedures.

ILLINOIS STATE TRAINING SCHOOL FOR BOYS, ST. CHARLES

One example of an upgraded Illinois correction facility is this medium-security facility serving several hundred boys with extensive academic and prevocational programs, as well as medical, dental, religious, recreational, psychiatric, psychological and social services. It is the largest facility for delinquent youth in the state. In an effort to overcome this disadvantage, it has been divided into smaller operational units with separate staffs and program identities, housed in clusters of cottages. Each such unit develops its own statement of rehabilitation goals and methods of achieving them. Intensive use is made of group living experiences, student council programs and planning and advisory roles in policy-making, along with more traditional forms of individual and group therapy.

Overall, the school's physical education and recreation program is operated under the direction of the Recreation Division, staffed by a director of recreation, an assistant director, an occupational therapist and a staff of physical education instructors. Facilities include a gymnasium and indoor swimming pool, 12 combination basketball, badminton and volleyball all-weather courts located near the cottages, 13 softball diamonds with backstops, a football field, a running track, a baseball field and four tennis courts that double as ice skating rinks during the winter months.

In addition to formal physical education, health and first aid instruction, the Illinois State Training School at St. Charles sponsors the following recreational activities:

1. Varsity sports competition with other schools or boys' clubs for highly skilled participants.
2. Intramural competition, including leagues and tournaments in all seasonal sports, carried on among the cottages.
3. Weekly swimming participation and instruction in small groups for nonswimmers.
4. Weekly movies of first-run features and talent shows by service organizations, colleges or other entertainment groups.
5. Ice skating during the winter and roller skating during the summer, using outdoor facilities.
6. Monthly birthday parties, special holiday parties (including trips to neighboring communities or special activities) and special events for Halloween, Labor Day, Thanksgiving and other holidays.
7. A hobby shop program, including lanyard, leather, clay, raffia and other craft activities.
8. Individual units may also sponsor special interest clubs; among the activities provided have been swimming, chess, Spanish, guitar lessons, physical fitness, tailoring and horseback riding.
9. Drum and Bugle Corps and other musical activities.

Although each of the units provides a somewhat different approach to treatment, the following statement is typical of the institution's recreational philosophy:

The Rehabilitative Environment.   It is the intended purpose of this Unit to create an accepting, warm, non-threatening, humane, and enriched environment in which the delinquent youth can learn that the world is not overwhelmingly hostile and alien. However, unlike the therapeutic setting in which the neurotic child or adult would likely be placed, this environment is not to be permissive. It is to be highly structured. A sense of authority is to be consistently maintained. The consequences of the delinquent youth's behavior, whether positive or negative, are to be clearly defined. An integral part of this environment is the creation of learning situations in which the delinquent youth can:

1. Ventilate his anger constructively.
2. Modify undesirable behavior and learn age-appropriate means to satisfy his desires and wants.
3. Learn the rewards of socially desirable behavior and deferred gratification of needs.
4. Experience the rewards of close, non-delinquent interpersonal relationships.
5. Correct distorted perceptions so that he can deal more effectively with the demands and stresses of life.[30]

Recreation in Nebraska's Institutions

Another state which has made a serious effort to evaluate and strengthen the role of leisure programming in its penal institutions is Nebraska. Here, the state legislature appointed a committee to investigate the kinds of activities offered and

---

[30]*Statement of Rehabilitative Objectives and Approaches, Unit III.* Departmental Manual, Illinois State Training School for Boys, St. Charles, Illinois, 1971, p. 2.

the attitudes and functions of four subgroups of the state institutions (administration, guards, recreation staff and inmates) with respect to recreation. In general, there was little support for recreation or understanding of its values. There was a wide diversity of opinion as to the amount of time which should be allotted to organized recreation and the kind of policies which should govern it. Based on this study, a number of new recreation positions were created with higher salaries. More adequate facilities and equipment were also provided. In addition, it was determined that in-service education programs on recreation would be provided for the four subgroups mentioned above, in order to improve the recreation program's effectiveness.[31]

LINCOLN CORRECTIONAL CENTER

One example of the progress made in Nebraska is the State Department of Correctional Services' new facility in Lincoln to serve younger male offenders. It replaces an antiquated structure. The center is organized in five housing units in order to separate offenders, promote security and aid rehabilitation. One of the prime considerations in designing the center was the facilitation of programs. Recreation facilities in the new Lincoln Correctional Center include a gymnasium with a regulation-sized basketball floor and markings for other court games, and indoor and outdoor areas for weightlifting, basketball, volleyball, handball and racquetball, softball, tennis, flag football and jogging. Additional recreational facilities include a music room, "reading" and law libraries, a stage for drama and music presentations, and hobby/crafts areas. Each housing unit also has four lounge areas with a pool table, television set, table games and vending machines.

The center has a staff of six recreation professionals, including a manager, two assistant managers, and three supervisors, who offer a varied and balanced program, including sports, games and creative and social activities. Murphy and Von Minden describe other characteristics of this program:

Periodic efforts are made to solicit input from the offenders regarding activities and events they would like to see included in the program. Survey instruments are administered to gather data to (assist) in making program decisions. . . . Offenders (are not assured) that their desires will all be incorporated into the program; safety and security must be primary considerations.

. . . the recreation staff has effectively used community and regional performers; rock bands, the Lincoln Civic Orchestra, theater groups, various traveling shows, and band and choral groups from local schools and colleges. A strong effort is made to bring in a program of this type at least once a month, and more frequently during the special seasons such as Christmas . . .

The Center also invites various athletic teams to compete with teams from the inside . . . (such as) intramural teams from local colleges and universities and municipal recreation leagues (as well as various) law enforcement agencies and the state highway patrol.[32]

---

[31]Ron Mendell and Thomas Kidd: "Nebraska Legislature's Study of Penal Institutions." *Journal of Physical Education and Recreation*, April 1981, pp. 54, 58.
[32]William D. Murphy and Scott Von Minden: "Hard Time and Free Time." *Journal of Physical Education and Recreation*, April 1981, p. 50.

Selected offenders are approved for recreation participation, such as sports competition with municipal athletic leagues, outside the walls of the institution. In addition, the recreation staff trains some inmates to be program assistants (team coaches, officials and timers), to help maintain athletic facilities, to plan holiday recreation events, and to assume other leadership roles. These responsibilities are viewed as an important aid in the positive socialization of the center's young residents. Murphy and Von Minden conclude that the recreation staff at the Lincoln Correction Center does not regard the recreation program as a magic avenue to rehabilitation. However, they are convinced that

> . . . offenders who experience nothing but hard time are less amenable to counseling, direction, and behavioral change than those offenders whose free time is spent in a positive manner. . . . Recreation will continue to serve as a bridge between hard time and free time for those offenders who wish to use it.[33]

There are numerous other examples of excellent recreation programs in youth correctional facilities around the United States and Canada; earlier editions of this text gave detailed descriptions of two such programs in Ohio and California.[34] It should be recognized, however, that such positive uses of recreation are in the minority; most recreation programs in penal or correctional institutions are extremely limited. Too often, administrators are unwilling or unable to allocate sufficient funds to support recreation activities; they see them in a narrow light—as a means of dispensing rewards or penalties. Guards frequently resent or resist leisure activity as a potential danger which interferes with their primary function of maintaining security. Even within institutions for girls and women, which one might expect to be somewhat more enlightened and less violent, programs tend to be minimal.

Programs in Girls' and Women's Facilities

To illustrate, one survey of women's penal institutions in the United States, Canada and Puerto Rico found that a number of prisons or reformatories had no organized programs at all. Of 17 responding institutions, only six had formal educational requirements for the director of recreations; in others, degrees were not required and staffing responsibilities were heavily assumed by male guards or female supervisors. The survey found that activities tended to be *active games,* such as softball, volleyball, badminton, croquet, basketball, tennis, horseshoes and tumbling, and *quiet activities,* such as cards, bingo and shuffleboard. It was concluded that the women's penal institutions with the most clearly defined purposes and

---

[33]*Ibid.,* p. 52.
[34]See second edition of this text, 1978, pp. 270–275.

with leadership assigned to specific recreation directors tended to have the most extensive and well-organized programs.[35]

In a more recent report, Williams describes his findings in a national study of recreation services for women incarcerated in state penal institutions. He found that even where new and more attractive facilities have been built for women, they

---

... perpetuate the philosophy, the operational methods, the hardware, and the repression of the state penitentiary. The facilities are surrounded by concertina fences, and the women's movements are monitored on closed circuit television. Inmates sit endlessly playing cards, sewing or just vegetating.[36]

Williams studied 31 state correctional institutions which housed women offenders in separate prison facilities; he examined their programming, personnel, facilities and funding sources. In general, he found that prison officials accepted the value of recreation services, although the facilities, staffing and actual programs were often extremely deficient. On the basis of his findings, he developed a number of study recommendations calling for expanded budgets and programs, increased use of community-based indoor and outdoor facilities, in-service training and staff development for all personnel in prisons, heavy emphasis on the young adult population, state-wide coordination of recreation services in correctional and penal settings and specialized degree programs in correctional recreation in college and university recreation departments.[37]

NEED FOR IMPROVEMENT OF CORRECTIONAL PROGRAMS

Despite the positive examples cited here, it should be stressed again that the majority of correctional institutions do *not* provide adequate recreational programs or, for that matter, adequate rehabilitation services overall. This situation is particularly true of prisons for adult offenders. One authority has characterized the nation's prison systems as a "total failure." He describes the criminal justice program as a "perpetual-motion machine" in which police arrest felons and send them into the courts, which send them into prisons, which in turn send them out into the streets to be re-arrested:

---

[35]Diane Peoples and Russ Walkup: *Survey of Women's Penal Facilities.* Unpublished report, Ohio Reformatory for Women, Maryville, Ohio, 1970.
[36]Larry R. Williams: "Women's Correctional Recreation Services." *Journal of Physical Education and Recreation*, April 1981, p. 55.
[37]*Ibid.*, p. 58.

We do no more for the criminal in jail than we do for animals in the zoo. We cage them and feed them. The average citizen has seen prison purely and simply as retribution. The uglier and grimier and older the prison, the more it has seemed to the average citizen to be a fine and splendid prison.[38]

What is needed is a widespread revolution in public attitudes and the infusion of large sums of money to replace vengeance with rehabilitation in the correctional system. If this does not happen, jails will continue to be nothing more than "warehouses for contaminated goods," and prison riots, crime and the rate of recidivism will continue unabated.

This point of view is strongly supported by Ramsey Clark, who stresses that it is essential to develop entirely different approaches to law enforcement and corrections. He urges the following priorities:

1. A philosophy of avoiding detention wherever possible through prevention efforts, community treatment, and probation supervision.
2. Recognition that the needs of each individual are different. Corrections programs should be carefully tailored to individual needs.
3. The creation of new substantive rights of persons convicted of crime that would require government to fulfill basic human needs in the following areas:
   (a) health and social services;
   (b) safety from assault, forced homosexuality, corporal punishment or solitary confinement;
   (c) communications, including the free access to family, friends, advisors and attorneys, and the right to write and read freely;
   (d) improved educational and vocational training programs; and
   (e) job placement services.
4. The creation of new procedural rights for prisoners.
5. An intensive effort to move offenders to the community where they will live, making use of the following:
   (a) improved probation and parole programs; and
   (b) a network of work-release, pre-release guidance, and halfway houses, with small, unmarked community facilities that will assist discharged or paroled prisoners in making the transition to responsible and law-abiding community life.[39]

Only if such programs are developed will it be possible to overcome the weaknesses of our corrective and penal system that are so destructive to human life and dignity. Within such programs, recreation must play an increasingly strong role by contributing to the rehabilitation process and helping offenders return successfully to their communities. What steps need to be taken in this direction? Obviously, the fundamental basis for any meaningful redirection or improvement of recreation

---

[38]"Murphy Attacks Nation's Prisons as 'Total Failure'." *The New York Times*, January 29, 1972, p. 33.
[39]"A Nickel for Rehabilitation." *The New York Times*, September 30, 1971, p. 46.

services would have to be an administrative philosophy that identifies the primary goal as preparing inmates to return successfully to the community, rather than simply punishing them for past crimes. Recreation programs would have to have adequate facilities and equipment, qualified leadership and cooperation from administrators to permit prisoners to participate in a variety of activities. Unlike many institutions today, where most prisoners are limited to reading, listening to the radio, playing cards, a daily session in an exercise yard and an occasional movie or other form of mass entertainment, the opportunity would have to be provided for challenging individual and group activities. Such activities might include the following:

Outdoor Recreation

The California Youth Authority has successfully experimented with small groups of youthful offenders who take extended wilderness trips in the Mojave Desert high country of the Lassen National Forest. Hiking more than 100 miles, using rock climbing and rappelling, the young wards gained greatly in self-confidence and the ability to deal with others responsibly. These trips have included three-day "solo" survival experiences, encounter sessions using transactional analysis and other experiences which engendered maturity and self-confidence in the participants. Obviously, not all prisoners could be trusted in such a situation; however, with carefully selected participants, programs of this type have an immense potential.

Theater Arts

A number of prisons have encouraged dramatics because it is rewarding in its own right and entertains the entire prison population. Recently, some theater groups have been formed to present works written by convicts themselves out of their own experience. One such group is "The Family," which began with eight inmates at the Bedford, New York, Correctional Facility who became involved in group therapy experiences such as theater games, exercises, role-playing and psychodrama, in which inmates acted out traumatic scenes from their own life. The prison theater workshops gave rise to a dozen new plays presented in homes for unwed mothers, drug rehabilitation centers and even leading professional theaters in the East. Ultimately, "The Family" became a touring professional company of 150 actors and stage technicians in the outside community.

Another example of outstanding prison theater was developed at San Quentin Prison in California, where a professional company of former inmates called the Barbwire Theatre has received funding from the U.S. Department of Health, Education and Welfare and the National Endowment for the Arts. In addition to performing, the Barbwire Theatre provides intensive training in acting techniques for inmates who show interest in drama and sponsors literary competitions among inmates and awards prizes for the best-written short story, essay, poetry and play.

The Barbwire Theatre's first production, *The Cage*, has toured the United States, including a run at Washington, D.C.'s Arena Stage.

A number of successful playwrights and actors on the professional stage today had their first experience in prison theater programs like those described here. Other prisons have experimented successfully in fine arts, music and creative writing.

Co-educational Prisons

The typical prison or correctional institution is established on a one-sex basis— all men or all women. This single sex environment tends to create an atmosphere of extreme tension; often homosexuality is widespread, with many younger or weaker inmates being forcibly seduced or violently gang-raped. Correctional institutions or state youth camps have often scheduled co-educational recreation activities in an effort to overcome some of the effects of such segregation, and a number of prisons have experimented with conjugal visits, in which small apartments are set aside and prisoners live for brief periods of time with their visiting families. Recently, several state and federal prisons have been restructured on a co-educational basis. For example, Framingham State Prison in Massachusetts now accepts both male and female minimum-security prisoners, who may transfer from other state prisons. Although it is far from a country club, inmates at Framingham can dine together, go for strolls in the prison courtyard and enjoy dinner dances, grooming classes, fashion shows, a pool paid for by the inmates and other recreation opportunities. Prisoners agree that this experimental arrangement has helped to reduce much of the tension normally found in penal institutions. The superintendent comments that although the public accepts this approach chiefly as a means of reducing prison homosexuality, in her view the co-ed approach is simply more realistic:

She reasons that the residents are going to have to cope with a man-woman world when they get out, and that learning to get along with the opposite sex inside the four walls will help with their adjustment to society once they are released.[40]

Prevocational Experience

Another important aspect of recreation programs in prisons and correctional institutions is that they may be structured to provide useful experience in recreation leadership, so that inmates, when discharged, are able to move into recreation aide

---

[40]Judy Klemesrud: "Men and Women in One Prison: 'Realistic' Idea Is Given a Try." *The New York Times*, June 20, 1974, p. 44.

positions in community or therapeutic agencies. Obviously, there are numerous opportunities for them to take on direct leadership responsibilities; Cipriano urges that these be combined with short-term training programs in job competencies in the institution itself, along with a coordinated effort to identify appropriate job opportunities in the outside community and to help place qualified individuals in these positions. Many normal job opportunities are virtually closed to ex-convicts because of their records; on the other hand, their backgrounds can be invaluable in helping them work with problem youth, with drug addicts or in other socially oriented programs.

Arjo and Allen provide a number of examples of leisure-related fields of employment in which an inmate may gain skills within the institution that may lead to part- or full-time work after discharge. These include (a) sports officiating or leadership; (b) designing and maintaining athletic and other recreational areas and facilities; (c) maintaining and repairing equipment; and (d) recreation and leisure programming in selected settings.[41]

Leisure Counseling

A final important aspect of recreation service for youth and adults who have been committed to correctional or penal institutions is leisure counseling. In a study of 50 male clients of the Pennsylvania Board of Probation and Parole, Panik and Mobley found that the most popular leisure activities of these individuals, prior to their conviction, were watching television, drinking and other tavern-related activities.[42] Ninety-eight per cent of the clients committed the act for which they were convicted (including such crimes as murder, arson, robbery and sex offenses) during leisure time. It was concluded that a program of group leisure counseling for probationers and parolees should be instituted, both to give the parole agent a better understanding of the leisure patterns of these clients and to help guide them in appropriate directions. Excellent rapport was established in these counseling sessions; attendance was high, and planning was initiated to develop a more complex counseling project, with experimental controls to measure its impact on recidivism.

McCall suggests that what is needed is a broad approach, called "leisure restructuring." This involves both the delivery of leisure services for their own sake and an added process that includes leisure education, values clarification, needs assessment, leisure counseling and skills acquisition. In this approach, the leisure services staff member should work closely with other institutional programs and personnel, such as academic and vocational education, psychological counseling, security and administration, to help the prison's recreation program become a meaningful therapeutic tool.[43]

A specific form of deviant behavior in our society related to leisure-time use is

---

[41]Raymond L. Arjo and Lawrence R. Allen: "Vocational Implications of Leisure." *Journal of Physical Education and Recreation*, April 1981, pp. 48–49.

[42]Martin A. Panik and Tony A. Mobley: "The Bottle and the Tube: Leisure for the Convicted." *Parks and Recreation*, March 1977, pp. 28–30, 54–55.

[43]McCall, *op. cit.*, pp. 38–39.

drug abuse. It ranges from casual experimentation with so-called soft drugs to intensive and regular use of hard drugs.

RECREATION AND THE TREATMENT OF DRUG ADDICTS

The problem of drug abuse and addiction has increased tremendously in the Western world over the past three decades, particularly among the young. Although estimates vary greatly, there was convincing evidence in the 1970's that a majority of the students in many schools and colleges in the United States were at least occasional users of marijuana. Government surveys in 1976 reported a continued rise in the use of marijuana; one third of all high school seniors reported themselves as current users.[44] The use of other, "harder" drugs, such as heroin, cocaine and LSD, was reported to have remained unchanged over the previous two years.

A survey of more than 1000 high school students in New York City and its suburbs and dozens of interviews with parents, drug counselors and teen-agers themselves conducted by *The New York Times* " . . . clearly indicates that today's young people are more immersed in the drug culture than any before them have been, and at a far younger age."[45]

It is evident that the use of drugs has become a major problem for American youth from all levels of society. Heroin, once chiefly used by blacks in urban ghettos, has now made inroads in fashionable suburban communities. Its users are increasingly younger. No social group is immune to this risk. Two articles on the same page of *The Philadelphia Inquirer* reported in June 1982 that the son of a famous American evangelist had committed suicide shortly after being ordered by the court to receive drug counseling and that the son of a Supreme Court justice had been arrested and arraigned on charges of selling cocaine as part of a possible multimillion-dollar drug deal. Another article on the same page reported that thousands of alcohol and drug abusers in 16 major United States cities would no longer be able to receive treatment because of $200 million in budget cutbacks for federal assistance programs under the Reagan administration.[46]

Although most adults tend to be shocked by the growing statistics on drug use among children and youth, the fact is that adults themselves are extremely heavy users of tranquilizers and other legal, or prescribed, stimulants. Many millions of adults are "hooked" on cigarettes or alcohol. Teen-agers frequently comment that for them "pot" is no different from their parents' martini cocktails. Indeed, it seems clear that for many, drug-taking represents a form of leisure activity, a way of hav-

---

[44]"U.S. Survey Finds Rise in High School in Use of Marijuana." Associated Press Dispatch, November 23, 1976.

[45]Anna Quindlen: "Teen-Agers Call Illicit Drugs One of Life's Commonplaces." *The New York Times*, July 19, 1981, pp. 1, 38.

[46]See three articles: "Son of Oral Roberts Dies in Apparent Suicide," "Justice Stevens' Son Charged in Drug Sale," and "Cuts in Drug Program Hurt Major Cities, Survey Finds." *The Philadelphia Inquirer*, June 11, 1982, p. 10-A.

ing fun, of avoiding boredom. One mental health authority suggests that "for people who are chronically unhappy, drugs bring some relief from a world without purpose."

Hechinger suggests that among middle-class youth, drug experimentation is the "chain reaction of a combination of permissive homes with the speed-up of youth's experiences in an affluent society." The early onrush of adolescence encourages youth to experiment with partying, dating, sex, smoking, drinking and, before long, glue-sniffing and marijuana. "As old thrills wear off, the search is on for new ones."[47] In the armed forces, it has been concluded that alcoholism among senior noncommissioned officers and drug abuse among young draftees stem from boredom.

Resistance to constructive, organized programs and the choice of escape through drugs frequently is seen in those who "put down" the "establishment" and prefer instead the illicit lure of narcotics or alcohol. Realistically, the sensation gained from drug use provides pleasure which is far more overwhelming than that which other activities might yield.

Goode concludes,

The simple fact is, marijuana is fun to smoke. . . . In my own study of marijuana users, pleasure emerged as the dominant motive for continued use. Almost 70 per cent said that sex was more enjoyable high. Almost 90 per cent said that the simple act of eating became more fun. Almost 90 per cent said that listening to music was a richer, more exciting adventure. . . . Marijuana has become, and will continue to be, increasingly, a *recreational* drug, and for larger and larger numbers of young (and not so young) people. This will not disappear, and it will not abate; drug "education" campaigns are doomed to failure. . . . Outlawing fun has always been a tough job.[48]

Beyond these explanations of drug use, there also is a new understanding of the nature of sensation-seeking as a driving form of human motivation. Many individuals are impelled by the need to dare and to risk, and to get the kind of "high" which comes from dangerous forms of recreation—such as skydiving or hang-gliding—or from substance abuse. One leading psychologist at the University of Pennsylvania, Richard Solomon, points out that addiction itself is a natural and widely found form of animal and human behavior. He comments that,

---

. . . the same principle that produces junkies and alcoholics also produces social attachment, love, thrill seeking, power seeking, over-eating and other forms of addiction. The theory's kicker: each addiction eventually produces its opposite; pleasure turns to pain, and pain to pleasure.

At the start drugs are highly pleasant. You get a big "rush" and euphoria. But as tolerance builds up, the rush disappears and the threat and pain of withdrawal begin to take command. We think that every event in life that has a strong effect also has an opposed process that fights it.[49]

---

[47]Fred Hechinger: "Drugs: Threat on Campus." *The New York Times,* April 10, 1966, p. E-7.
[48]Erich Goode: "Turning on for Fun." *The New York Times,* January 9, 1971, p. 27.
[49]John Leo: "A Painful Theory on Pleasures." *Time,* November 10, 1980, p. 112.

Conflicting Views on Marijuana

As indicated earlier, probably the most popular drug today is marijuana. According to a 1982 report in *Time* magazine, more than 25 million Americans spent some $24 billion in 1980 for the illegal privilege of regularly smoking marijuana. Another 25 million have tried the drug at least once, making it the most widely used illegal substance in the country. A major reason, according to *Time*, is the tenacious belief of marijuana smokers that the occasional "joint" does little, if any, harm.[50]

There continues to be considerable controversy about the actual effects of marijuana. A growing body of experts have concluded that this form of drug use is nonaddictive and actually less dangerous than many other stimulants, including alcohol. A comprehensive report, issued by the National Governors Conference and prepared under a grant from the Federal Law Enforcement Assistance Administration, concluded that moderate or infrequent marijuana use did not appear to pose a significant health hazard and urged that harsh laws penalizing the possession of "pot" be repealed. Numerous authorities have suggested that casual marijuana use is quite similar to social drinking; there is no evidence that it leads to involvement with more serious drugs.[51]

On the other hand, there is evidence of numerous psychotic reactions to marijuana use. There appear to be marked behavioral changes associated with the use of marijuana among some subjects. Wikler writes of a group of subjects involved in a pharmacological experiment:

During the first few days, they exhibited euphoria, bursts of spontaneous laughter, silly behavior, and difficulty in concentrating. Later, they showed loss of interest in work, decreased activity, indolence, non-productivity, and neglect of personal hygiene. . . .[52]

Similarly, a number of medical authorities have documented the damaging effects of marijuana, particularly with adolescents, the age group most open to experimentation with drugs, with the highest rate of usage and most vulnerable to its effects. One doctor urges that legal sanction *not* be given to marijuana, because of its

---

. . . adverse psychological effects: hallucinations, paranoid reactions, depressive reactions, acute psychotic reactions, spontaneous flashbacks and chronic withdrawn reactions (i.e., the so-called amotivational syndrome). All of these adverse responses have been noted and recorded in scientific journals, but receive little or no recognition in the lay media. . . . Since we cannot, ethically, use adolescent subjects for deliberate experimentation, we must rely on clinical observation and on

---

[50]"Another Sort of Smoke." *Time*, March 8, 1982, p. 73.
[51]"Study Finds Marijuana No Hazard." Associated Press Dispatch, March 31, 1977.
[52]Abraham Wikler: "Marijuana *Is* Dangerous." *The New York Times*, April 3, 1971, p. 29.

reports from foreign countries, where cannabis has been widely used, and for countless generations. A review of the world literature is replete with confirmation of our admittedly limited American clinical experience.[53]

The most authoritative study on marijuana use is reported in a long-awaited
188-page document issued in 1982 by the Institute of Medicine of the National
Academy of Sciences. While the study made clear that there was as yet insufficient
evidence on whether marijuana causes irreversible, long-term health damage, there
were sufficient findings to conclude that its use was a matter of serious national
concern. Specifically, the study found that marijuana has major behavioral effects:
it hampers short-term memory, slows learning and distorts judgment, sometimes
inducing panic and confusion.

The National Academy of Sciences report also confirmed that chronic heavy
marijuana use may lead to cancer of the respiratory tract and seriously impair the
lungs; it also impairs the reproductive and immune systems.[54] There also is the
widely held view (although it is not supported by scientific evidence) that many
young people move from experimentation with marijuana, glue-sniffing, "uppers"
and "downers" and other soft drugs to involvement with harder and more dangerous narcotics. Without question, it is essential that every effort be made to stem the
tide of drug use in American society.

Recreation in Drug Treatment Centers

There are a number of different forms of care for drug addicts. One method is
the so-called British system, based on the premise that heroin addiction is a sickness,
not a crime. This approach makes drugs available, by prescription, to formally registered addicts and is intended to meet the needs of those who are unwilling to
undergo a cure or enter an institution—thus minimizing the commercial exploitation of the drug addict's needs.

A second approach to the problem of heroin addiction is the methadone maintenance program. This involves switching an addict from heroin to methadone, a
synthetic substitute that costs relatively little for a day's dosage. Methadone eases
heroin withdrawal and blocks heroin's euphoric effects. It is addictive in itself, however, and many legal and medical authorities resist substituting one form of addiction for another. On the other hand, methadone is much less dangerous than heroin
and permits the addict to lead a relatively normal life.

Another popular approach to working with drug addicts has been the small,
controlled therapeutic community, like Synanon, begun in California and extended
throughout the country, or New York's city-run Phoenix and Horizon House. Such

---

[53]Doris H. Milman: "Of Marijuana, Health and the Law." *The New York Times,* June 2, 1977.
[54]"Another Sort of Smoke," *op. cit.*

residential centers are run largely by former addicts; they first detoxify and then attempt to rehabilitate the drug user by restructuring his ego and life pattern. They accept only those who have proved their determination to kick the habit, and they strive to increase the addict's self-understanding and self-regard through frequently brutal group-encounter sessions.

The traditional method of institutional care has been the special hospital, or hospital unit, such as the two federal narcotics hospitals at Lexington, Kentucky, and Fort Worth, Texas. Most of these programs are more conservatively run. Having been ordered there by the courts, their patients are less highly motivated for change; records indicate that over 90 per cent of those discharged from such institutions eventually return to heroin.

Finally, there are a variety of treatment centers connected to mental health hospitals or outpatient programs, part of state mental health systems or municipal or voluntary hospitals. Many of these are residential, while others provide a variety of "crisis" or continuing treatment services for addicts living in the community. In almost all cases, they use a variety of treatments including individual and group therapy, remedial education, vocational training and placement and other social services—including recreation.

The nature of recreation service in drug addiction centers is heavily influenced by the typical personality patterns of drug users. Characteristically, they tend to have extremely low self-esteem, be overly dependent on others and have a very low threshold for frustration. Their defense and adjustment mechanisms are often juvenile; they demand immediate gratification, have little sense of time and are unable to plan effectively for the future.

Like other social deviants, drug users typically engage in few organized, constructive recreational activities. Although they may have been involved in sports or social programs at an earlier time, they usually relinquish such interests when they become heavily addicted. Their lives revolve about the drug culture. They associate with other addicts; getting and using drugs becomes their chief preoccupation. Those who work with addicts in drug treatment programs comment that they tend to be extremely passive in their use of free time and usually resist structured programs.

The goals of recreation in treatment centers for drug users should be

1. To contribute to the overall rehabilitation of the addict by encouraging the development of more varied interests and talents so that the need to turn to drugs for pleasure or release will be lessened.
2. To encourage personality changes that will strengthen the addict's self-concept and ego controls and provide a sense of worth and accomplishment.
3. To contribute to the overall therapeutic environment by providing a relaxed, tension-free atmosphere and by encouraging group activities that can break down barriers among participants and encourage communication between participants and staff members.

A key factor in such programs is the need for the recreation specialist to establish a relationship of mutual trust and respect with the addict under treatment. It may take days or weeks for this to develop, but it is essential that the recreation worker become accepted as a trustworthy person who has the addict's needs as a primary concern. Young and Hutchison write,

The therapeutic recreation program revolves around a ''core'' of planned group activities. Enough variety is provided in group programming to give each individual patient a chance to find his sphere of interest and to function at his particular level of comfortable interaction with others. Because the attention and interest span of the post-addict tends to be limited, specific recreative activities are provided in periods of from thirty minutes to one hour in length. The number of activities per day, and the number of times an individual patient is involved in a given activity per day or per week depend on the center's population at a given time. Activities that allow for various combinations of patient-staff ratio are scheduled according to the individual patient's current level of dependency.[55]

They stress that it is important not to place too much pressure on the addict during the initial stages of treatment. Although the physiological trauma of withdrawal may be over, the addict is still fighting a psychological battle to remain off drugs. At this point, many addicts find it difficult to accept specific rules related to attendance and participation; excess pressure may be counterproductive.

Typically, programs may include both voluntary and required participation in group and individual activities. At the Ridge Hill Rehabilitation Center, a residential facility for drug addicts operated by the New York State Drug Abuse Control Commission, the daytime program involves required participation in such activities as sports and physical fitness, arts and crafts, music, table games and trips. In the evening and on weekends, there is voluntary participation in many of the same activities, with closer interaction between staff members and residents in small-group activities and counseling sessions.

Gradually, as clients become more involved in activities, a shift in the addict's attitude and level of participation takes place. When this is observed, leadership approaches are changed:

. . . a gradual increase of pressure from the staff, and involvement in situations where the post-addict takes more responsibility — and risks greater chance of failure — are introduced into the individual program plan. At this point, the recreation specialist becomes primarily a supportive figure. He spares no effort to ease the transition from a dependent attitude and existence to a semi-independent or independent level of functioning.[56]

LEADERSHIP RESPONSIBILITIES

Throughout this process, the recreation leader working with addict groups must operate much less as a direct, authoritarian leader of activities and much more as a nondirective counselor and friend, a catalyst who gently encourages and makes changes in behavior and attitudes possible.

The recreation specialist must function as a professional member of the treatment team. He or she should be fully involved in interdisciplinary staff meetings

---

[55]Elliott G. Young and Ira Hutchison: ''Prescription Recreation: A Bridge to Community Living for the Narcotics Addict.'' *Recreation in Treatment Centers*, September 1964, p. 60.
[56]*Ibid.*, p. 61.

and should work closely with psychiatrists, psychologists, unit counselors, vocational rehabilitation specialists and other personnel to exchange information and share in planning to meet the needs of each patient. Furthermore, the recreation leader should be active in promoting community programs designed to serve addicts and discharged patients.

RECREATION AND THE TREATMENT OF ALCOHOLICS

Although the public has been greatly disturbed by the growth of drug abuse in recent years, alcoholism represents a much greater threat to society. There are an estimated ten million alcoholics in the United States today who cannot control their drinking and have serious personal, social or vocational problems stemming from it. It was reported in 1975 that

---

According to the National Institute on Alcohol Abuse and Alcoholism, 1.3 million Americans between 12 and 17 have serious drinking problems. About one-third of our high school students get drunk at least once a month. Arrests of teenagers for drunken driving have tripled since 1960; 60 per cent of the people killed in drunken driving accidents are now in their teens.[57]

Overall, according to the American Medical Association, an average of 35,000 Americans are killed each year in automobile accidents in which alcohol is involved. Alcohol now ranks as the third major cause of death in the United States; it has been estimated that the life span of the alcoholic is 12 years shorter than that of the nonalcoholic. Excessive drinking not only is a major health risk but also is often linked to the loss of jobs, marital breakdown and other personal problems. Recent research has shown that drinking is closely associated with other forms of delinquency among young offenders.[58] Seventy per cent of patients with a diagnosis of antisocial personality are likely to subsequently become alcoholics. In particular, many alcoholics suffer from secondary depression.[59]

Nature of Alcoholism

Alcoholism is the subject of numerous misconceptions and stereotypes in our society. The popular way of thinking about alcoholism is that it represents a form

---

[57]"School Study Calls 28% of Teen-Agers 'Problem' Drinkers." Associated Press Dispatch, November 20, 1975.
[58]Nick Heather: "Relationships Between Delinquency and Drunkenness Among Scottish Young Offenders." *British Journal on Alcohol and Alcoholism*, Second Quarter, 1981, pp. 50–61.
[59]Frederick Petty and Henry A. Nasrallah: "Secondary Depression in Alcoholism: Implications for Future Research." *Comprehensive Psychiatry*, November-December 1981, pp. 587–595.

of immoral behavior or weak character and that the typical alcoholic is a "skid row" type—a disheveled, helpless vagrant or bum. In reality, the American Medical Association has identified alcoholism as a complex disease "with biological, psychological, and sociological components" that takes numerous forms.

Alcoholism affects all levels of society, including many extremely successful and hard-working men and women. Studies have shown that in some populations, the incidence of alcoholism is actually higher among more economically successful individuals. It is peculiarly linked to the work world; heavy drinking is encouraged by the very nature of many jobs that require business entertainment and heavy travel and carry a high degree of tension. Society as a whole is extremely ambivalent about drinking. On the one hand, we decry and discourage it, particularly in excess; on the other hand, it is a built-in part of most adult social occasions, and it is a mark of maturity to be "able to hold one's liquor" or "drink like a man." Drinking is important throughout culture. When people pledge loyalty and friendship, a drink is often shared. The drinking of alcohol is an accepted ritual at such occasions as betrothals, weddings, christenings, banquets and receptions. It is taken for granted as a way to relax, a way to relieve self-consciousness and loosen the tongue. Most people drink chiefly to produce the kind of pleasant relaxation and glow that comes from a mild concentration of alcohol in the bloodstream. Indeed, in some therapeutic settings, such as nursing homes, the practice has developed of having modest cocktail parties or beer sessions, at which residents may have a drink or two under controlled circumstances.

Although it is popularly thought of as a stimulant, alcohol is a depressant of the central nervous system and particularly its inhibitory mechanisms. It tends to reduce tension and anxiety and often results in exaggerated behavior, such as aggression toward others, loud joking, crying or extremely extroverted behavior. It may be considered a psychoactive, or mind-altering, drug, as well as an addictive substance. Sessoms writes of the "alcoholic personality" as one who suffers from extreme feelings of inadequacy and anxiety, and is excessively dependent upon others for support and direction.[60] For such individuals, drinking becomes a quick and effective way to "escape from reality," a temporary and destructive mechanism that brings an artificial sense of pleasure and satisfaction.

Navar and Nordoff agree, pointing out that

For the alcoholic, drinking has become a means of coping with stress. As stress builds, an individual must take some action to obtain relief in order to achieve a state of balance. The alcoholic has learned that consuming alcohol brings a sense of relief. However, that sensation is short-lived, as drinking produces more problems and thus more stress. A state of balance or well-being is not reached. The alcoholic has attempted to use alcohol as a change agent. The person must find another change agent of a healthier nature to reach a state of balance or well-being.[61]

---

[60]H. Douglas Sessoms: "Recreation and the Alcoholic and Drug Addict." *In* Thomas A. Stein and H. Douglas Sessoms: *Recreation and Special Populations.* Boston, Holbrook, 1977, p. 180.
[61]Nancy Navar and Jacquelyn A. Nordoff: "Recreation as a Change Agent for the Alcoholic." *Journal of Physical Education and Recreation*, May 1975, pp. 36–37.

There have been numerous approaches to curing people of alcoholism in the past; these have included imprisonment (alcoholism is a crime in many states and is typically linked to the commission of many other crimes), psychoanalysis, use of antiabuse or aversion therapy, group therapy and behavior modification. Alcoholics Anonymous, a nonprofessional, self-help organization, along with its companion organizations Al-Anon and Al-a-Teen, has been extremely helpful for many thousands of alcoholics. It is a fundamental tenet of alcoholic rehabilitation that people who have this disease simply cannot drink at all, even in minor amounts (although some recent findings suggest that many former alcoholics have become social drinkers, imbibing in moderation).[62]

Recreation and Alcohol Rehabilitation

A landmark research study in this field by Sessoms and Oakley found that patients in a state alcoholic rehabilitation center in North Carolina differed sharply from the general population in their leisure involvements.[63] Typically, they engaged most in those activities that required a minimum of skill and equipment and demanded little personal commitment. A heavy stress on work and spectator activities and a generally passive attitude toward leisure and recreation, particularly outdoor recreation, characterized those studied. Much of the recreation of the typical alcoholic is built around drinking—and the alcoholic tends to stay away from places where drinking is not possible.

Any approach to helping in the rehabilitation of the alcoholic through recreation must accept the nature of his or her personality—often dependent, compulsive and lacking in confidence and self-esteem. The recreation program must seek to build self-understanding and self-acceptance, as well as important group skills. The alcoholic's lifestyle must be modified by providing new and different satisfactions that give the individual a different kind of "high," without liquor. Sheridan suggests that an effective recreation program for alcoholics, while obviously not a panacea by itself, should have the following values (in effect, these supplant the "payoffs" formerly derived from alcohol):

1. Socialization with a minimum of tension and anxiety.
2. Alternative methods of dealing with feelings of frustration, anxiety, anger, depression, etc.
3. Fun or escape from life situations which cause tension.
4. Relaxation.
5. Adventure and the opportunity to express oneself creatively.[64]

---

[62]"Alcoholism: Is There Normal Drinking?" Report by RAND Corporation, in Associated Press Dispatch, June 10, 1976. It should be noted that more recent findings, in 1982, have raised a serious question about the earlier study, and reaffirm the view that alcoholics *cannot* drink socially.
[63]H. Douglas Sessoms and Sidney R. Oakley: "Recreation, Leisure and the Alcoholic." *Journal of Leisure Research*, Winter 1969, pp. 21–31.
[64]Paul M. Sheridan: "Therapeutic Recreation and the Alcoholic." *Therapeutic Recreation Journal*, First Quarter, 1976, pp. 14–17.

To accomplish these ends, recreation should be used as a significant tool to fill the patient's leisure with constructive, enjoyable and nonthreatening activity. Emphasis should be placed on helping each individual to overcome feelings of inhibition and guilt and to relax, behaving spontaneously and freely in a socially accepted and nondestructive manner. Leisure counseling is also a much needed part of this program, for both individuals and small groups, so that clients may understand the role of leisure in their lives and develop values, attitudes and resources to use it most constructively. Finally, Navar and Nordoff point out that the family ties of many alcoholics have deteriorated because of drinking, and the therapeutic recreation program should attempt to involve the family and reintegrate clients under treatment with their close relatives.

A uniquely successful approach to the treatment of alcoholics in California has strongly emphasized sports and physical fitness. These activities have several important values: (a) they help the client rebuild and take pride in a body that may have seriously deteriorated during years of excessive alcohol intake and poor nutritional support; (b) they provide an opportunity for the alcoholic to develop self-discipline and enthusiasm through participation in competitive events; and (c) they raise the alcoholic's sense of self-worth and status in the eyes of others. A vivid example of how such activities may promote the rehabilitation of the alcoholic is shown in a successful Alcoholic Olympics which has been carried on for the past several years, with widespread participation and community support.[65]

RESIDENTIAL PROGRAMS FOR DISTURBED AND DEPENDENT YOUTH

A final category of institutional therapeutic recreation programs related to social deviance may be found in residential programs serving neglected, emotionally disturbed or socially maladjusted children and youth. Often, such youngsters come from families who have not provided adequate care and guidance. Typically, although they may not have been adjudged delinquent, they have been unsuccessful in school and have developed severe emotional difficulties. For many, delinquency and a later criminal life are probable unless they are cared for at this critical point in their lives in a stable, nurturing environment.

In such residential settings, recreation supplies the means for normalizing the daily living routine by providing the opportunity for the full range of recreational, cultural and social activities that children living in the community have—or should have. Youth-care institutions of this type may be sponsored by a variety of agencies.

An excellent illustration of such facilities is the Dobbs Ferry Children's Village in Dobbs Ferry, New York. Children's Village, founded in 1851, has been a pioneer in the field of child care since its inception. It was among the first institutions serving indigent and homeless children to establish a mental health clinic on campus;

---

[65]Kurt Freeman and Ronald R. Koegler: *From Skid Row to the Olympics.* Castaic, California, Institute of Creative Leisure, 1978.

to employ a staff psychiatrist; to develop a therapeutic environment that integrated casework, child care, education and recreation; and to prescribe individual treatment programs for all young residents.

Recreation is offered on several different levels: *leisure education, after-school group activities, individually chosen workshops* and *voluntary participation in campus-wide activities* (see p. 130). Children's Village offers an extensive program of sports, musical and dramatic activities, hobbies, trips and special events. In addition to these regularly provided activities, it has experimented with a number of unique programs that have been extremely successful in involving children with limited recreational backgrounds and interests.

One of these programs has involved nature activities. Children's Village operates an extensive nature study and hobby program, including 32 different organized activities, such as the study and observation of mammals, reptiles and amphibians, plants, birds, and insects and other arthropods. While studying mammals, for example, the children collected nearly 30 assorted skulls and portions of skeletons, usually of skunks, raccoons, opossums and birds, found in the woods adjacent to the village. They restored and mounted these artifacts and became involved in field trips and in a variety of other experiences related to natural science and animal life.

The institution also maintains an extensive winterized zoo, with a variety of birds, domestic animals and small wild animals. Many of the children are involved in the care of these animals; this experience has been found to be of great value in working with emotionally disturbed children, who often have difficulty in relating to their peers and in accepting other types of responsibility.

A second major project of the Children's Village has been the development of unique outdoor recreation areas. Working under the direction of professional staff members, children have built an elaborate Indian village, with tepees, totem poles, archery ranges and similar facilities. Materials were bought from government-surplus stocks or were donated. The Indian village has become the site of many interesting activities related to Indian lore, including arts and crafts, tests of courage, music, dance and other programs based on Indian rituals. In addition to this project, children have also built a space center, an army camp center, a pioneer fort and a Western town. Each of these facilities is used for various outdoor recreation activities, including camping out, pageants and similar program features.

At Children's Village, recreation is fully accepted as an important aspect of the institution's overall program in terms of status on the treatment team, qualifications and salaries of recreation staff members and similar criteria. For this situation to be maintained, the director of recreation services must be certain that every effort is made to identify new and more meaningful potential services, that the help of other disciplines is brought into planning programs and developing treatment plans, that needed research is carried on and that all programs are carefully evaluated. Among the unique features of Children's Village is its continuing effort not simply to deal with the child in the institution but to work with families through counseling, group therapy sessions and other supportive services, to re-establish an environment to which children can return successfully. Recreation plays an important role in this process, in terms of both helping to familiarize parents with the community resources available to them and counseling residents at the village about community opportunities and helping them establish favorable affiliations when they return to their families or foster homes.

COMMUNITY RECREATION PROGRAMS
AND DELINQUENCY

In addition to residential corrections centers which are needed for hard-core offenders, community-based corrections will require a number of specialized types of facilities and programs. These may include halfway houses, pre-release centers and multi-service programs for youth that provide drug counseling and vocational and other needed forms of assistance.

Beyond these, many public recreation and park departments have as a major purpose the prevention and "cure" of juvenile delinquency. Since its inception in the early decades of this century, the recreation movement has used slogans such as "keep the kids off the street" or "give them something useful to do" as explanations of their social goals. This has been particularly true in large cities, where youth problems have been severe. Few recreation departments have been successful in this effort, however, for the following reasons:

1. Most obviously, delinquency is the result of a variety of factors, such as family instability, slum housing, poor education, limited vocational opportunity or the lack of other vitally needed social services. Within this context, it is unrealistic to believe that recreation, by itself, can significantly deter delinquent activity. However, it can and should be an important part of total community efforts to serve the socially deviant.
2. Most recreation departments and agencies do *not* make a special attempt to serve delinquent or predelinquent youths. Often they view this as a difficult task that they are not equipped to handle. In many cases they bar disruptive and antisocial youth from their facilities, thus making it impossible to serve them meaningfully.
3. Usually, antisocial and gang youth reject organized activities and are unwilling to become part of the formal structure of community agencies. In part, this is because they do not wish to be controlled or because their high-impulse, hedonistic values do not permit them to conform to the rules and limitations inherent in youth programs, team sports and the like.

In some cities, gangs may use community centers as hangouts—often discouraging other participants from entering. However, it is rare for them to be meaningfully involved in such programs. Instead, in most communities, special youth boards or commissions or antipoverty organizations—where these exist—have been the only formal agencies to work with delinquent youth.

Guidelines for Working with Problem Youth

How *can* the public recreation department or voluntary agency that is concerned about working with delinquent or predelinquent youth do so effectively?

1. It is essential to view recreation, at the outset, as a positive and meaningful form of community service. Unless it is seen and supported in this light, it cannot be successful in any form of significant social programming.

2. In working with problem youth, it is not possible to plan programs at a high level of authority and simply present them with the results. Instead, it is essential

to involve youth *fully* in the planning and development of programs. This may be done by having representatives from various gangs or neighborhoods join together in a recreation center council to plan programs and formulate agency policies.

3. Gangs generally are thought of negatively—and it is true that they often are responsible for various forms of crime in urban slums. However, gangs also represent an understandable need for group affiliation, for status and even for self-protection in ghetto areas. In some cases, minority-group gangs have driven drug pushers out of their neighborhoods or have accomplished similar desirable goals. It is essential to recognize their existence and attempt to work with them positively rather than to try to eradicate them.

4. Recreation programs designed to serve antisocial youth often fail to attract them because they are not interesting or challenging enough. Such programs *must* be well planned and staffed and should involve exciting goals and experiences. They may include trips, cultural programs, activities that have career-development potential, and—when possible—activities that have a degree of risk or danger about them. Activities like skiing or tobogganing, horseback riding or underwater exploration, which "test" manhood, have been used successfully with such youth. Their particular value is that they may sublimate the urge to take part in dangerous, unlawful activities by providing an equally challenging, but socially acceptable, leisure outlet.

5. Community center programs designed to meet the needs of delinquent youth *must* provide more than recreation. They should also include educational or remedial educational programs, vocational training and placement, psychological counseling services, drug abuse programs and similar activities. All this can be woven into the overall program of an agency that is primarily geared to offer recreation services.

6. In any long-range program intended to reduce delinquency, it is essential to reach children between the ages of 6 and 12. Often, the patterns of antisocial behavior are set as early as age 6 or 7. By age 8 or 9, children are involved in criminal activity and antisocial gangs. Therefore, every effort must be made to work regularly with children at this age, to reduce antisocial group involvement and to recognize and refer to appropriate agencies those children who have severe individual problems of adjustment. As much as possible, parents should be drawn into this effort.

7. Programs in centers need to be more carefully organized and structured. In many community centers in low-income areas, there is a constant flow—in and out—of unregistered participants. Often activities are carried on in a completely casual way, with informal games and music being the heart of the program. Instead, it is desirable to have a registration system so that only center members may enter, with rules set by the youth council itself as to the basis for membership. Programs should be scheduled and carefully directed to encourage the maximum participation in organized activities.

8. A final guideline applies to those youth who are *not* willing to enter community centers at all and who have no regular contact with adult leaders or youth workers. These are unaffiliated gang youth who hang out in the neighborhoods, are frequently school dropouts and are often responsible for incidents of gang violence or sporadic criminal activity. For such youth, a special "outreach" approach is required.

THE ROVING LEADER APPROACH

A number of cities have adopted an approach under which special youth workers—usually individuals who have themselves grown up in slum neighborhoods and may have been involved in gangs—are assigned the task of making contact with unaffiliated youth. They are usually detached from organized programs and go out into the street, neighborhood hangouts or other places where problem youth may be found.

In Washington, D.C., roving leaders typically work directly with several hundred gang youth, as well as others who are sporadically associated with gangs. They receive on-the-job training in group-work techniques, street-corner contact methods, community resources and psychological counseling. The goals of these workers are both short-range and long-range.

Their short-range objectives are to (a) reduce the severity and frequency of offenses, such as gang warfare, murder and theft; (b) redirect behavior into more desirable channels; and (c) help adolescents make use of available community resources. Their long-range goals are to help gang youth become more fully integrated in the "major culture" and to change their social values and life patterns so that they may become responsible, law-abiding and gainfully employed citizens.

Since they are often attempting to reach extremely hostile and alienated individuals who come from broken homes, have arrest records or have been confined to correctional institutions and are wary of adult contact, leaders often must work for months and years to establish rapport with target gangs. They seek to get to know them, gain their confidence, counsel and assist them and ultimately guide them in the constructive directions previously described.

Although this may be seen primarily as a social-work function, it has been assigned to the Recreation Department in Washington and other cities, because the recreation program has the broadest capability for reaching and involving large numbers of youth in the community. In addition, recreation *is* an important aspect of the Roving Leader program. For example, programs offered by Washington's detached workers have included trips to amusement parks, theaters, art galleries and soccer, football, baseball and basketball games; picnics; fishing; nursing aide and census-taking projects; bowling; skating; and talent shows. Camping and boat and airplane rides are also offered.

The roving leader approach is being used in an increasing number of large cities. It has been encouraged by the U.S. Office of Education's Division of Manpower Development and Training, which funded the Office of Recreation and Park Resources at the University of Illinois, in cooperation with the National Recreation and Park Association, to promote and research the roving leader concept.

Such programs are examples of how recreation may serve preventive as well as treatment needs—in the community as well as in institutions. Obviously, the problem of working with deviant groups is much less costly, both in human and financial terms, if it can be done before patterns of serious antisocial behavior are clearly established. The treatment process in institutions is too often ineffective when antisocial attitudes and deviant behavior patterns have become deeply ingrained. Youth often leave correctional institutions more fully committed to a life of crime than they were when first committed. The cost of residential programs for deviant or dependent youth is extremely high, ranging up to $25,000 to $30,000 per child per year in some states. One publicly funded addiction treatment facility costs $45,000 a year per patient. Clearly, a major thrust of all community youth agencies, including therapeutic recreation service, must be to prevent antisocial behavior at its start.

In many cities, police departments join forces with other voluntary or public organizations, through Police Athletic Leagues or police youth bureaus, to provide recreation activities and youth centers. In some instances, special projects have been mounted with funding from the Federal Law Enforcement Assistance Administration to combat juvenile delinquency. One such program, carried out by the Youth Services Program of the Dallas, Texas, Police Department, appears to have been strikingly successful in reducing the re-arrest rate among juvenile offenders who were involved in a police-sponsored sports and physical fitness program.[66]

The long-range trend in youth services appears to be away from institutional care and toward community-based programs, either in foster care or small-group homes or intensive services provided for youth living with their families on a semi-probationary status. The New York State Division for Youth's Cooperative Placement Program has made intensive efforts to involve local voluntary agencies in youth care programs and has moved assertively to end the practice of caring for dependent children and youth (known as PINS, or Persons in Need of Supervision) in state training schools. It seems likely that this trend will continue to grow throughout the United States. Much richer and more effective programs of youth recreation must come from the communities themselves to serve problem youth.

Some large cities have developed a broad range of youth services, including centers, city-wide youth councils and special events. These include programs designed to appeal to the current interests of youth and to provide a degree of physical risk or challenge that makes them especially exciting for youngsters who might otherwise become involved in gangs. Related programs are wilderness camps involving Outward Bound–type challenges, including rock-climbing, rope courses, forestry work and survival activities.[67]

As we become increasingly aware of the mounting financial and human costs posed by juvenile delinquency and adult crime—with steadily swelling prison populations—it seems clear that many new forms of prevention and rehabilitation will be developed in the years ahead. Therapeutic recreation must continue to be an important element in such treatment and prevention programs.

Suggested Topics for Class Discussion, Examination Questions or Student Papers

1. What are some of the basic factors underlying juvenile delinquency, as a form of social deviance, that make constructive and well-planned recreation programs essential in correctional institutions?

---

[66]T. R. Collingwood and Mike Engelsgjerd: "Physical Fitness, Physical Activity, and Juvenile Delinquency." *Journal of Physical Education and Recreation*, June 1977, p. 23.
[67]See, for example, Kenneth I. Lingle: "Alternatives for Youth at Risk—Outdoor Experiences for a Special Population." *Camping Magazine* and Fund for Advancement of Camping, May 1980, pp. 15–26.

2. Although there is much more interest today than in the past in providing recreation in correctional and penal settings, most such programs are extremely limited. What are the major obstacles to improving recreation in such institutions? How might these be overcome?

3. Describe the roving leader approach as a technique used by recreation departments to combat socially deviant gang behavior. What are its strengths and limitations as a form of community service?

4. How can recreation serve both as a preventative and as a form of treatment in community and institutional programs for alcoholics and drug addicts? In your reply, deal with the nature of the addictive personality and the substitution of recreation for drugs or alcohol as a means of meeting psychosocial needs, or getting "high."

11

Community Services for the Disabled

This chapter focuses on the role of community organizations in providing special programs to serve the disabled. It describes the scope and focus of such agencies and presents guidelines for expanding their efforts.

FOCUS OF COMMUNITY-BASED THERAPEUTIC RECREATION

It is the purpose of community-based recreation or social service agencies to serve disabled persons who live with their families or in other settings in which they have a degree of social independence. The great majority of aged, mentally retarded and physically disabled individuals are not institutionalized. They may, however, require modified or specially designed programs or environments to meet their recreational needs.

Mainstreaming as a Goal

As earlier chapters of this text have shown, a major thrust of educational, recreational and other social services for the disabled over the past two decades has been to maximize their opportunities to reach their fullest potentials as human beings—and to do so whenever possible in integrated settings. Hayes summarizes the slogans and goals with respect to integrating the disabled in society that have been widely accepted in the human service field during this period: "Mainstreaming! Normalization! Integration! The least restrictive environment! Maximizing one's potential! Equal opportunity! Humanistic approach!"[1]

On its most basic level, mainstreaming implies bringing the disabled into full

---

[1]Gene A. Hayes: "Philosophical Ramifications of Mainstreaming in Recreation." *Therapeutic Recreation Journal,* Second Quarter, 1978, p. 5.

participation in various aspects of community life, side-by-side with the nondisabled population. The concept of mainstreaming is summed up in Section 504 of the federal Rehabilitation Act of 1973:

No otherwise qualified handicapped individual in the United States . . . shall, solely by reason of his handicap, be excluded from the participation, be denied the benefits of, or be subjected to discrimination under a program or activity receiving federal financial assistance.

Although integration of the disabled with the nondisabled is a highly desirable goal, it is not always a feasible one. In the field of education, for example, the passage in the mid-1970's of the Education of All Handicapped Children Act, which required that all states receiving federal aid provide "free and appropriate" education for the handicapped, gave a tremendous stimulus to those who sought to end educational isolation of the disabled. Yet, as Hechinger points out, some disabilities are far more receptive to "mainstreaming" than others. Many children with physical disabilities such as blindness, deafness or limited mobility

. . . are endowed with high intellectual and motivational qualities that enable them to overcome their handicaps. . . . Children with varying degrees of retardation pose substantially different problems. Some may benefit from being integrated into nonintellectual activities, such as sports, shop and other nonverbal subjects. But their sense of defeat and frustration might be heightened rather than diminished in intellectual competition with their non-handicapped peers. Children with serious emotional problems may not only disrupt ordinary educational procedures but also arouse anger and antagonism in their classmates. Here too, however, the degree of the emotional disturbance should be seriously considered.[2]

Similar considerations prevail in planning recreation services for the disabled in the community. The administrator of a community-based therapeutic recreation program jointly sponsored by three Michigan cities asks,

Does mainstreaming eliminate the need for special recreation programs for the handicapped? Can all handicapped individuals participate in and benefit from a mainstreamed recreation program? Does mainstreaming really work? As a community recreation professional who is responsible for programming for special populations, I have asked myself these questions many times.[3]

---

[2]Fred M. Hechinger: "Bringing the Handicapped into the Mainstream." *The New York Times*, April 25, 1976, p. ES-15.
[3]Michael Mushett: "Is Mainstreaming for Everyone? Concepts and Issues as Experienced in One Program." *Therapeutic Recreation Journal*, Fourth Quarter, 1978, p. 31.

While it is appealing to think of the disabled as people "just like other people, with the same needs, desires and abilities," the fact is that their disabilities may be so severe that they are simply not capable of fully integrated participation with others. As an example, when many large residential institutions for the mentally retarded moved numbers of clients into community-based supervised group homes and apartments, a high percentage of these individuals were in the moderately to severely retarded range—with IQ's of 30 to 45. Such persons often have such limited social skills that it would simply not be feasible for them to attempt to enter community recreation programs requiring a higher level of behavior.[4]

Disabled individuals may be divided into three broad categories, whatever the specific nature of their impairment:

1. Those whose limitations are so severe that they require completely segregated programs and social groupings. They may be unable to participate in activities for the nondisabled, or they may be rejected by the nondisabled or excluded by sponsoring authorities. In the latter case, therapeutic recreation specialists should seek to determine whether there is a legitimate basis for the exclusion or segregation, or whether it should be challenged.
2. Those whose disabilities prevent them from taking part in integrated programs in some areas of activity but who can readily share in other programs. Children with severe physical impairments might not be able to play in sports leagues with nondisabled children without experiencing repeated failure and rejection. On the other hand, they might engage very successfully in activities such as arts and crafts or dramatics on a fully integrated basis.
3. Those who are able to take part with a considerable degree of success in varied activities with the nondisabled. Efforts should be made to integrate such individuals as fully as possible with the overall population.

For many individuals, it is possible to gain social and physical skills and self-confidence, and move from segregated programs into integrated groups. As an example, disabled children may become involved first in a day camp serving those with impairment on a segregated basis. Gradually, they may be able to attend a sleep-away camp and, ultimately, to take part in camping programs that serve both the disabled and the nondisabled. Antozzi cites a number of examples of integrated camping for physically handicapped and nonhandicapped populations which showed how both groups benefited from the experience—although not without difficulty. For example, in a pilot project conducted by the New York Association for the Blind, which integrated sighted persons with the visually disabled,

---

... much aggression, non-acceptance and inhibition was observed throughout the duration of the project. However, toward the conclusion of this three-week experience, social stigmas broke down, friendships developed and a greater understanding and perception of each other's world transpired between the handicapped and non-handicapped.[5]

---

[4]"The Closing of Pennhurst: Will Society Be Ready?" *The Philadelphia Inquirer*, March 20, 1978, p. 1-A.
[5]Robert Antozzi: "Mainstreaming: Social Ramifications of Integrated Camping for Physically Handicapped and Normal Populations." *Therapeutic Recreation Journal*, Fourth Quarter, 1979, p. 35.

On the other hand, one extensive study of camping for the disabled found that segregated camps had a positive effect on self-concept. Handicapped children in the segregated setting generally felt more competent than handicapped children in an integrated camp.[6] Obviously, the process is a complex one; it cannot be approached simply by expressing idealistic but impractical beliefs about the values of main-streaming. Collard and Charboneau-Klein sum up by pointing out that the mutual acceptance and interaction of disabled and nondisabled individuals is a widely accepted goal of mainstreaming:

> Yet, a broader definition considers mainstreaming to be a developmental, step-by-step process. This process entails careful planning to develop a disabled person's skills and decision-making abil-ities, to initiate interagency cooperation, to train staff, to educate able-bodied consumers and the community . :. In other words, we are mainstreaming not people, but "the system."[7]

The purpose of all community-based recreation programming for the disabled is to provide the most appropriate and richest kind of leisure experience for each individual—to contribute to his or her growth and personal development. Inde-pendent living and integration with the nondisabled is a major although not always achievable goal. Usually, the sponsors of such programs fall into the following categories.

Sponsors of Community Services for the Disabled

PUBLIC RECREATION AGENCIES

These include public recreation or recreation and park departments, school dis-tricts, youth service agencies, community service departments in housing projects, publicly sponsored libraries, museums and other agencies which provide recreation for the general public. Included may be programs in which the disabled participate without any special planning, identification or modification of activities or equip-ment, provided they are able to achieve a degree of success and satisfaction on this informal basis. Specially designed programs intended to serve the disabled and established for this purpose are also included. More and more, such special recrea-tion programs are becoming collaborative efforts involving the joint sponsorship of two or more public agencies or the cooperation of public and private or voluntary groups.

---

[6]*Ibid.*, p. 38.
[7]Kathleen Collard and Ethel Charboneau-Klein: "A Catalyst to Change." *Therapeutic Recreation Journal*, Fourth Quarter, 1979, p. 27.

ORGANIZATIONS CONCERNED WITH DISABILITY

As described earlier, a considerable number of national organizations with local or regional chapters promote programs designed to meet the needs of individuals with special disabilities. If they do not provide such services directly, they often cooperate with other agencies that do by providing funding, technical advisement, volunteers or other forms of support.

SERVICE ORGANIZATIONS

In most American communities, there are a variety of service organizations or civic clubs committed to providing or assisting programs that meet social needs. Fraternal or service organizations, such as the Elks, Moose, Kiwanis and Oddfellows, and veterans' organizations, such as the Veterans of Foreign Wars and the American Legion, frequently sponsor programs serving disabled children and youth. In addition to such organizations, other voluntary organizations in the recreation field, such as the YMCA or YWCA and Boys Clubs or Girl Scouts, frequently mount special programs for the disabled.

SPECIAL AGENCIES

In a few cities, special agencies have been established that have as their primary purpose the provision of recreation to varied groups of disabled persons. One such agency, the San Francisco Recreation Center for the Handicapped, is described later in this chapter.

COMMUNITY COUNCILS OR BOARDS

In order to develop systematic recreation services to meet the leisure needs of disabled persons, community councils or boards have been formed in a number of major cities. Such councils usually serve to promote public awareness of the needs of the disabled, to identify existing programs and to make recommendations, develop support and coordinate new services.

The range of services offered is extremely wide. They may include any or all of the following:

Social clubs for mentally retarded or physically disabled youth and adults.
Day camps or residential vacation camps for those with varied disabilities, including the aged.
Special facilities, such as playgrounds, parks or community centers, designed to be suitable for those with physical handicaps.
After-care programs for discharged mental patients, former drug addicts or other persons who require sheltered social settings in their transition to community life.
Volunteer services for homebound individuals with severe disabilities.

PUBLIC RECREATION PROGRAMS FOR
THE DISABLED

In a number of major cities, as well as in many smaller communities, public recreation or recreation and park departments offer comprehensive programs to serve the leisure needs of the physically and mentally disabled.

In Seattle, Washington, an extensive program is offered under the direction of a full-time therapeutic recreation specialist employed by the Recreation Division of the municipal Park Department. The schedule of special programs in Seattle includes such elements as

1. Monthly meetings for disabled children in various recreation centers around the city, usually on Friday or Saturday afternoons. These meetings are continued throughout the year and involve varied club and recreational activities.
2. Swimming lessons for disabled children, given in ten-week series during the fall. The lessons are specially designed so that there is at least one instructor for every two or three children. Beginners, or those who cannot support themselves in the water, are taught individually.
3. A summer day camp for disabled children 6 years of age or older. These are held in three three-week sessions at several camp and park locations in Seattle and King County. Activities include nature crafts, music, games, singing, creative dramatics, sports, cookouts and hiking.

Other programs in Seattle include groups organized by the Cerebral Palsy Workshop and the Washington Association for the Retarded. There is a special bowling league for the retarded and wheelchair basketball for the orthopedically disabled, as well as a basketball league for deaf adult participants. A major portion of the leadership is provided by volunteers, with the assistance of a central volunteer bureau and a number of service agencies in the community.

Many other cities offer comparable programs. For example, the Los Angeles Park and Recreation Department provides programs for blind adults, multiply disabled youth, the physically disabled and the mentally retarded.

The Chicago Park District has special programs for the disabled in 15 of its major centers, providing assistance to Alcoholics Anonymous, the mentally retarded or perceptually handicapped, the deaf and blind and discharged mental patients and their families.

The Ill and Handicapped Division of the Greensboro, North Carolina, Parks and Recreation Commission provides 18 different programs for the mentally retarded, cerebral palsied, blind, orthopedically handicapped, emotionally disturbed and other disabled individuals. Special programs are provided for nursing homes, and a six-week summer day camp serves a substantial number of disabled children with music, nature activities, games, sports and crafts.

The Memphis, Tennessee, Park Commission, in cooperation with a nonprofit Memphis organization called Handicapped, Inc., has established a year-round comprehensive recreation program for the disabled. It is housed in an outstanding redesigned building equipped to serve the mentally retarded, blind, deaf and other special groups. The program serves all age levels with a wide range of activities, trips and camping programs and is assisted by over 2000 volunteers yearly.

Similarly, the Washington, D.C., Recreation Department has built an excellent multi-million dollar facility to serve the district-wide recreation needs of the disabled. Over the past two decades, Washington has pioneered in community recreation service for the disabled. One of its unique contributions during the early 1970's was to employ a substantial number of disabled youth and adults, including those with such conditions as retardation, visual disability and orthopedic impairment, as recreation leaders and bussing aides in its own summer programs.

The involvement of municipal recreation and park departments in programming for special populations has been facilitated in a number of cities that have established umbrella-like human services departments. Such departments incorporate a number of important social services for different population groups—the socially or economically disadvantaged and the disabled—which makes it possible to deliver services efficiently. For example, the Huntington Beach, California, Community Services Department offers a wide range of recreation activities for senior citizens in the community—along with medical, legal, tax, voting, home maintenance, meals-to-the-home and other vital services for the aged.[8]

Continuum Approach in Municipal Recreation

As institutional therapeutic recreation programs have adopted more sophisticated approaches to serving the disabled, more and more community-based agencies have done the same. In Cincinnati, Ohio, for example, where a Division of Therapeutic Recreation was created as part of the city's recreation department, the approach has shifted from an informal emphasis on serving the disabled as part of overall integrated programming where possible, to a much more highly structured "continuum" approach.

Under Cincinnati's system, potential participants are assessed and classified under four levels:

Level I includes children and youth lacking sensory-motor or self-help skills sufficient for independent involvement in program activities; they are carefully evaluated and individual treatment plans are developed to improve such skills.

Level II is designed for children with basic sensory-motor and self-help skills, who are prepared to begin learning basic activities and skills that require socialization capability.

Level III includes moderately retarded teen agers with adequate behavior and socialization skills, who are ready to learn much more advanced recreation skills, in areas such as bowling, archery, softball or canoeing.

Level IV involves more advanced participants; here the role of the Division of Therapeutic Recreation is to act as facilitator, trainer, consultant, liaison and advocate.[9]

[8]See *Annual Report*, City of Huntington Beach, California, Community Services Department, 1981.
[9]Catherine Burdett and Mary E. Miller: "Mainstreaming in a Municipal Recreation Department Utilizing a Continuum Method." *Therapeutic Recreation Journal*, Fourth Quarter, 1979, pp. 41–47.

In general, the division personnel found they encountered resistance or apathy in response to their attempts at integrating the disabled from varied groups—the supervisory and general recreation staff, the public, social service agencies, parents and potential participants. After these initial reactions, attitudes gradually became more favorable in response to a variety of information and direct-contact techniques.

Role of State Agencies

Some state departments of parks and recreation, health and welfare or other human services have strongly promoted service to the handicapped at the local level. For instance, the Division of Parks and Recreation of the North Carolina Department of Natural Resources and Community Development has enthusiastically endorsed the sponsorship of recreation programs for special populations by municipal and county departments. The division has published a detailed manual on the subject that includes summaries of federal and state laws, administrative aspects of programming for the disabled and program guidelines for different special populations, such as the physically disabled, visually impaired, hearing-impaired, mentally retarded and aged.[10]

Community Recreation for the Disabled in Canada

In recent years, both local municipalities and provincial governments in Canada have assumed a growing responsibility for providing community recreation opportunities for special populations. In Vancouver, British Columbia, for example, the number of elderly persons served in municipal recreation programs during a recent seven-year period rose from 21,414 to 108,269 annually; participation figures for disabled children in summer programs increased from 781 to 2519 during the same span. The city park and recreation department offers "meals on wheels" services to shut-ins, serves disabled elderly persons in community center day-care programs and offers weekly recreational activities to mental health patients living in city-licensed boarding houses. In Winnipeg, Manitoba, and in the city of Montreal, similar programs have been initiated to serve mentally retarded children, the physically disabled and aged persons.

In 1975, Haist reported the findings of a survey of municipal recreation services for special groups in the Province of Ontario. Based on an analysis of all Ontario communities with a population of 5000 or more, it found that

---

[10]Drusilla F. Welborn: *Recreation Programs for Special Populations for Public Park and Recreation Department.* North Carolina Division of Parks and Recreation, September 1978.

Eighty-seven of the 169 municipalities surveyed (51.5 per cent) indicated that they were providing recreation services for at least one of the four special groups: the mentally retarded, the physically handicapped, the emotionally disturbed, and the learning disabled.

Forty-five per cent of the municipalities surveyed provided recreation services for the mentally retarded, compared with 29 per cent for the physically handicapped, 13 per cent for the learning disabled, and 8.3 per cent for the emotionally disturbed.[11]

Obviously, such figures do not provide an in-depth picture of the range or qualities of the services provided; in addition, the survey's finding that only eight (4.7 per cent) of the municipalities surveyed had staff members who were responsible for working with the disabled suggests that many such programs are of a limited or superficial nature. In general, Haist found that recreation programs for special populations tended to be offered more in larger cities with a population of 50,000 and up.

A number of Canadian provinces have begun to vigorously promote leisure services for the ill and disabled. In Alberta, for example, the provincial government has established a Recreation Services to Special Groups Branch that

. . . provides consultative services, information, Provincial, Area and Regional Workshops, and financial assistance to various clientele to facilitate greater recreational opportunities for the mentally and physically disabled, pre-school and school-age children, senior citizens and those in correctional systems, while making the public aware of the existence and needs of these individuals and groups.[12]

As part of its overall effort, the branch has supported a planning and research program, as well as the production of public relations materials (such as films, slides and tapes) designed to promote outdoor recreation for senior citizens, sports for the physically disabled, hospital recreation and, most of all, favorable public attitudes toward the disabled individual's place in community life.

ORGANIZATIONS CONCERNED WITH SPECIFIC FORMS OF DISABILITY

Many voluntary community organizations concerned with specific disabilities, such as blindness, mental retardation, cerebral palsy or orthopedic disability, provide recreation service as a part of their total program of rehabilitation and social

---

[11]Doris Haist: "A Survey of Municipal Recreation Services for Special Groups in Ontario." *Recreation Review*, August 1975, pp. 29–50.
[12]*Recreation Services to Special Groups Branch*. Manual, Provincial Department of Parks, Recreation and Wildlife, Edmonton, Alberta, April 1975, p. 5.1.

assistance. In many cases, the national organization carries on research, develops guidelines or materials in this area or provides other forms of funding assistance. Usually, when direct programs of recreation sponsorship are offered, it is by local chapters or organizations in the cities themselves.

Although it is not possible to provide examples drawn from each of these organizations, an excellent illustration may be found in the work of the Lighthouse, a service center operated by the New York Association for the Blind. This voluntary, nonsectarian, nonprofit agency serves legally blind, visually impaired persons (many of whom are multiply disabled) with a year-round program. Its clientele consists of approximately 3300 persons ranging in age from 6 months to 90 years; they are of all races, creeds and socioeconomic backgrounds.

Its overall services include the following:

1. Medical, including a Low Vision Clinic
2. Rehabilitation, including evaluation of needs, orientation and individual training in mobility
3. Social services: admission, referral consultation and case work, with respect to personal and economic problems, welfare status and similar problems
4. Music school
5. Library service
6. Recreation and camping
7. Transportation
8. Men's and women's residences
9. Lighthouse Industries, including a sheltered workshop
10. Craft shop
11. Child development center
12. Nursery school
13. Reader's service
14. Food service

The objectives of the Recreation and Camping Division include the following: (a) providing recreational counseling in order to help clients develop a personal philosophy of recreation that meets their needs and skills for participation; (b) providing information about available community opportunities for recreation; (c) using recreation to assist in the personal development, social adjustment, health and appearance of participants; and (d) promoting participation in independent, self-directed programs.

Activities are offered for five different age groups or categories of visually disabled persons, ranging from children of nursery-school age to older adults. They include a wide variety of both active and passive activities, such as arts and crafts, bowling, trips, table games, dancing, dramatics, swimming, newspaper work and such special events as parties, festivals, carnivals and fairs. The Lighthouse operates its own 14-story building, with such recreation facilities as bowling alleys, a swimming pool, a social hall, an auditorium, lounges, crafts shops, a play roof for younger children and two summer camps for residential camping.

Mental retardation is another field in which specialized voluntary community organizations make a strong contribution. For example, in Toronto, Canada, the mental retardation movement has been the fastest growing area of social service of its type since the late 1940's. Today, the gross operating budget of the Metropolitan Toronto Association for the Mentally Retarded is close to $2 million, with funds gathered from public sources, the United Appeal and parents' fees. There are four full-time recreation staff members who supervise 50 different recreation programs throughout the metropolitan Toronto area with volunteer assistance. Elsewhere in this text, the work of numerous other voluntary agencies serving specific types of disabled populations is described. Without question, such groups make a tremendous contribution to meeting the needs of the disabled in community life.

Service Organizations

Fraternal, civic and service organizations like the Elks, Moose, Lions, Oddfellows and Kiwanis have traditionally taken a strong responsibility for providing special programs for the disabled. In the past, when comparatively few services were offered by public recreation departments, these organizations cooperated closely with health and welfare agencies to co-sponsor recreation programs. For instance, the Lions of North Carolina have joined with the North Carolina Association for the Blind to develop Camp Dogwood, a camp and vacation facility for visually handicapped residents of that state, at a cost of approximately a half million dollars.

There are numerous other examples of such organizations, along with civic groups and youth associations, such as the Scouts or Y's, that assist or sponsor programs for the disabled. In Ottawa, Canada, the YM-YWCA operates physical recreation programs for the disabled, including weekly swim sessions for children with asthma, learning disabilities or other physical impairments. Other special programs are operated for blind adults, those with psychiatric disabilities and similar special groups. Many other Y's operate similar programs. One particularly innovative example of outreach programming is found in Westchester County, New York, where the YWCA has conducted an activities program (including crafts, creative writing, music, cooking, grooming and exercise) and an after-care program for women in the Women's Correctional Facility, Valhalla, New York.

In both the United States and Canada, Boy and Girl Scouts have made a strong effort over the past decade to serve physically and mentally disabled children and youth. In the United States, it has been estimated that there are 59,000 disabled Scouts, including "blind, deaf, crippled, spastic, and even lepers." New York City alone has 150 "special handicapped" scouting units, involving about 2000 boys out of a total of 80,000 Boy Scouts in the city. An equal number of regular units include some disabled boys in their programs. In one troop, the volunteer scoutmaster is learning sign language to communicate with the boys who cannot talk:

Only two of the 10 Boy Scouts in Troop 198 can talk, but they have learned personal fitness, know how to tie knots and have studied firemanship. They have earned their family skill award by helping to clean up communities, and they will soon attain the Tenderfoot Badge. Next they will start on the Community Merit Badge.[13]

---

[13]"Boy Scouts Reaching Out for Handicapped Members." *The New York Times*, February 9, 1976, p. 31.

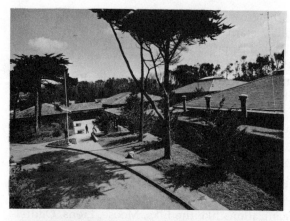
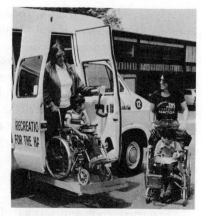
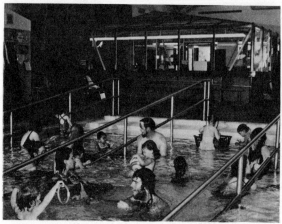
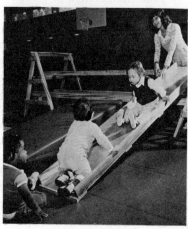

The Recreation Center for the Handicapped in San Francisco has an outstanding new facility, including a specially designed swimming pool, excellent transportation resources and a gym with varied play equipment. (Bill Cogan, Photographer.)

Special Agencies for Therapeutic Recreation

In a limited number of cities, centers have been established under private sponsorship to provide recreation for the mentally and physically disabled.

A leading example is the Recreation Center for the Handicapped, Inc., in San Francisco, California. This nonprofit corporation has pioneered in providing therapeutic recreation service in the San Francisco Bay area since 1952, when it was founded as a demonstration project to meet the needs of the disabled. It provides year-round recreation and camping programs for children, youth and adults. Most are severely handicapped—many in wheelchairs, on crutches or even bedfast. Others have severe speech impediments, visual handicaps or hearing loss. This program, directed by Janet Pomeroy, a noted authority in the field of therapeutic recreation service, began with six severely handicapped adults; today it has an enrollment of approximately 1600 of all ages and every level and type of disability.

For years, the bulk of the Center's programs were carried on in the Fleishhacker Pool Building, a previously unused, publicly owned structure on the Great Highway in San Francisco that was converted to include two large social halls, a craft room, music room, library, multi-purpose rooms, stage, offices, kitchen, gymnasium, indoor swimming pool and four activity rooms. This building, which was made available by the San Francisco Recreation and Park Department, has now been replaced by an impressive new facility built in the mid-1970's to serve the disabled. Outdoor activities are also provided on a day-camp site adjacent to the Center and at Lake Merced—a nearby zoo, playground and beach. Resident camping is provided at La Honda, approximately 60 miles from San Francisco.

FUNDING

The Center began with completely private funding and still relies heavily on contributions. Its Board of Directors raises a major portion of the budget from individuals, civic and fraternal organizations, fund-raising campaigns, shows, benefits and rummage sales. However, the San Francisco Recreation and Park Department, the Community Mental Health Service and the Department of Social Services subsidize a portion of the Center's budget. It has also received as many as five federal grants at a time to provide care for previously institutionalized, mentally retarded persons and children receiving day-care services and to support a physical fitness program serving all participants. Fees are paid by the families of participants who are able to afford them. The Center's total annual budget is $1.8 million.

TRANSPORTATION

Participants of all ages are transported from their homes to the Center and back each day, including those in wheelchairs, on crutches and on portable cots. Nine specially equipped buses are in operation six days a week, from 8 A.M. to 11:30 P.M., with transportation planned by a full-time coordinator, and 14 bus drivers—specially selected for their skill in working with severely retarded and disabled participants—working on day and evening shifts.

Whenever possible, parents provide transportation for their disabled children; furthermore, volunteer aides accompany children on the daily bus trips. In addition to the traveling to and from the Center, many special trips are scheduled throughout the year to nearby sites of interest.

With the growth of enrollment, it has become necessary to expand the services of the Center in other locations. Today, it has reduced the need for additional facilities and transportation and made it possible to serve large numbers of disabled persons at low cost by conducting programs in neighborhood social halls, housing project meeting rooms, Y's and youth clubs and other recreation and park facilities. Special services are provided for severely disabled persons in their homes—including withdrawn elderly individuals or severely retarded children and youth who are unable to interact within the Center program.

PROGRAM SPONSORSHIP

The immense effort required to plan and carry out this program would not be possible without the help of an active Board of Directors, composed of both lay and professional persons representing public and private institutions in such fields as recreation, education, medicine, welfare and business. The Board works through committees that deal with finance and budget, program, personnel, publicity, speakers' bureau, transportation, parent auxiliary, building construction, equipment and supplies and by-laws.

STAFF

The paid staff includes recreation program supervisors, a coordinator of volunteer services, a social worker and a number of recreation leaders and specialists in various activity areas—along with a business manager, clerical staff and dietary and housekeeping personnel. Each year, a number of graduate and undergraduate college students serve full-semester internships at the Recreation Center for the Handicapped, along with a number of classes from various California colleges whose students carry out field work assignments there.

Program participants are separated into small groups, according to such factors as age, degree of retardation or physical impairment, social independence and mobility. A substantial proportion of the participants are multiply disabled children and youth who have not been accepted in any school. During a recent five-year period, almost half these participants improved so markedly that they were able to be accepted in city schools for the retarded or in special classes in regular schools. In addition to this group, many previously institutionalized teen-agers and adults have gained sufficient confidence and leisure skills to be able to "graduate" into community-sponsored recreation and park programs.

The activities provided cover a broad range of recreation services, including arts and crafts, music, dance, games, sports, drama, trips and a variety of special events. Increasingly, camping and nature-oriented activities have been introduced. Programs for integrating even the most severely disabled with nondisabled children, teens and adults are offered regularly at the Center. In addition, integrated programs are conducted at other community recreation and camping facilities under the direction of the Center's staff.

The Recreation Center for the Handicapped has based its program on recognition of a critical need that was not being met. Janet Pomeroy writes

For the handicapped who attend the Center, recreation has been found to be the only activity experience available to most of them. Some children and teens attend school but many do not. A few adults attend workshops, but the vast majority have been judged to lack the ability for work training or job experience. . . . their days are filled with emptiness and recreation has been seen as the only possible outlet for their energies.[14]

[14]Janet Pomeroy: "Recreation Unlimited: An Approach to Community Recreation for the Handicapped." *Journal of Physical Education and Recreation*, May 1975, p. 30.

Table 11-1   San Francisco Recreation Center for the Handicapped: 30-Year Summary[15]

	1952	1982
Enrollment		
Number	6	1600
Age groups	Young adults	Infants through elderly
Disabilities	Primarily cerebral palsy	All disabilities—32 different types of disabling conditions
Programs		
Number	12 per month	75 per week—350 per month
Hours	192 per month	12 per day—300 per month
Volunteers		
Number	3	150 per week
Parents' Auxiliary		
Number	10	450
Staff		
Number	2	80 full-time 56 part-time
Departments		
Recreation	1	Program—7 divisions
Business	0	Support Services—5
Transportation		
Number of buses	None—use of taxicabs, Red Cross and volunteer drivers	12 vans and buses 5 station wagons
Mileage	720 miles per month	38,000 miles per month
Housekeeping		
Number of meals served	12 per month	3 meals per day 4100 meals per month
Financing	Small grant-in-aid from a foundation	City, state, federal and private donations
Facilities	One room	Main recreation building, swimming pool complex and gymnasium building with garage—a total of 48,000 square feet. Use of a wide variety of community facilities for outreach and mainstreaming, i.e., schools, Recreation and Park, churches, housing authority complexes and residential homes.

[15]*Special Report of San Francisco Center for the Handicapped,* June 1982.

As a consequence, parents, social agencies and the disabled themselves have turned to the Center's programs, in part as a point of entry into the community service system and in part simply to fulfill their full range of social, emotional, physical and intellectual needs. In addition to purely recreational services, a day-care program and nutritional, referral and educational services have all been provided to clients, and close relationships are maintained with other social and rehabilitative agencies in the community. Recreation is seen as both an end and a means and is presented as an important developmental experience for all clients.

The Recreation Center for the Handicapped is unique in the United States in terms of its variety and scope. Despite the fact that it owes much of its success to the energy and interest of its founder, Janet Pomeroy, it should be possible for other cities throughout the nation to develop similar centers through large-scale citizen support and the development of the kinds of recreation opportunities for the disabled that are now available in San Francisco. The Center's growth since its inception is shown in Table 11-1.

Community Councils or Boards

A final type of administrative structure for programs serving the disabled is a council or board with representatives from a variety of agencies and professions primarily concerned with providing programs for the disabled. The author has described in another text the unique work of the Greater Kansas City Council on Recreation for the Handicapped.[16] That description is repeated here because it provides an excellent model for other communities to follow.

The Recreation Division of the Welfare Department of the Kansas City government for a number of years conducted summer programs for orthopedically disabled, diabetic, cardiac and cerebral palsied children. In the early 1950's, it established day camps for the deaf and hard of hearing and the orthopedically disabled.

In 1955, a Supervisor of Special Recreation was appointed to establish a year-round comprehensive program of recreation—initially for the orthopedically disabled, of whom there were estimated to be about 14,000 within the Kansas City metropolitan area. Before developing the program, the following agencies were approached for consultation and advice: the United Cerebral Palsy Association, the National Foundation for Infantile Paralysis, the Jackson County Society for Crippled Children, the Kansas City Board of Education, Goodwill Industries, the Muscular Dystrophy Association, the Arthritis and Rheumatism Foundation, the Multiple Sclerosis Association and others.

It was found that 11 different day and overnight camping, Scouting, club and swimming programs were already being sponsored for the disabled by various organizations in the metropolitan area. However, the following important needs were revealed:

---

[16]See description of Kansas City plan in Richard Kraus: *Recreation Today: Program Planning and Leadership.* Santa Monica, California, Goodyear, 1977, pp. 216–218.

1. The majority of orthopedically disabled youths and adults in the city were not being served by the programs offered.
2. There were many adults who were able to leave their homes but who felt they were too disabled to join regular social groups, as well as teen-agers who had gone as far as they could in school but could not find work and therefore had lost all meaningful social involvement.
3. Many homebound children and adults were left completely on their own in terms of recreational pursuits.
4. Existing programs were so limited in budget and staff that they could not satisfactorily meet the needs of those they attempted to serve.

In an effort to meet these needs, a Greater Kansas City Council on Recreation for the Handicapped was formed—to serve not only the physically disabled but also those with emotional or social limitations. Encouragement and support came from a nearby Veterans' Administration hospital which sought to improve opportunities in the community for its discharged patients. Other organizations that joined the Council—in addition to those first involved—included the YWCA, American Red Cross, the Junior League, the Boys Clubs, the Visiting Nurses' Association and others. The Council worked closely with the Recreation Division in establishing policies and procedures, planning programs, helping to recruit and train volunteers, stimulating interest and participation in the program by referring disabled persons to appropriate groups and providing clerical and office assistance. Among its first steps was the establishment of a comprehensive insurance plan to protect program participants and sponsors.

Through the years that followed, the Greater Kansas City Council on Recreation for the Handicapped developed a program that included the following elements:

1. A visiting program for homebound children and adults to help them discover new interests and abilities in games, crafts, puppetry, collections, instrument playing and other hobbies. This program relied heavily on volunteers.
2. A club program for orthopedically disabled adults which stressed their assuming the leadership themselves. Activities included weekly meetings, parties for holidays and special occasions, square dancing, group singing, movies, hobbies, dramatics and games.
3. A similar program for orthopedically disabled teen-agers, with activities suited to their interests.
4. A training program in home recreation activities for orthopedically disabled children, which was given to parents of such children or to other interested adults. In a series of ten sessions, workshops and discussions dealt with ways of minimizing disability, modifications of recreational activities and other forms of assistance.
5. Television programs directed to the orthopedically disabled. The programs encouraged them by presenting "write-in" tournaments and contests, interviewing disabled persons who had special hobbies and teaching crafts and games. The programs also helped to educate the public about the needs and capabilities of the disabled.

In addition, outdoor programs during the summer months included overnight camping for children with cardiac conditions, diabetes, cerebral palsy or blindness and day camping for children who were deaf or hard of hearing, orthopedically disabled or mentally retarded.

The Kansas City Council on Recreation for the Handicapped served a valuable coordinating function by (a) making surveys of community needs for therapeutic recreation and carrying out other research projects; (b) acting as a referral agency for disabled individuals; (c) stimulating public interest; (d) enlisting the help of community groups and the public; and (e) recruiting and training professionals and workers in this field. During the 1970's, the Recreation Division merged with the Park Department, forming a joint Department of Parks and Recreation. It continues to serve special populations with adapted sports and social programs, including various family activities.[17]

Jointly Operated Programs

A final type of community-based therapeutic recreation service that may have elements of all the preceding is the jointly operated program. This may involve two or more public agencies cooperating to provide recreation for the disabled, two or more voluntary or service organizations or other combinations.

As an example of the first type, the Nor-West Regional Special Services Program in northern Westchester County, New York, was among the first joint efforts by several adjacent units of government to provide varied services for the disabled, which the agencies could not do independently. The towns of Cortlandt and Yorktown, the city of Peekskill and the village of Ossining planned and initiated a therapeutic recreation program with matching funds from the County Mental Health Board. Under this joint sponsorship, Nor-West has provided swimming, bowling, crafts and movement education, a canteen, special events, trips, Scouting and similar programs for the physically disabled, mentally retarded, learning-disabled and emotionally disturbed (including discharged mental patients). The program is directed by a full-time professional supervised by a board composed of the superintendents of each of the communities involved, who, in turn, act as liaisons with their own governing boards.

Another type of structure is one in which colleges or universities with recreation curricula sponsor programs for the disabled in cooperation with community groups. Temple University in Philadelphia has conducted a special project titled, "A Coordinated Approach to Community Recreation Services for Multiply Handicapped Adults," under a grant designed in part to help disabled individuals develop favorable leisure attitudes and involvements. The university's Developmental Disabilities Office and Recreation and Leisure Studies Department, in cooperation with several community agencies (Woodhaven Center, Haverford State Hospital, Elwyn Institute, Interact Group Home, Programs for Exceptional Children and the Frankford YWCA), have conducted leisure awareness sessions, workshops, social programs and other activities to serve the mentally retarded, as well as those with other disabilities.

---

[17]Letter from Bonnie Bratcher, Director of Special Programs, Kansas City Board of Parks and Recreation, June 1982.

Rural Leisure-Service Cooperative

Another example of cooperative planning designed to meet the needs of special populations in a predominantly rural area is found in Chico, California. A survey carried out by the National Institute on New Models for Community Recreation and Leisure for Handicapped Youth found that of the responding communities, none with a population under 50,000 had leisure services for special individuals. Thus, many citizens of rural communities who are developmentally disabled, physically handicapped or emotionally ill are severely deprived of recreational opportunities.

In the greater Chico area the DO-IT Leisure Cooperative was organized to provide a continuum of sequentially planned social integration experiences for the disabled. The Cooperative provides specialized services for individuals with severe levels of disability, as well as transitional adjustment and normalization programs for more capable participants. Like the Recreation Center for the Handicapped, it is supported by private donations, matching funds from the local recreation department, contractual funds, community fund-raising efforts and state and federal grants. It shares facilities with the local state university, public schools, park and recreation departments and other private, voluntary and commercially-owned organizations.[18]

Recognizing that in many smaller communities or rural areas no one agency is likely to have the financial resources, trained staff and facilities required to serve the disabled adequately, this cooperative structure appears to offer an excellent model for many similar areas.

GUIDELINES FOR AGENCIES PROVIDING THERAPEUTIC RECREATION SERVICE

Community agencies which provide recreation services for the disabled must (a) determine needs, priorities and capabilities; (b) develop programs; (c) provide trained leadership; (d) maintain an effective public relations and community relations program; (e) finance programs; (f) operate needed transportation services; and (g) plan and develop facilities to serve the disabled. Each of these administrative functions is described in the following section.

Surveying Needs, Priorities and Capabilities

It is essential to get a clear picture of the existing need for therapeutic recreation service within a given community before attempting to plan programs. In gen-

---

[18]Jerry Root, Carol Stensrud and Gary Quiring: "Rural Leisure Services for Special Populations," *California Parks and Recreation*, February-March 1978, pp. 12–13.

eral, it is necessary to determine the number of persons with disabilities and then assess the ability of existing programs to serve these individuals.

There are three possible ways of determining the extent of disabilities in a given area. Allan writes,

The first is the abstract method of applying a formula based on the estimated or known national figures for specific types of disabilities, or the composite figures and percentages for broad classes of disability from national or regional surveys, applied to the local population. The second is the pooling of available data from local agencies and services to form the basis for an "educated guess" on the total disability picture. The third method is the house-to-house survey or canvass type of personal contact, carried out on either a broad or limited segment of the community.[19]

The community survey is generally regarded as the most useful of these approaches, because it provides a more accurate picture of actual needs than the other methods. Also, it may serve as an important first step in developing community interest and a nucleus of individuals and agencies to carry the work further. As described by Warren, here are the major steps to be followed in carrying out a community survey:

1. **Determine Scope and Size of Survey.**   It is important to determine in advance the size of the service area, the number of people to participate in the study, the amount of time available, and the degree of detail required in the survey.

2. **Sponsorship of the Survey.**   Appropriate sponsorship not only lends prestige to the survey but also provides effective guidance, funding and authority. If no single sponsoring organization is suitable, it may be desirable to form a special sponsoring group or council.

3. **Cost of Survey.**   It is necessary to estimate, in advance, the costs of the survey, including personnel needs, supplies, equipment, transportation and printing costs. This estimate should be realistic, and if different co-sponsoring groups agree to share the costs, this arrangement should be clearly spelled out.

4. **Organization.**   A typical pattern is to develop an overall survey committee, which selects its own chairman, and a number of sub-committees. The survey committee should represent the major interests of the community, as well as those with special interest in therapeutic recreation, and with appropriate technical skills. In a large-scale survey, it may be necessary to hire a professional researcher, or team of experts, to head up the study.

5. **Volunteers.**   In any survey which involves large-scale interviewing or canvassing, it is helpful to be able to count on volunteers. These may be drawn from interested parents, representatives of service organizations, college students, or similar groups.

6. **Survey Instruments.**   Forms for the collection of data should be carefully developed, or adapted from previously used instruments. If they have not been used before, they should be pilot-tested to determine their validity, ease of administration, and general usefulness. Complete accuracy in the collection, tabulation and presentation of all data is imperative.

7. **The Survey Report.**   The survey report should cover the work of the entire survey team, integrating the findings of various sub-committees. It should outline the need for therapeutic

[19]W. Scott Allan, in: *Community Planning for the Rehabilitation of Persons with Communication Disorders.* Washington, D.C., National Association of Hearing and Speech Agencies, 1967, p. 45.

recreation service, the target populations, the existing programs, and both short and long-range recommendations both for policies and specific projects in this area.[20]

In addition to surveys of this type, it is also advisable to consult with individuals or agencies serving the disabled. Public school administrators, special educational services for the disabled, visiting nurse services, hospital-based recreation and social work personnel, doctors, public health departments and organizations working with the disabled can all provide much information.

If the plan is to develop program services for a specific population, inquiries may be directed at that population. Mitchell, for example, describes the planning process followed in Washington, D.C., in developing a comprehensive community-based recreation program for the mentally retarded. After an initial survey had disclosed some 7000 retardates in the District, she writes,

---

In order to assess the availability of persons in this group for the program, 500 of the 7,000 were sent a brief questionnaire. The 500 names were selected at random and represented a cross-section of the retarded population. Other factors considered were the families' economic conditions, place of residence, and ages of the retarded children. The results of this sample indicated that the bulk of those questioned would be interested in programs in the morning and early afternoon, and those currently enrolled in other programs would be available for Saturday programs. It was evident that many of the retarded were concentrated in certain geographic regions of the District. The original 500 names, plus an additional 1,000 names were located by address on an overlay of the District. . . . the resulting map showing both postal zones and recreation regions enabled us to locate the children in terms of their accessibility to the playgrounds and community centers which could provide special programs.[21]

As an example of how a municipality or organization may use surveys to determine current practices and needs, the city of Miami, Florida, recently carried out an innovative project called "Opening Doors to Leisure." Its purpose was to develop community awareness of and accessibility to the city's park and recreation facilities. The first component, a publicity campaign, involved color movies, slide shows, new guides to park and recreation offerings and an ongoing mass media program involving television, radio and newspapers. The second component coordinated the public transportation system to promote the use of parks and recreation facilities. In addition, a special park transportation system called "Park Breeze" was developed, using new wheelchair buses and vans for the nonambulatory and other persons unable to use or afford the public transportation system. To provide a data base for this project, the Park and Recreation Department used a questionnaire to survey park users about their means of transportation, as well as to locate the barriers which prevented some residents from using the parks.[22]

---

[20]R. I. Warren: *Studying Your Community*. New York, Russell Sage Foundation, 1955.
[21]Helen Jo Mitchell: "A Community Recreation Program for the Mentally Retarded." *Therapeutic Recreation Journal*, First Quarter, 1971, p. 4.
[22]*Opening Doors to Leisure*. Miami, Florida, Department of Leisure Services Newsletter, February 1981, p. 1, and letter from Albert Howard, Department Director.

Program Development

In planning a recreation program to serve the disabled, whether it is to be for a broad range of impairments or for a single, clearly defined group, several steps must be taken:

1. A careful survey of need, as indicated in the preceding section, carried out with both the number and type of disabled persons and the potential sponsors of programs clearly identified.
2. In order to indicate the possible directions the program might take, programs serving similar populations in other communities should be observed and the professional literature explored for specific guidelines and examples. In addition, consultants and authorities on therapeutic service, or on the disability itself, might be asked to make recommendations.
3. At this point, it might be advisable to call a meeting of interested parents or relatives to answer such questions as: "What are the recreational needs of their children?" "What types of activities would be most desirable?" "Would the parents themselves be willing to volunteer as program aides or provide transportation?"

The purpose and scope of the program would have to be defined. Decisions would be made with respect to (a) whether the program would be separate from programs for the nondisabled or linked fully or in part; (b) whether it would be open to all types of disabled persons or designed for one or more specific disabilities; (c) whether the program would use regular community recreation facilities or facilities designed for the disabled; and (d) the time schedule that would be most suitable for the program.

When these basic guidelines are determined the next step is to plan programs. The most suitable activities are chosen and fitted into a schedule, based on the following factors:

1. Appeal of activity: whether it would be enjoyed by participants as any group of nondisabled persons might enjoy it.
2. Suitability for age level: the activity should be appropriate for the age of participants.
3. Within range of capability: the activity should be one that can be carried on by disabled persons with a reasonable degree of success.
4. Therapeutic benefits: where possible, activities should be chosen that are valuable in terms of the particular disability or disabilities of the participants.
5. Suitability in terms of other factors: number of participants in group, needed facilities and equipment, staff numbers and leadership skills available.

In general, it is desirable to schedule certain regular activities that require little new instruction. At the same time, each session should involve some opportunity for new creative development or learning. There should be a reasonable balance between physical, mental, creative, social and other activities. As much as possible, disabled children should be treated like those with no physical or mental impairments and encouraged to help themselves, rather than rely on adult leaders or volunteers for assistance. Participants should be drawn into planning and leadership roles whenever possible.

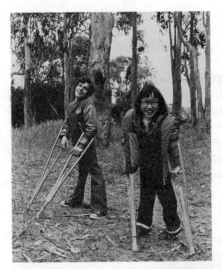
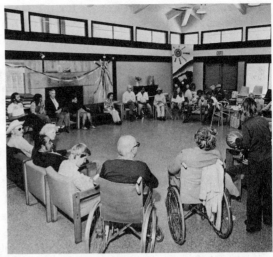
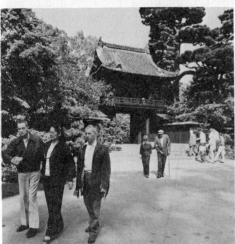
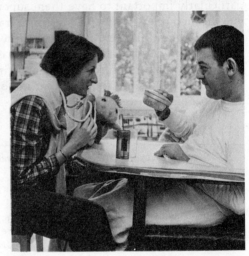

Clients at the Recreation Center for the Handicapped explore the wooded day-camp area, meet to plan a special trip, and visit Golden Gate Park. Services include teaching self-help and independent living skills to homebound clients. (Bill Cogan, Photographer.)

Providing Trained Leadership

Whenever possible, it is desirable to have professionally educated leaders with a background in therapeutic recreation service in key supervisory and leadership positions. Pomeroy, for example, provides a detailed statement of the duties, training and experience requirements for three levels of leadership personnel (Center Director, Program Director and Senior Leader) as they have been developed at the

San Francisco Recreation Center for the Handicapped.[23] These include graduation from a recognized college or university with a degree in recreation, group work or a related field and a minimum number of years of experience in responsible leadership or supervisory positions in recreation.

Although Pomeroy points out that, as a general rule, recreation leaders successful in working with the nondisabled are also able to work effectively with the disabled, it seems clear that those who have had basic courses in therapeutic recreation concepts and methods, are familiar with medical terminology and practices in the field of rehabilitation and have had previous clinical experience with the disabled are likely to be most effective. Based on the recent growth of college and university departments with programs in therapeutic recreation, it would appear appropriate today to employ graduates of such programs for all professional-level positions in community recreation for special populations. The same expectations in employing personnel in institutions (such as registration with the National Therapeutic Recreation Society on an appropriate professional level) should apply in community situations. When workers are employed on sub-professional levels, it is particularly important to have them supervised by qualified specialists and to provide needed orientation and in-service training by experts in the field.

Apart from formal qualifications, the traits expected of leaders in therapeutic recreation are similar to those expected of all leaders in this field. They must be emotionally stable, secure, patient, imaginative, enthusiastic, fair and responsible. Pomeroy also outlines several other important qualifications for therapeutic recreation leaders:

---

1. They must accept disabled persons fully as individuals who have the same basic needs, desires and problems as all other people.
2. They must be sympathetic to each participant's disability, but must not permit themselves to indulge in pity.
3. They must be patient and ingenious in helping adapt activities so that the severely disabled can take part in them, and must be able to inspire and encourage them to persevere.
4. They must recognize and be able to meet the specific, immediate social and recreational needs of participants, setting goals that allow a reasonable degree of achievement and pleasure.
5. They must be willing to help the disabled participants help themselves, rather than do everything for them.
6. They must be willing to do menial tasks such as feeding and lifting the disabled, assisting with toileting, and handling wheel chairs and portable beds. Pomeroy indicates that in many settings, "matrons" or "orderlies" are used for such tasks, but that when it is necessary to carry them out in community recreation programs, they are best handled by recreation staff members, with the help of additional staff and volunteers.[24]

---

[23]Janet Pomeroy: *Personnel Handbook, Recreation Center for the Handicapped.* San Francisco, 1970, pp. 5–22.
[24]*Ibid.*, pp. 14–16; see also Pomeroy: *Recreation for the Physically Handicapped, op. cit.*, pp. 52–59.

CLASS ADMIT CARD

NAME _Jean Paine_

STUDENT NO. _046-34-3093_

ITEM NUMBER _0661_

COURSE TITLE _THRE 116_

GEN. FUND _____ COMM. SERV. _✓_

AUTH. SIGN. _Jarnette Small_

DO NOT ADMIT STUDENT TO CLASS
WITHOUT AUTHORIZING SIGNATURE.
PLEASE RETAIN UNTIL YOU RECORD
FINAL GRADES.

As indicated elsewhere, the ratio of staff to participants must necessarily be much higher in community programs for the disabled than in programs for the general population. It is essential that, in addition to professional leaders, substantial numbers of nonprofessional aides or volunteers be involved in such programs.

Public Relations and Community Relations

This is one of the key areas of responsibility in planning and carrying out community recreation programs for the disabled. The goals of public relations include the following:

1. To arouse concern and public awareness of the need for recreation for disabled persons in the community.
2. To encourage volunteers to serve in existing and new programs and to stimulate financial support for programs.
3. To create a climate in which municipal government and other voluntary agencies will support programs of therapeutic recreation.
4. To inform disabled persons and their families of recreation opportunities in order to encourage their registration and participation.
5. To report program accomplishments and development to the community.
6. To share information regarding therapeutic recreation with other health, welfare, and social agencies that serve the disabled.

Depending on the specific population which must be reached, the following media are useful:

Printed materials: newspaper stories and features; magazine articles; newsletters and brochures; annual reports and other printed reports.
Visual and other outlets: television and radio programs; exhibits and displays; bulletin boards; speeches, motion pictures and slide talks.
Special events: open houses, tours, programs to which the press and public are invited.

A well-designed public relations program makes use of each of these methods. Newspaper stories are obviously most useful for conveying timely information, particularly publicity designed to encourage attendance at events or to provide information about functions, fund-raising drives or other newsworthy matters. It is important to develop favorable contacts with newspaper editors and feature writers and to prepare professionally designed releases that are simple, clear and factual; they should emphasize the human relations aspect of programs and special projects.

Newsletters and brochures reach more specific audiences of parents, disabled youth and adults, other professionals and municipal officials. Usually, they describe the total range of therapeutic recreation services in the community and encourage participation in specific activities, day camps, clubs or other programs. They may range from inexpensive and brief mimeographed one- or two-page leaflets to carefully printed and attractive full-color brochures.

Visual media, such as television, motion pictures, slide talks or radio programs, are more difficult to arrange than printed publicity but can produce effective results. Therapeutic recreation program directors should constantly be alert to the possibility of getting television or radio news coverage of interesting events or of scheduling panel programs or other informational "spots" on the mass media. As in the case of newspaper and magazine editors, it is important to cultivate the interest and support of radio station or television program directors. They will best be able to judge the newsworthy quality of events or possible features which are brought to their attention.

Speeches, slide talks or similar presentations are useful in reaching audiences of high school or college students, Parent-Teacher Associations, service and civic clubs and similar groups.

It is not enough to publicize the existing program in the hope that it will receive adequate coverage in the media. The program director who is alert to public relations possibilities will deliberately *plan* events of an unusual nature which lend themselves to promotion: displays, exhibits, performances, open houses, tours, field days and similar ventures are particularly newsworthy and of interest to the public.

Since the preparation of releases, radio or television scripts, brochures or films requires expertise, it is important to get competent staff assistance on such efforts. Frequently, skilled volunteers may be willing to contribute their services. A professional writer or film-maker may prepare releases or articles, radio or television features or even informational films about the program. College and university departments of film-making or television may also make such projects class assignments.

Community relations are obviously associated with the need to develop community support for therapeutic recreation programs in the form of advisory councils and planning groups, neighborhood teams, task forces and similar efforts. It is essential to get citizens' reactions in planning and to obtain the cooperation of all interested individuals and organizations if a community-based therapeutic recreation program is to receive the fullest possible support.

Financial Support

The process of fiscal management is a complicated one; it is covered in detail in books on recreation and park administration. It includes the process of budget planning and approval, maintaining fiscal controls and auditing procedures and similar functions; it is not dealt with here in detail.

It is important, however, to recognize the unique problem of community-based recreation programs in obtaining adequate financial support. Such programs are inevitably much more expensive than programs that serve the nondisabled. They require a more intensive level of staffing, special equipment, transportation, facilities and other costly services if they are to be effective. How can the needed funds be raised? Pomeroy suggests the following sources.[25]

---

[25]*Ibid.*, pp. 97–108.

VOLUNTARY GROUPS

Service clubs, parent auxiliaries, Parent-Teacher Associations, United Chest or United Crusade and similar organizations may all contribute funds to programs serving the disabled.

FOUNDATIONS

National or local foundations often are willing to provide funds for developing facilities or for establishing demonstration projects. Usually, they will support an ongoing program for a limited period of time—such as two or three years—and will then expect other sources of funding to be found. In some cases, they may be willing to provide a portion of continued funding year after year for a special program.

INDIVIDUAL GIVING

Many organizations conduct their own fund drives annually. These may include mail solicitations of individuals, companies or organizations, door-to-door campaigns or fund-raising solicitation through churches or similar organizations. They may be carried on for a limited period of weeks at Christmas or another appropriate season or may include a variety of fund-raising events, such as carnivals, cake sales, bazaars, charity balls, dinners or theater parties throughout the year. In addition, some organizations make a concentrated effort to encourage large-scale individual gifts, legacies and bequests from wealthy donors or families.

GOVERNMENT CONTRACTS AND GRANTS

Some agencies, like the San Francisco Center for the Handicapped, have been successful in negotiating contracts with municipal government to provide needed services for the disabled. Such contracts may be with recreation and park departments (which in effect subcontract this particular function to a voluntary agency) or may be provided by a department of welfare, youth services or aging. Other grants may be obtained from county or state welfare departments, social rehabilitation agencies for the blind or mentally ill and similar sources. Federal funding, as in the case of day-care programs, may be obtained on a matching basis through the Department of Health and Human Services (Title IV of the Social Security Act) or other sections of recent federal legislation supporting special education programs.

FEES AND CHARGES

A final important source of funding may be through fees charged to the families of participants. Reasonable fees may be established for day camping, residential camping and similar services. It is essential, however, that scholarships be provided for those unable to pay such fees, to avoid excluding participants from low-income families.

Whether the sponsoring department is a public or voluntary agency, it is essential that fund-raising be recognized as a high priority and that every possible avenue of obtaining grants and needed subsidies be explored. Volunteers may be interested in assisting with fund-raising. A financial or fund-raising subcommittee may be established, which systematically develops a financial plan, does research on possible grants and subsidies, develops proposals and sponsors fund-raising events. Business executives, bankers and other financial experts are useful on such committees, partly because of their personal expertise and partly because they have the contacts in the business and government world that are essential in fund-raising.

Transportation Services

Transportation is often the chief stumbling block that prevents many individuals from taking part in community-based programs. Thompson describes a number of major problems encountered in transporting homebound adults to a special recreation demonstration project:

1. Untrained or uncooperative drivers
2. Uncomfortable vehicles (with unpadded seats, for example)
3. Vehicles late for pick-ups
4. Jostling of patients
5. Lack of portable steps
6. Overcrowding of vehicles
7. Poor planning by transportation management
8. Lack of ramp for wheelchairs
9. Unheated vehicle (winter)
10. Improper handling of wheelchairs[26]

Private vehicles can be used to transport the mentally retarded, mentally ill or aged persons who do not have serious physical disabilities. In some cases, volunteers are used to man such programs through car pools. This approach tends to be somewhat unreliable, however. Proper insurance coverage is essential, and additional volunteers must go along with the disabled persons being transported. Buses and taxicabs may also be used on a contract basis. Although expensive, this alternative may offer a more reliable solution to the problem.

In some communities, service organizations such as the Kiwanis, Lions and Elks

---

[26]Morton Thompson: *Meeting Some Social-Psychological Needs of Homebound Persons Through Recreative Experience: Project Report.* New York, National Recreation Association, 1962.

provide transportation services; in others, the American Red Cross Motor Corps provides cars and trained drivers. Whenever commercial services are used, drivers must have appropriate licenses and be fully aware of the responsibilities involved in carrying the disabled. Drivers must understand the special needs of the disabled, and it is important for them to know first aid procedures and be able to handle emergencies that may occur.

The task of transporting those who are severely physically impaired and wear heavy braces, use crutches or are in wheelchairs or portable cots is obviously much more difficult. Special vehicles must be provided, with fuller space, special steps to assist the ambulatory, ramps for wheelchairs or lifting devices to assist loading and unloading. A number of car manufacturers have designed special vehicles for this purpose.

Whatever form of special transportation is provided, the role of the driver is extremely important. Pomeroy describes the responsibilities and needed qualities of such drivers, as outlined in the job description code of San Francisco's Recreation Center for the Handicapped. Drivers must have

---

1. *Knowledge of:*
   The California State Motor Vehicle Code and the Education Code, particularly as they relate to the operation of vehicles in transporting children
   Geography of the local area
   Safe driving practices
   Basic preventive maintenance of automotive equipment

2. *Ability to:*
   Operate a large and small bus with patience and skill
   Make minor mechanical adjustments of automotive equipment
   Understand and carry out oral directions
   Get along well with children
   Maintain a calm, even disposition
   Exercise mature judgment in relation to driving and child care
   Maintain a semblance of order on the bus
   Handle large children and adults with heavy braces

3. *License:*
   A valid Class "B" chauffeur's license
   Red Cross first aid certificate

4. *Experience:*
   Two years of successful full-time paid experience in driving commercial or heavy-duty vehicles. Experience with children. Safe driving record and current driver's license.[27]

Precise policies should be established for all aspects of the transportation program. Schedules for pickup and delivery should be worked out in full detail and maintained as accurately as possible. Generally, this is easier to do in small towns or suburban areas than in large cities where congested traffic conditions and parking difficulties make the transportation problem even more difficult to solve.

---

[27]Pomeroy: *Recreation for the Physically Handicapped, op. cit.,* p. 140.

Planning Facilities for the Disabled

In general, the facilities used by recreation programs for the disabled are of the same type as those used for the general population. Parks, playgrounds, community centers, day camps and similar facilities are widely available and, in most cases, able to accommodate the disabled with comparatively little modification. It is generally desirable for programs serving the disabled to use existing facilities, since they enable disabled participants to mingle with the nondisabled.

When programs involve severely disabled persons, it is obviously necessary to make sure that halls, rest rooms, entrances and similar locations are constructed so that they can readily be used by those in wheelchairs, on crutches and in braces. In some communities, elaborate playgrounds and day-camp sites have been constructed for use by the disabled. Some authorities have questioned this practice, particularly when it leads to a segregated pattern of use by the disabled—thus defeating attempts at mainstreaming them with the nondisabled population. In some cases (see p. 287), facilities have been built to serve both the disabled and their families or other nondisabled individuals, which makes much greater sense.

A number of innovative designers have developed facilities that go beyond a routine concept of recreational use to provide a much fuller range of developmental and growth experiences. For example, the town of Hempstead, New York, has constructed an Environmental Resource Center on the Atlantic Ocean at Lido Beach Town Park. This facility provides year-round recreational opportunities for those with varied disabilities, both children and adults, as well as the nondisabled population. It was constructed to serve the town's ANCHOR Program (Answering the Needs of Children with Handicaps through Organized Recreation), with about 750 participants. McGrath describes the planning emphasis given to environmental activities in the Center's program:

. . . (in addition to) music, arts and crafts, physical exercise, field and court games, aquatics, special events such as Christmas shows and family picnics, field trips, home economics and hygiene, and cultural activities . . . it is expected that environment-related activities will be substantially increased (such as):

Interpretation of the economy of Long Island and New York in terms of animal life, erosion, plant life, etc.

Horticulture, including gardening

Animal husbandry — care, feeding, and raising of animals

Outdoor recreation skills — bait and fly casting, fly tying, resource management, camping skills, riflery, and laboratory techniques

Special events — nature projects (building bird houses, conservation programs), hikes, fishing, trips, flower shows, pet shows, fishing contests, and hobby shows and activities[28]

The Environmental Resource Center utilizes large garden plots worked by the participants, nature trails related to the ecological systems of the seashore, three

---

[28]Ray McGrath: "Environmental Resource Center—Making the Outdoors Available to the Handicapped." *In* Larry Neal, ed.: *Leisure Today: Selected Readings.* Washington, D.C., American Association for Leisure and Recreation, 1975, p. 92.

camping units for platform tent camping, a large Center building, outdoor shelter areas, beach access at three locations, special curbing and sitting walls to guide the blind, hard-topped game areas and pathways and a playground designed to be a progressive obstacle course.

It is essential that more such facilities be built to provide enriched play and learning experiences for the disabled in a specially designed setting. In addition, *all* community recreation facilities must be remodeled, where necessary, to provide reasonable opportunities for the disabled. It goes without saying that, today, all *new* facilities being constructed to serve the general public must be made accessible for the disabled.

LEISURE COUNSELING

Basically, two kinds of populations must be considered in planning community recreation services for the disabled. One is the population living at home, with either physical or mental disabilities, that has some form of impairment as a continuing condition of life and that requires appropriate opportunity for leisure involvement either as a supplement to other family or work involvements or as a primary form of commitment. The other population consists of those who have been hospitalized or are in a special school, rehabilitation center or other residential facility and who are in the process of returning to the community. Often, this group must relearn old skills, make new contacts and develop both confidence and "know-how" in re-establishing a healthy, full leisure life.

For both groups, leisure counseling is a key element in their becoming successfully involved in community-based recreation programs. For all groups, as McDowell points out, such counseling is essential to remove blocks or difficulties which may interfere with the individual's capability for creative use of leisure. Through observation, testing and counseling which analyzes the source of difficulty, a better understanding of such maladaptive factors as the following is achieved:

. . . guilt, obligation, anxiety, fear, social isolation, procrastination, boredom, uncertainty, flightiness, or obsessive compulsiveness, to name a few. This approach attempts to promote awareness, understanding, and clarification of the individual's self (attitudes, beliefs, values, personal resources) so that alienation from leisure is minimized.[29]

Having established a more positive outlook and constructive attitudes toward participation, the leisure counseling process must clarify leisure goals for the individual, identify potential community resources and follow through with a sequence of referral, contacts, help with transportation if necessary and assistance in estab-

---

[29]Chester F. McDowell, Jr.: "Leisure Counseling: Professional Considerations for Therapeutic Recreation." *Journal of Physical Education and Recreation*, January 1976, p. 27.

lishing a solid base of recreational participation. In some cases, as indicated in an earlier chapter, this may involve first participation in a protected or "special" environment and then satisfying and successful involvement in an integrated program. It should be stressed that leisure counseling is not designed only for the disabled. For example, Overs, Taylor and Adkins describe an experimental project designed to help individuals in later middle age (55 years and older) prepare constructively for retirement and increased leisure time through avocational counseling.[30]

Similarly, Magulski, Faull and Rutkowski describe a computer-based approach to leisure counseling developed by Milwaukee, Wisconsin, Public Schools Division of Municipal Recreation and Community Education. In addition to serving large numbers of disabled persons in sheltered environments (such as prison inmates, hospital patients and alcoholics) or in the community (such as the aged or mentally retarded) the service has also been made available to people already in the mainstream of life who want to raise the quality of their lives through leisure participation.[31] It appears, then, that leisure counseling must continue to develop as a key service to all groups—and particularly the disabled—in community recreation programs.

In conclusion, this chapter has outlined a number of examples of community-based recreation programs and approaches for the disabled which supplement other examples provided throughout this text. The final chapter deals with the important role of research and evaluation in programming for the disabled.

Suggested Topics for Class Discussion, Examination Questions or Student Papers

1. Develop a model program of therapeutic recreation service for a municipal recreation and park department. Show how this program might be linked to institutions or voluntary agencies serving varied disabled populations, as part of a continuum-of-service approach.

2. Carry out a direct analysis of a community agency providing comprehensive services for a specific form of disability, such as the mentally retarded or cerebral palsied. Use visitation and observation to determine how recreation is provided or assisted by this agency; then make recommendations for its improvement.

3. What is the rationale for having a nonpublic agency, such as the San Francisco Recreation Center for the Handicapped, assume major community responsibility in this area, with varied forms of public funding? What are the advantages and disadvantages of such an approach?

4. Mainstreaming of the disabled has become a major thrust in many community agencies. Develop a set of policies designed to bring about this objective, and discuss the circumstances in which it may not be a realistic goal.

---

[30]Robert P. Overs, Sharon Taylor and Catherine Adkins: "Avocational Counseling for the Elderly." *Journal of Physical Education and Recreation: Leisure Today*, April 1977, pp. 20–21.
[31]Michael Magulski, Virginia Hirsch Faull and Barbara Rutkowski: "The Milwaukee Leisure Counseling Model." *Journal of Physical Education and Recreation: Leisure Today*, April 1977, pp. 25–26.

12

Evaluation and Research in Therapeutic Recreation

Within any field of social service, it is essential to determine the effectiveness of programs and to develop a foundation of knowledge which will strengthen both professional performance and the general image and understanding of the field. The two terms generally applied to such efforts are *evaluation* and *research*.

These processes are related in that both rely on standardized instruments and systematic investigative procedures to gather information that will be useful in formulating theory and improving professional methods. They differ, however, in the following respects:

MEANING OF EVALUATION

Evaluation is usually regarded as the process of determining the effectiveness of programs, leadership or other elements of professional service in achieving predetermined goals. The quality of a program may also be evaluated according to accepted standards within a field. Evaluations make use of a number of research techniques, of both a quantitative and a qualitative nature. Generally, evaluations examine specific agencies or situations.

Patient or Client Evaluation

In the field of therapeutic recreation, a second specific use of the term "evaluation" applies to the examination of patients or clients. They are systematically and regularly examined through interviews, observations or check-lists and rating scales to determine their interests, needs, disabilities and capabilities. Information gathered in this way leads to the planning of therapeutic programs and the prescription of appropriate areas of participation for patients and clients.

MEANING OF RESEARCH

Research is usually thought of as an organized search for knowledge. Its objective is to discover answers to questions through the application of scientific procedures of measurement. It may simply involve examining what *is*—that is to say, a given phenomenon or institution as it exists—or may involve establishing certain artificial conditions or circumstances, which are then systematically observed. Research generally falls into two major categories: (a) so-called *pure* research (sometimes called *fundamental* or *basic* research), which is concerned with conceptual or theoretical questions that do not have immediate practical value; and (b) *applied* research, which is intended to provide useful information. *Statistics Canada* has developed definitions of these two categories, based on a formulation by the Organization for Economic Cooperation and Development:

Basic Research Original investigation undertaken in order to gain new scientific knowledge with the primary purpose of contribution to the conceptual development of science. Basic research yields hypotheses, theories and general laws. . . .

Applied Research Original investigation undertaken in order to gain new scientific knowledge with the primary purpose of applying such knowledge to the solution of practical or technical problems. It is required either to determine possible uses for the findings of basic research or to select the appropriate method of achieving some predetermined objective. It develops ideas into operational forms.[1]

Like evaluation, research may gather both quantitative and qualitative information. Although it may involve a wide variety of measurement designs, customarily it includes the following steps: (a) a concise formulation of a problem or hypothesis; (b) the development of an investigative procedure (usually referred to as a study design) appropriate to the problem; (c) data gathering; (d) scoring, analysis and interpretation of data; and (e) presentation of conclusions and recommendations for possible action or further study.

IMPORTANCE OF EVALUATION AND RESEARCH

Why are these two processes important to the field of therapeutic recreation service? The most obvious reason is that they provide information that can be useful in developing recreation programs and services.

Beyond this practical need, however, it is obvious that any field *must* rely on more than the judgment of its practitioners as a basis for operation. The entire field of recreation service demands a fuller understanding of the dynamics of play, the

---

[1]"Research Definitions." *Recreation Review,* March 1973, p. 12.

meaning of leisure in society, the attitudes and expectations that underlie participation and the significance of recreation as a form of social service or government responsibility.

Wilson points out that community recreation standards have been developed over the past two decades and have been accepted by regional, state and federal agencies—often as the basis for funding assistance. Typically, local communities must be part of comprehensive regional planning and must be in compliance with state and regional planning recommendations or standards.[2] Mobily and Iso-Ahola stress the fact that recreation professionals, like other professionals involved in public service, are

> . . . expected to make well-informed, competent decisions. To assist in this end, the manager seeks reliable and valid information upon which to base judgments and decisions. . . . The results of assessment and evaluation cannot make decisions for the administrator, but the information gained through surveys, physical accessibility studies, interviews, or various other techniques can provide valuable data to help the manager choose the best course of action.[3]

Within therapeutic recreation service, the role of recreation as therapy, its goals and outcomes, its methodologies and its relationships to other rehabilitative functions demand thoughtful analysis.

Example of Need for Evaluation and Research: Leisure Counseling

To illustrate, Compton, Witt and Sanchez suggest that research and empirical evidence with regard to leisure counseling are sadly lacking. Although this form of service has become increasingly popular and widely practiced in recent years, there are many problems of terminology, procedures and focus. Few attempts are made to measure the actual gains of participants in leisure counseling programs. They conclude,

> Until research is conducted which shows the link between selected counseling methodologies and intended outcomes, leisure counseling will lack credibility and a firm base of support that goes beyond bandwagon enthusiasm. One difficulty is that counseling methodology in general is such a subjective process that exact specification of outcome and methods producing specific results is often difficult. In an era that demands accountability, however, skepticism will have to be met with better evidence than testimonials.[4]

---

[2]George T. Wilson: "Evaluating the Results of Community Recreation." *Journal of Physical Education and Recreation*, October 1980. p. 39.
[3]Ken Mobily and Seppo Iso-Ahola: "Mastery of Evaluation Techniques for the Undergraduate Major." *Journal of Physical Education and Recreation*, October 1980, p. 39.
[4]David Compton, Peter A. Witt and Barbara D. Sanchez: " . . . Leisure Counseling." *Parks and Recreation*, August 1980, p. 35.

Numerous other examples might be cited of the specific need for effective research and evaluation in therapeutic recreation services. During the early decades of the development of the recreation profession, it was commonplace to suggest that *no* significant research was being carried on in recreation, and that its evaluative procedures were lacking in validity and meaning. Today, this is not the case. With the assistance of government and foundation grants, the growth of recreation programs in colleges and universities and increased efforts by professional organizations in this field, remarkable strides have been made in developing meaningful programs of evaluation and research.

EVALUATION IN THERAPEUTIC RECREATION

Evaluation in therapeutic recreation may be done in the following areas: (a) evaluation of an entire department, including all relevant elements; (b) evaluation of a program's effectiveness in meeting specific goals and objectives; (c) evaluation of patients' or clients' needs and interests or progress within given program areas; (d) evaluation of staff performance; (e) evaluation of facilities; and (f) evaluation of entire institutions or agencies.

A number of distinct approaches to evaluation have been developed and presented as alternative models, including the following:

Evaluation as Professional Judgment. In this form of evaluation, an expert appraises a program or agency on the basis of his or her subjective views. Or, an evaluation panel or task force of respected professionals does the evaluation, as in the case of an accreditation review of a hospital or curriculum.

Evaluation as Measurement. This method relies on quantitative data and statistical analysis; it is often part of systems management and planning. While it may provide a rational basis for decision-making, according to Howe, it is nonhumanistic and tends to overlook values as a basis for judgment.

Evaluation as Congruence Between Performance and Objectives. In this method, performance objectives are carefully defined, and the evaluative process consists of measuring as efficiently as possible the degree to which the objectives are realized. This type of evaluation is a good way of determining productivity and accountability, although it may not always be possible to determine whether objectives *are* achieved.

Transaction-Observation Evaluation. This type of evaluation is based on developing a detailed picture of what has occurred in a program or process; it relies on case-study interviews and observations by trained evaluators.[5]

Of these various approaches to evaluation, two are found most frequently in

---

[5]Christine Z. Howe: "Models for Evaluating Public Recreation Programs: What the Literature Shows." *Journal of Physical Education and Recreation,* October 1980, pp. 36–37. *See also* Dan H. Kennedy and Herberta M. Lundegren: "Application of the Discrepancy Evaluation Model in Therapeutic Recreation." *Therapeutic Recreation Journal,* First Quarter, 1981, pp. 24–34.

the therapeutic recreation field. The first relies on the use of *standards and criteria,* which represent guidelines for organizing a program and providing services. The second attempts to measure the program's success in *achieving stated objectives,* by identifying the actual outcomes of a program or agency project. Both of these approaches are described in the following section.

The Evaluation Process

Too often, people or programs are evaluated in sketchy, informal or subjective ways. Based simply on an "impression" or on attendance figures, judgments are made on rating sheets or other evaluation forms. The best kind of evaluation is based on careful, systematic observation carried out regularly and keyed to clearly stated goals, objectives or other criteria. Evaluation should seek to be quantitative as much as possible—that is, stated in terms of ratings that can be scored, to give a meaningful final index of quality or a profile that demonstrates strengths and weaknesses.

Normally, ratings should avoid "yes or no" scoring and such questions as "is a program successful?" or "is it a failure?" Instead, evaluation seeks to measure gradations of quality or performance. Thus, ratings might include such possible choices as "always, often, sometimes, never" or "excellent, very good, good, fair, poor," with each response given an appropriate number value. On the other hand, they might be couched in descriptive phrases like "Places heavy emphasis on acquiring new skills," "Gives moderate emphasis on acquiring new skills" or "Seldom encourages children to learn new skills." In general, each institution or program must develop its own evaluative instruments, since no standardized tests of this kind have been widely developed to cover the broad range of programs in therapeutic recreation.

A key element in such evaluative procedures is the ability of the observer to make intelligent judgments. There are four types of raters:

SELF-EVALUATION BY PRACTITIONER

Although it is certainly valuable to encourage self-evaluation, usually the person responsible for a program is not able to examine his or her program objectively. In any case, it is usually desirable to get other viewpoints and critical reactions.

EVALUATION BY PARTICIPANTS

Those who take part in a program may be asked to judge whether in their views its goals are being met. Often, such reactions may be extremely helpful in an evaluation process. Certain groups, such as the mentally retarded or the mentally ill, may not be able to make effective judgments in their areas, although their opinions or wishes may be helpful in other ways.

EVALUATION BY OTHER PROFESSIONAL PERSONNEL

Other staff members in the same institution, who are thoroughly familiar with the work of the recreation department, may be asked to evaluate its effectiveness. The other professionals might be nurses, doctors or social workers.

EVALUATION BY OUTSIDE EXPERTS

Outsiders, such as leading therapeutic recreation specialists from other institutions, college teachers, professional consultants in this field or state officials, might carry out this type of evaluation. In some cases, a thorough evaluation process might include each of these elements.

Often there is disagreement as to the comparative effectiveness of "inside" versus "outside" evaluators. *Insiders* (that is, those who are employed by the agency) obviously have the advantage of being familiar with the program, and they are available without additional expense. On the other hand, they may be biased or self-protective and may not be able to see the program and its outcomes objectively. *Outsiders*—visiting experts or panels of evaluators—are generally unbiased and can be chosen for their rich experience and expertise. However, it may take them a long time to find out all the necessary details of a program. Also, it may be costly to employ them unless they are volunteering their services.

A final useful source of evaluators in therapeutic recreation may be the parents of those served. Wyatt and Hunt point out that parents of children attending a camping program for the mentally retarded may be excellent evaluators because of their ability to determine the long-term effects of the program and their closeness to the clients, who would be likely to trust and confide in them.[6]

Evaluation of Program or Department

An evaluation may be made of a therapeutic recreation program or department that has been either in action over a period of time or set up a short while before on an experimental basis. A useful set of standards for the evaluation of recreation services in residential institutions was developed by Berryman and associates as part of a three-year study of therapeutic recreation service supported by a grant from the Children's Bureau of the U.S. Department of Health, Education and Welfare.[7] This document provides a systematic means of looking at a total program, based on 55 different standards grouped under several major categories and supported by illustrative criteria. Examples of several standards and illustrative criteria follow:

---

[6]William J. Wyatt and Sharon K. Hunt: "Using Parents as Evaluators of a Therapeutic Recreation Camping Program for the Retarded." *Therapeutic Recreation Journal*, Fourth Quarter, 1976, pp. 142–147.
[7]Doris L. Berryman, Project Director: *Recommended Standards with Evaluative Criteria for Recreation Services in Residential Institutions.* New York, New York University School of Education, 1971.

Philosophy and Goals

Standard 1.   The therapeutic recreation services offered are based on a written philosophy of recreation as it applies to the residential treatment center.

Criteria

a. The statement is in accord with the philosophy, purpose, and policies of the agency and has been approved by its administrative authority.

b. Within the department, provisions are made to acquaint all recreation staff members and volunteers with this statement.

Administration

Standard 5.   Structure. Recreation services are administered by a professional department as an integral part of the institution's overall functional structure.

Criteria

a. Administrative authority and responsibilities are clearly delineated in writing.

b. Responsibility for recreation services is assigned to professionally qualified staff.

c. The department administrator participates in interdepartmental meetings.

Personnel

Standard 13.   Personnel Practices. The institution has written personnel policies and practices which are periodically reviewed by its governing body and revised as necessary.

Criteria

a. There is a written statement of personnel policies and practices.

b. A copy of the statement is given to each employee as well as kept on file in the department.

Programming

Standard 37.   Needs and Interests of Residents. Recreation Services are designed to meet the needs, competencies, capabilities and interests of individuals and groups and take into account individual treatment objectives.

Criteria

a. There is an established method for assessing the needs, interests, competencies and capabilities of residents which includes:

1. an interview with each resident; and/or

2. access to pertinent medical, psychiatric and other information concerning each resident.

b. Resident committees are utilized in planning the activities program where feasible.

Areas, Facilities, and Equipment

Standard 45.   Design and Layout. Recreation areas and facilities are designed and constructed or modified to permit all recreation services to be carried out to the fullest possible extent in pleasant and functional surroundings accessible to all residents regardless of their disabilities.

Criteria

a. Recreation staff and appropriate outside consultants are consulted in the designing or modification of all recreation areas and facilities.

b. Recreation areas and facilities meet local legal requirements concerning safety, fire, health, sanitation, etc., codes.

Evaluation and Research

Standard 54.   Evaluation of Recreation Services. The recreation department has established procedures for evaluating recreation services in relation to stated purposes, goals and objectives.

Criteria

a. The recreation department maintains adequate records concerning the residents. These records include:

1. periodic surveys of their interests;

2. periodic surveys of their attitudes and opinions of the recreation services;

3. extent and level of each individual's participation in the activities program;

4. where appropriate, progress reports are maintained

> b. An appropriate time schedule is established for each type of evaluation. (Some aspects of recreation services will be evaluated annually, some periodically, some after each event, etc.).[8]

This is only a partial list of the standards and criteria developed by Berryman and a panel of experts. For example, the separate standards under the heading of Personnel include the following: personnel practices; job descriptions and classification system; salary ranges; hours of work; fringe benefits; hiring, assignment and promotion of employees; recruitment; evaluation of performance; workload; staffing; supporting services; orientation program; staff development; responsibilities of director; supervision; contribution to the profession; consultation; use of volunteers; and statements of suggested qualifications on several job levels.

Evaluation in the Accreditation Process

Another example of evaluation may be found in the accreditation process initiated in 1975 by the Council on Accreditation of the National Recreation and Park Association. The overall purpose of this process is to (a) serve the public by promoting and maintaining high educational standards; (b) assist college and university officials in attaining defensible goals of recreation education; (c) foster continual self-study and improvement of professional preparation programs; and (d) encourage experimentation to improve professional education and services in recreation, leisure services and resources.

In order to standardize accreditation procedures, evaluative criteria have been developed in the following major areas: Philosophy and Purposes; Faculty; Students; Research; Public Service; Organization and Administration; Areas, Facilities, Equipment and Instruction Resources.[9] In addition, detailed standards and evaluative criteria are provided for both undergraduate and graduate curricula. Procedural guidelines outline the sequence through which a given institution many apply to the Council for accreditation, complete a Self-Study Evaluation Report, be visited by an Accreditation Team and so on.

The accreditation process has been made more meaningful by the publication of a set of competencies needed for both undergraduate and graduate professional emphasis in therapeutic recreation. The undergraduate emphasis, for example, includes the following competencies, which serve as a useful means of evaluating a college or university's curriculum and overall operation:

Knowledge of illness and disability with implications for recreation programming, i.e., physically handicapped, mentally ill, emotionally disturbed, developmentally disabled, penally incarcerated, and aging.

[8]*Ibid.*, pp. 11–12, 17, 33, 37, 43.
[9]*Standards and Evaluative Criteria for Recreation, Leisure Services and Resources Curricula: Baccalaureate and Master's Degree Programs.* Arlington, Virginia, National Recreation and Park Association, Council on Accreditation, October 1975.

Knowledge of specific service delivery systems related to treatment and rehabilitation, i.e., medical models, leisure education models, etc.

Knowledge of administrative policies and procedures associated with treatment and rehabilitation settings.

Understanding of specific facilitation and counseling techniques predominantly used with special populations.

Knowledge of specific needs of special populations, and activity modification techniques needed to adapt activities to individual needs.

Knowledge of procedures used in formulating individual and group assessment, prescription, and evaluation plans with special populations.

Understanding of principles used for recording and reporting client information in treatment and rehabilitation settings.

Understanding of administrative principles related to community recreation programs for special populations.

Knowledge of facility design and equipment modification related to accessibility and mainstreaming concepts.

Knowledge of institution to community service continuum designs.

Knowledge of both normal and abnormal growth and development as traditionally taught in related fields, including: special education, psychology, sociology, anatomy/physiology/kinesiology.

Ability to apply the unique practices and principles of therapeutic recreation in authorized practicum experiences commensurate with the approved NTRS guidelines for field placement.[10]

On the graduate level, competencies suggested in the Accreditation Standards and Evaluative Criteria include (a) the ability to conceptualize and articulate major professional issues related to therapeutic recreation; (b) demonstrated involvement in professional growth experiences other than academic, such as professional memberships, workshops or conferences; (c) in-depth knowledge in a minimum of two disability groupings; (d) the ability to conceptualize, design, implement and evaluate therapeutic recreation programs; and (e) an in-depth knowledge of activity analysis and its application for assessment and prescription of programs for special populations.

Such specific criteria are extremely useful in evaluating a college or university therapeutic recreation curriculum, in terms of whether it is providing undergraduates or graduate students with essential competencies in their chosen area of specialization. It should be pointed out that such evaluative tools cannot be developed by a single individual—no matter how competent or authoritative. Instead, they must be the product of teams of qualified practitioners and educators who share their viewpoints and expertise.

Evaluation in Therapeutic Camping

Another example of the use of evaluation in therapeutic recreation programming is found in the manual *Evaluating the Camp Experience* prepared by Vinton and

---

[10] *Addendum to Accreditation Standards and Evaluative Criteria: Competencies Needed for Undergraduate Professional Emphasis in Therapeutic Recreation.* Arlington, Virginia, National Recreation and Park Association, Council on Accreditation, October 1976.

Farley as part of Project Reach at the University of Kentucky.[11] Evaluative information is gathered from campers and staff members to measure the camp's success in achieving specific objectives. Recommendations are developed on the basis of the conclusions of this self-study process. The manual uses a "discrepancy evaluation" approach, which measures the discrepancy, or gap, between stated objectives and actual program outcomes.

Although a number of distinctly different program or agency evaluation models have been identified in the literature, it is possible to blend several different approaches in an ongoing evaluation process. For example, Miller describes a method for auditing activity programs in long-term care facilities:

The most desirable method of program assessment would be to include a combination of outside consultant and inside evaluators (including staff, residents, families and volunteers). All concerned groups should participate in periodic assessments to be aware of current social, physical and emotional needs as the patient population changes. Audit methods might employ in-depth interviews, case studies, check lists and rating scales. Full participation by interested persons will ensure cooperation in implementing an activity program designed to improve the quality of life in the long-term care facility.[12]

Evaluation of Program Elements

A more limited type of evaluative procedure involves the appraisal of a simple type of program service. Here, any given program element, such as sports and games, arts and crafts, social activities or other events, may be evaluated by asking such questions as the following:

"Does it contribute to overall program goals of the institution?"
"Does it attract participants; is it regularly attended and popular with patients?"
"Is is administratively feasible—that is, can it easily accommodate schedule, staff and facility demands?"
"Does it contribute to specific treatment needs of individual patients?"

In addition, evaluation may focus on the programs provided for a specific *population*, in a particular *unit* or other *special setting* or using a unique or *experimental method*. If it is a routine procedure designed to measure and improve the effectiveness of an ongoing program, it should legitimately be considered evaluation. If, on the other hand, it is concerned with measuring a program set up specifically to test the effectiveness of certain techniques or program methods, it should be regarded as a form of research.

Evaluation of specific programs tends to be carried out on two levels: (a) by

---

[11]Dennis A. Vinton and Elizabeth M. Farley, eds.: *Camp Staff Training Series, Module 6.* Lexington, Kentucky, Project REACH, University of Kentucky; the American Camping Association; and Hawkins and Associates, 1979.

[12]Dulcy B. Miller: "Suggested Methodologies for Auditing Activity Programs in Long Term Care Facilities." *Therapeutic Recreation Journal*, Third Quarter, 1975.

1. What is the average number of week-nights per week that activities are conducted? _____

2. What is the average number of activities per night? _____

3. Where are activities conducted? Wards _____ Rec Building _____ Gym _____ Off-grounds _____ Other _____

4. What is the average number of staff working per evening? _____

5. What is the average number of volunteers working per evening? _____

6. Is evening duty rotated among staff? Yes _____ No _____

   If "Yes," are activities provided Sat. morning _____, afternoon _____, evening _____; Sun. morning _____, afternoon _____, evening _____.
   If "No," do you regularly provide activities weekends? Yes _____ No _____
   If "Yes," what is the average number of evenings each staff member works per week?

7. Do you regularly provide activities weekends? Yes _____; No _____
   If "Yes," are activities provided Sat. morning _____, afternoon _____, evening _____; Sun. morning _____, afternoon _____, evening _____

Figure 12–1. Questionnaire on night, weekend and holiday therapeutic recreation programs. (Modified from State Department of Public Welfare, Office of Mental Health and Mental Retardation, Harrisburg, Pennsylvania, 1970.)

gathering statistics on attendance or participation, staffing arrangements, costs and similar data and making judgments based on them; and (b) by attempting to assess, in a more analytical way, the actual quality of the program or its demonstrable success in terms of patient or client service and outcomes. As an example of the first approach, Figure 12–1 indicates questions on a report used in the Pennsylvania State Department of Public Welfare. It is intended to assess practices with respect to night, weekend and holiday programming in state mental hospitals and schools.

A second report form used by the same department seeks information on therapeutic recreation participation by patients within six categories: (a) mass activities; (b) off-grounds activities: (c) ward activities; (d) interest group activities; (e) individual activities; and (f) recreation therapy groups. Frequency of participation, as well as total and average hours of involvement, and similar information are gathered through such instruments to assist in overall review of the program.

Evaluation of Patients' or Clients' Needs, Interests and Participation

The second major method of evaluating program effectiveness would be to assess the extent to which goals are being met—rather than simply gathering facts and figures about services provided and amounts of participation. Evaluation of outcomes is most reliable when based on careful observation of patients' or clients' involvement and behavorial change. There are several steps in this process: (a) assessing their needs and interests; (b) developing recommendations for program involvement; (c) implementing recommended plan; and (d) evaluating, based on systematic observation and feedback.

The therapist may use forms such as those shown in Chapter 6 (see pp. 211, 219) to gain a comprehensive picture of the individual's past interests and hobbies, and those he or she might like to carry on within the present treatment program. Many community agencies use an "intake" form to gather information about the patient's or client's degree and type of disability, in addition to his or her skills, life circumstances and other relevant information (Fig. 12–2).

In addition to such information, the therapeutic recreation specialist might use an observation form, which is helpful in assessing the individual's social behavior. One example of a range of possible behaviors is shown in Figure 12–3. A much more systematic form has been developed by Parker, Ellison, Kirby and Short for use in short-term, acute-care psychiatric settings.[13] This instrument, called the Comprehensive Evaluation in Recreational Therapy Scale (CERT Scale), requires careful observation over a period of time. It measures aspects of appearance, physical performance and group behavior, including such specific elements as the ability to take part in structured or unstructured activities, to relate meaningfully to others, to play appropriate sexual roles, to handle conflict situations, to tolerate frustration, to apply judgment and to make decisions. Although these might appear to be difficult abilities to judge or measure objectively, the percentage of agreement between therapists who rated a large number of patients was extremely high, averaging over 90 per cent. In most cases, staff members of different institutions or agencies tend to make up their own assessment instruments, but the CERT Scale has been used successfully in a number of different settings.

In some cases, institutional recreation staffs have employed a variety of techniques to gain a rounded picture of patients' or clients' needs, interests and capabilities. For example, in the Penetanguishene, Ontario, Mental Health Centre in Canada, the patient evaluation process includes a series of sessions, with (a) concealed observation of the individual taking part in evening group activities; (b) videotaped interview between the assessor and the client, dealing with his or her attitudes about recreation and prehospital interests and social involvement; (c) administration of a psychological projective test, the Guilford-Zimmerman Temperament Survey, and a printed Interest Survey; (d) a second interview between the assessor and the patient, including use of a game or other activity in which the subject may be involved; (e) observation of the individual taking part in regular group activities, with the client and assessor interacting around the framework of a game; and (f) other sessions involving observation, group interaction and a final interview in which the assessment program is discussed and the client indicates his or her reactions to it.[14]

---

[13]Robert A. Parker, Curtis H. Ellison, Thomas F. Kirby and M. J. Short: "The Comprehensive Evaluation in Recreational Therapy Scale: A Tool for Patient Evaluation." *Therapeutic Recreation Journal*, Fourth Quarter, 1975, pp. 143–152.

[14]For a fuller description, *see* Richard G. Kraus, Gay Carpenter and Barbara J. Bates: *Recreation Leadership and Supervision, Guidelines for Professional Development*. Philadelphia, Saunders College Publishing, 1981, pp. 214–215.

Name _____   Date _____

       Last   First   Middle

Birthdate	Age	Race	Sex	Religion

Address _____

City _____

Telephone _____

Marital Status of Applicant (Circle One)
1. Never Married
2. Married
3. Widowed
4. Divorced
5. Separated

Emergency Information: _____

Name _____

Address _____

City _____

Telephone _____ Relationship _____

Other children in the home

Number of Boys ___ Ages _____

             Girls ___ Ages _____

Lives with Parents ☐ Guardian ☐

Name of Guardian _____

Parents	Occupation	Business Address	Telephone Number
Father			
Mother			

Diagnosis: _____   Cause _____

Special Handicaps (Check Degree)	None	Mild	Moderate	Severe	Comments
Emotional Disturbance					
Speech Impairment					
Impairment of Mobility					
Impairment of Hearing					
Impairment of Vision					
Epilepsy					
Suffers Motion Sickness					

Name of Doctor _____ Address _____ Telephone _____

Please Check Correct Box:	Yes	No		Yes	No
Needs toilet assistance			Can read		
Uses public transportation with assistance			Can write		
Uses public transportation with no assistance			Can dress self		
Can make self understood with words			Can feed self		
Can make self understood with motions					
Can understand simple word commands					
Can understand motion commands only					

Note: In addition to above sections, the form also asks for detailed information regarding the applicant's educational background, transportation needs, social worker (if any), available financial assistance and family income. It concludes with parental consent and photographic release forms and a space for general comments regarding the applicant's needs and admissions decision. Accompanying it is a separate medical report form to be filled out by a doctor.

Figure 12–2. Participant application form. (Adapted from Participant Intake Form, San Francisco Recreation Center for the Handicapped, 1974.)

Date: _____ Weekly Session No.: _____ Participant's Name: _____

Topic: _____ Group Leader: _____

Categories of observable participation	Level of Performance				Comments
	Never	Occasionally	Often	Most of the time	Give illustrations of behavior, including both positive and negative examples.
Appears isolated and uninvolved in midst of group					
Listens passively					
Shows interest but responds only when called on					
Speaks voluntarily on occasion but only to group leader					
Speaks to others but without reference to self					
Reports personal experiences with some insight					
Seeks information					
Speaks with support of others' feelings					
Establishes relationships with others					
Clearly expresses feelings and personal ambitions					
Other behavior (explain)					

12-3. Chart for recording patient participation in group sessions (Adapted from Patient Behavior Assessment Form, Bellevue Hospital, New York, 1975.)

In addition to information gathered through such procedures, the entire treatment team, including medical and nursing staff and other therapists or social service personnel, may contribute their views of the patient's or client's needs, interests and capabilities. Specific psychological or physical needs, which serve as the basis for prescribing, recommending or contracting for activity, may also be indicated.

Techniques for assessing play and recreational behavior of patients and clients have become increasingly sophisticated in recent years. For example, Levy describes a number of methods of systematic observing and recording: (a) continuous recording or anecdotal reporting; (b) frequency count or event recording; (c) duration and interval recording; and (d) time sampling methods. Each of these techniques is useful in gaining a valid picture of play behavior. However, all depend heavily on the scientific definition and description of the play behaviors to be measured. Levy points out that there is no standardized list of behaviors, actions or situations and that no taxonomy of therapeutic recreation behavioral units has been established. Thus, any researcher who seeks to do this type of measurement must devise his or her own instruments, behavioral descriptions and observational techniques.[15]

In some cases, particularly under the *medical model* of therapeutic recreation service, there may be a direct prescription of activity to achieve treatment objectives. For example, if a patient or client is extremely withdrawn, shy or lacking in self-confidence, the prescription may be for group involvement in social activities. If the individual is extremely aggressive or hostile, competitive sports or other vigorous forms of activity may be indicated.

In other situations, instead of directly prescribing activity, the treatment team may help the patient or client come to an accurate realization of his or her own needs and select a program of activities to achieve certain mutually accepted goals. In some cases, specific behavioral goals may be designated and agreed upon by the therapist and patient or client. For example, in some behavior modification programs for disturbed or socially deviant individuals, the *contingency contracting* approach is used.[16] Simply described, this means that, based on the analysis of the treatment team, certain behavioral objectives are identified—in terms of either strengths to be built or deficits to be overcome. These might include such behaviors as (a) cursing or attacking others; (b) coming to sessions regularly and on time; (c) carrying out group responsibilities; (d) not coming to sessions "high" on liquor or drugs; or (e) performing work tasks effectively. Both the client and the therapist sign an agreement stating that if the objectives are attained, certain rewards will be granted; if not, certain negative reinforcers will be applied. Thus, as an ongoing part of the process, evaluation is carried on with immediate feedback.

In other situations, evaluation is more of a one-way process. In working with the mentally retarded or the brain-injured, for example, specific exercises or activity-related tasks may be prescribed, with a sequence of skills to be mastered. For

---

[15]Joseph Levy: "Behavioral Observation Techniques in Therapeutic Recreation/Play Settings." *Therapeutic Recreation Journal*, First Quarter, 1982, pp. 26–32.

[16]For descriptions of behavior modification and contingency contracting methods, *see* R. D. Jodrell and R. S. Fisher: "Basic Concepts of Behavior Therapy: An Experiment Involving Disturbed Adolescent Girls," *American Journal of Occupational Therapy*, November–December 1975, and R. R. Parlour: "Some Behavioral Techniques in Community Psychiatry," *American Journal of Psychology*, 29–79–91, 1975.

example, physical activities may be outlined in a step-by-step process, with each skill, its purpose and a criterion for measuring its performance listed in sequential order. In a Therapeutic Recreation Curriculum Manual developed at the Fairview Hospital and Training Center in Salem, Oregon, for example, goals and graded tasks are presented under five major headings: (a) Music and Dramatic Activities; (b) Physical Activities; (c) Arts and Crafts; (d) Social Activities; and (e) General Skills and Concepts. These in turn are broken down in the manual with a variety of sub-tasks presented under five levels of difficulty. For example, sequential tasks are identified under the heading of Group Interaction in the Social Activities area (Fig. 12–4A). In the manual, a rating system for assigning points to each sub-task and each overall activity area is presented. This approach provides a means of identifying desired tracks for improving performance of participants, monitoring performance and arriving at scores through which to appraise their progress over a period of time. The Progress Report Form used to sum up a client's total effort, as evaluated by the therapeutic recreation team, is shown in Figure 12–4B.

It should be pointed out that not all departments or institutions make use of such forms in the evaluation process. Touchstone points out that many place considerable reliance on methods like psychodrama or role-playing, which do not lend themselves to quantitative evaluation, and that in general, standardized instruments are not used widely in this field. This suggests that the evaluation process must be designed for a particular institution or agency or set of patients or clients, along with the unique objectives that have been established for a given situation. In some cases, the deliberate policy has been to *resist* elaborate or complicated evaluation report forms as unnecessary paper work. Instead, brief written, anecdotal statements appraising a patient's or client's behavior and progress within a program are required.

Evaluation of Behavioral Change

In some cases, recreation can provide the setting in which behavioral change can be evaluated. For example, at the Children's Village in Dobbs Ferry, New York, boys are regularly assessed using sociometric rating techniques to determine their popularity and acceptance by others. In addition, a number of other aspects of behavior are measured at regular intervals. These include such characteristics or behaviors as social isolation, need for contact with adults, tendency to become emotionally upset, expressions of anxiety and fear, ability to delay gratification and exhibition of unethical behavior. The findings, when analyzed, provide useful information not only about individual children, but also about groups living in separate cottages and about the overall school population.[17]

---

[17]Howard Millman: "Current Implications of Cottage and Sociometric Rating Research." *Children's Village Bulletin: Journal of Residential Treatment*, Dobbs Ferry, New York, May 1978, pp. 1–2.

Levels	I	II	III	IV	V
1.	Joins group and participates in all Level I activities upon request of instructor	Knows his own position within group formation and takes his turn	Recognizes other peoples' turns and positions within group	Knows his position within more complicated activities (e.g., *when to speak* in a play or *position* in a team sport)	Organizes and directs group game involving peers during *free time* on own initiative
2.	*Waits to take turn*	Communicates *ideas* and *needs* to instructor and peers in a *polite* and considerate manner	Listens to and accepts ideas of others within group	Gives appropriate encouragement to peers in activities	Participates actively and appropriately in group *discussions*
3.	Communicates ideas and needs to instructor	*Shares* play area and materials on his *own* initiative	Develops concept of *sportsmanship*; being good *winner and loser*	Displays good *sportsmanship* in all activities	Participates actively and appropriately in group *decision making*
4.	*Shares* play area and materials upon request of instructor	Accepts and *follows* rules of Level I and Level II activities	Understands and follows rules of Level I, II, and III activities	Understands and follows rules of Level I, II, III, and IV activities	Exhibits socially acceptable behavior when participating in community recreation programs

Note: Levels I through V represent increasingly advanced levels of performance. Some tasks or skills begin at a low level and continue up through the higher levels. Others begin initially at higher level.

Figure 12–4A. Group interaction tasks excerpted from Fairview Hospital and Training Center Manual. (Adapted from Barbara Mumford, Coordinator: *Therapeutic Recreation Curriculum Manual.* Salem, Oregon, Fairview Hospital and Training Center, 1973, pp. 3–4.)

Name: _____   Cottage: _____   Level: _____

Music and Dramatic Activities: Score
  a. Music expression   _____
  b. Rhythmic movement   _____
  c. Creative dramatics   _____
  d. Care and use of equipment   _____
  e. Receptive and expressive language   _____

                                         Sub-total _____

Physical Activities:
  a. Locomotor activities   _____
  b. Nonlocomotor activities   _____
  c. Group activities and individual-team sports   _____
  d. Care and use of equipment   _____
  e. Receptive and expressive language   _____

                                         Sub-total _____

Arts and Crafts:
  a. Eye-hand coordination and finger dexterity   _____
  b. Identification and discrimination   _____
  c. Expressive art   _____
  d. Care and use of equipment   _____
  e. Receptive and expressive language   _____

                                         Sub-total _____

Social Activities:
  a. Group interaction   _____
  b. Leadership and followership   _____
  c. Spectator skills   _____
  d. Care and use of equipment   _____
  e. Receptive and expressive language   _____

                                         Sub-total _____

General Skills and Concepts:
  a. Self-help skills   _____
  b. Number and time concepts   _____
  c. Travel   _____
  d. Care and use of equipment   _____
  e. Receptive and expressive language   _____

                                         Sub-total _____

                                         Total Score _____

There are four points possible for each item; the highest score possible is 100%.
  Rating Code: 4 = does correctly
               3 = attempts correctly
               2 = attempts incorrectly
               1 = does not attempt

Comments: _____
_____
_____

Figure 12–4B. Therapeutic recreation report form. (From Barbara Mumford, Coordinator: *Therapeutic Recreation Curriculum Manual.* Salem, Oregon, Fairview Hospital and Training Center, 1973, pp. 3–4.)

Evaluation of Staff Performance

In large institutions, it is generally the practice for supervisors to regularly evaluate their staff. Such evaluations are normally based on formal records that rate the employee on attendance, appearance, leadership qualities, organizing ability, control and discipline, initiative, judgment and responsibility.

These evaluations tend to be fairly mechanical, although they are a useful way of getting a numerical picture of staff performance. Another method is to rely on anecdotal records. A supervisor will observe a leader or therapist at work over a period of time and will write a descriptive account of his or her performance, including both strengths and weaknesses. This case record becomes the basis for supervisory conferences. Thus, the evaluation leads to improvement of performance, which should be its main justification.

Teague points out that formal employee evaluations tend to yield unsatisfactory results, in part because of resistance from the supervisors who are expected to administer them. This resistance, he writes, is usually attributed to the following causes:

> (1) a normal dislike of criticizing a subordinate, and very possibly having to argue about it; (2) lack of skill needed to effectively manage an appraisal interview; (3) mistrust of the validity of appraisal instruments; and (4) dislike in implementing a new procedure with its accompanying operational changes. . . . managers (express) real misgivings . . . when they are put in the position of 'playing God' . . . [18]

In part, the problem is that procedures measuring on-the-job performance and personality traits are routine and superficial. To make this process more effective, Teague suggests the development of more dynamic job descriptions and action plans which take into account human relationships within the agency. More varied and probing evaluation techniques and support mechanisms also are needed to assist both supervisors and employees in the personnel evaluation process.

Evaluation of Facilities

These evaluations may be carried out with a preestablished list of desirable facilities for a particular type of rehabilitative or therapeutic recreation setting, such as gymnasium, swimming pool, outdoor sports facilities, lounges, arts and crafts rooms and meeting rooms. Despite the fact that institutions vary widely, certainly it would be feasible to develop a *minimal list* as a standard for institutions.

Another way to evaluate facilities might be to establish questions that relate to their quality and usefulness. A checklist could be developed for various types of

---

[18]Michael L. Teague: "Performance Appraisal: A Bold Plan." *Therapeutic Recreation Journal*, First Quarter, 1980, p. 5.

facilities, such as the playground: Does it offer varied pieces of equipment for creative and active physical play? Is it aesthetically designed? Are health and safety guidelines followed? Does it permit participation by children on crutches, in wheelchairs or in braces? Does it meet the needs of various age groups? Has it been effectively maintained, and is maximum use being made of it?

Summing up this section of the text, evaluation must be regarded as an important tool in appraising the quality and effectiveness of therapeutic recreation programs or their component parts, or in assessing patient or client needs and interests to determine appropriate program involvement.

RESEARCH IN THERAPEUTIC RECREATION

Research is much broader than evaluation, both in its focus and in the methods employed. For example, evaluation generally deals in the here and now; it is concerned with directly observable phenomena, such as patient behavior, staff strategies or program outcomes. Research, however, may deal with the past as well as the present or future. Research questions may be conceptual; the answers might result in new models or understandings of professional processes and relationships. Data may be gathered in the field, in *real* situations, or from *artificial* environments and situations structured to impose a degree of control over elements in the area being investigated which would not be possible in a natural setting.

Research may deal with the *empirical*, involving real situations that can be observed and measured, or with *nonempirical* concerns, such as analytical or philosophical questions. It may be *nonobtrusive*, that is, careful not to influence what is being observed, or it may be *obtrusive*, deliberately altering the environment or introducing new elements into the situation. It may be *quantitative* or *qualitative* in its data-gathering procedures. Research may rely heavily on statistical analysis, or it may make use of anecdotal, descriptive reporting and analysis.

Types of Research Designs

In therapeutic recreation service, research designs include (a) *descriptive* research, which has several sub-types, including survey research, case studies, longitudinal and evaluative research; and (b) *experimental* research, which includes such sub-types as quasi-experimental, ex post facto and true experimental studies.

DESCRIPTIVE RESEARCH

As indicated, descriptive research aids in observing and measuring real situations, without altering them in any way. It tends to be of an applied or practical nature, rather than theoretical, and to be carried on in field situations.

Surveys.   Surveys are a sub-category of descriptive research; they tend to be the most common form of research approach in therapeutic recreation, as they are in the broad field of social research. Surveys are used to determine current conditions with respect to such elements as practices, participation, recreational choices and attitudes, employment and professional development, program content and a host of similar subjects.

The term "survey" implies taking a broad or comprehensive look, rather than a sharply focused one. Therefore, a survey is generally concerned with examining a number of programs, communities or organizations. or with gathering information about a large class of people, a region or even the entire country. Surveys make use of mailed questionnaires, interviews and polls, check lists, rating scales and similar techniques.

Case Studies.   This method customarily is used to examine a single program, institution, culture or other social group. It involves intensive study utilizing a variety of data-gathering techniques—observations, historical, documentary analysis. interviews and other methods. It may be of a comparative or cross-sectional type, in which two or more cases or subjects, or groups of subjects, are compared.

Longitudinal Design.   This usually involves the study of quantifiable data over a period of time. It differs from historical research in that it may involve the deliberate monitoring of an agency, a group of subjects or another situation over a period of time extending into the future.

Two related forms of research are: (a) the *time-series* study, in which information is gathered at regular intervals to determine change; and (b) *trends-analysis* studies, which make predictions based on past trends and the current situation.

EXPERIMENTAL RESEARCH

This is a form of obtrusive study design, in which the researcher typically applies new services, treatment procedures, equipment or other types of environmental changes and carefully measures the outcomes of such changes. Usually, it is carried on in an attempt to determine whether certain pre-existing hypotheses are correct and whether they can be supported by significant statistical findings. Experimental analysis may be carried on in the field or in a carefully controlled laboratory situation.

True Experimental Approach.   In the true experimental approach, the most scientifically valid form of research, the purpose is usually to investigate possible cause-and-effect relationships by exposing one or more experimental groups to one or more treatment conditions and comparing the results to control groups which have not been exposed to the treatment conditions. For the research to be valid, the subjects should be randomly selected, and rigorous conditions should be established to prevent other factors from influencing the cause-and-effect relationship.

Quasi-Experimental Research.   Because of the difficulty in imposing the necessary controls or in randomly selecting subjects, many studies are carried out without meeting the full requirements of true experimental research. Such studies are called quasi-experimental.

Ex Post Facto Research.   This involves the analysis of past events and the treatment of data to determine possible cause-and-effect relationships, without, however, having strict controls over the experimental situation or selection of subjects.

OTHER RESEARCH DESIGNS

Another major form of research used in various disciplines is *historical* research, which consists of reconstructing the past as objectively and accurately as possible, making use of primary sources of data. Historical research is most meaningful when it not only records what has taken place, but also examines it within the context of the social environment and period in which it occurred, and when it seeks to test hypotheses regarding events or trends of the past.

Several other research techniques in therapeutic recreation may involve *documentary analysis,* which consists of the careful study of documents, reports or other written information; *critical-incident method,* which is based on the in-depth study of one or more significant episodes or incidents; *field study,* a technique widely used in both sociology and anthropology, in which the researcher immerses himself or herself in an ongoing situation or environment and gathers information about it, using a variety of methods: *judge's appraisal,* a method of utilizing the expert judgment of a group of authorities; and *tests of behavior or performance,* which are normally used in experimental research.

Two other types of research which may be part of any of the designs just described are *correlational research,* which measures the relationship between two or more sets of variables, and *evaluative research,* which analyzes an existing program, process or service to determine how effectively it meets its objectives.

Examples of Published Research in Therapeutic Recreation

At an early point in the development of therapeutic recreation service, a number of key research questions were suggested at professional meetings. At the outset, these questions concerned the contributions of recreation to the treatment process for different types of patients and the needs of different types of patients. In addition, other research studies examined the use of "prescribed" versus "voluntary participation" programming, specific leadership techniques and the backgrounds of different types of patients.

Beginning in the late 1960's, with the establishment of the National Therapeutic Recreation Society and the *Therapeutic Recreation Journal* and the stimulus provided by other publications, such as the *Research Quarterly* and *Journal of Leisure Research* in the United States, and *Recreation Review* and *Leisurability* in Canada, the range of research subjects expanded considerably. Several broad areas of concern have emerged; a number of illustrations of studies carried out within each of these areas within the past 15 years are presented in the following section.

The examples presented here fall under the following major headings: (a) examinations of organized programs and surveys of professional practices; (b) studies of professional development in therapeutic recreation; and (c) analysis of special populations in relationship to recreation and leisure. The examples chosen are only a few of dozens of such studies carried out and reported in the literature in recent years; however, they are a fairly representative selection and give a picture of the research thrust in this field.

EXAMINATIONS OF ORGANIZED PROGRAMS AND SURVEYS OF PRACTICES

Recreation Services for the Mentally Retarded in the State of Kansas (1969). This study involved a large-scale survey intended to determine the scope and nature of recreation programs for mentally retarded children and youth in the state of Kansas and to develop a set of recommendations designed to improve programs and services.[19]

A Study of Therapeutic Recreation Services in Kentucky Nursing Homes (1970). This study examined the extent, nature and administrative arrangements of recreation programs provided for older persons in extended-care facilities in the state of Kentucky. As in similar reports, in addition to providing a statistical picture of existing services, the study concluded with recommendations for improved and expanded services.[20]

Availability and Utilization of Recreation Resources for Chronically Ill and Disabled Children and Youth in the United States (1970). This survey sought to determine the extent of recreation services offered to disabled children in a cluster sampling of nine Standard Metropolitan Statistical Areas and one Consolidated Metropolitan Statistical Area in the United States. It identified a variety of existing and potential recreation resources for children and youth, as well as major needs for development in this field.[21]

Recreation and Related Therapies in Psychiatric Rehabilitation (1973). This study examined practices and trends in various types of psychiatric treatment centers in the New York–New Jersey–Connecticut region, with emphasis on objectives, administrative structure, staffing, programming and leisure counseling in recreation and activity therapy. It sought also to determine the effect of "unitization" on psychiatric treatment centers and the influence of milieu therapy and therapeutic community approaches upon programming and leadership.[22]

An Examination of Weekend Recreational Patterns at the Mental Health Centre, Penetanguishene, Ontario (1973). This study sought to examine (a) the provision made for organized recreation programs on weekends in the institution under study and (b) the actual use of weekends by patients, including town or

---

[19]Gene A. Hayes: "Recreation Services for the Mentally Retarded in the State of Kansas." *Therapeutic Recreation Journal*, Third Quarter, 1969, p. 13.
[20]Martha Peters and Peter J. Verhoven, Jr.: "A Study of Therapeutic Recreation Services in Kentucky Nursing Homes." *Therapeutic Recreation Journal*, Fourth Quarter, 1970, pp. 19–22.
[21]John E. Silson, et al.: "Availability and Utilization of Recreation Resources for Chronically Ill and Disabled Children and Youth in the U.S." *Therapeutic Recreation Journal*, Fourth Quarter, 1970, pp. 1, 36.
[22]Richard G. Kraus: *Recreation and Related Therapies in Psychiatric Rehabilitation.* New York, Herbert H. Lehman College and Faculty Research Foundation, November 1972.

home-visiting privileges. The basic question was whether the recreation staff was responding creatively to the real leisure needs of patients.[23]

Recreation Services for the Handicapped in Canada (1974).   This was a large-scale survey of recreation services for the disabled in agencies, institutions and municipalities with populations over 1000 persons throughout Canada. It sought to determine the populations served, the nature of sponsorship, programming elements and particularly the degree of concern for the disabled in the communities studied.[24]

Survey of Municipal Recreation Services for Special Groups in Ontario (1975).   Somewhat similar to the preceding study, this survey examined programs provided by municipal recreation authorities in communities of 5000 or more residents, for four special populations: the mentally retarded, physically disabled, emotionally disturbed and learning-disabled. It examined the nature of special services, the role of recreation authorities, administrative problems and solutions and the degree of integration or segregation of the disabled in the programs reported.[25]

Camping for the Handicapped in Selected Camps in California (1975).   This survey examined the status of camping for disabled children and youth in 305 California camps and agencies accredited by the American Camping Association and the Western Association of Independent Camps. It studied the extent of such provision, the reasons why camps did not serve the disabled (if they did not), the nature of integration or segregation in camp life, special administrative or leadership adaptations in serving the disabled and, finally, the potential for increasing camping opportunities for the disabled in California.[26]

Study of Five Land and Water Conservation Fund Projects for Accessibility for the Physically Disabled (1976).   Using a 13-section checklist of items to determine the degree of accessibility and usability of recreation facilities and buildings for the physically disabled, this study examined five selected projects in Georgia that had received funding under the Land and Water Conservation Fund Act by the Bureau of Outdoor Recreation. Its primary purpose was to determine whether the minimum standards established by the American National Standards and Specifications in this area and required according to the Outdoor Recreation Grants-in-Aid Manual were actually being met.[27]

Survey of Therapeutic Recreation Service in Oregon (1981).   This study sought to gather operational details about funding, staffing, programming and those served, of all therapeutic recreation agencies in the state of Oregon. A unique outcome was that it reached many individuals working in the field who had not pre-

[23]D. C. Green, P. N. Byrne and J. M. Montagnes: "An Examination of Weekend Recreational Patterns at the Mental Health Centre, Penetanguishene, Ontario." *Recreation Review,* March 1973, pp. 12–23.
[24]Peter A. Witt: *Status of Recreation Services for the Handicapped.* Ottawa, Department of National Health and Welfare, 1974.
[25]Doris Haist: "A Survey of Municipal Recreation Services for Special Groups in Ontario." *Recreation Review,* August 1975, pp. 29–50.
[26]Susan C. Buchan: "Camping for the Handicapped in Selected Camps in California." *Therapeutic Recreation Journal,* First Quarter, 1975, pp. 38–41.
[27]Charlene D. Farmer: "A Study of Five Land and Water Conservation Fund Projects in Regard to Accessibility and Usability for the Physically Handicapped." *Therapeutic Recreation Journal,* First Quarter, 1976, pp. 27–30.

viously been involved in professional society membership, and motivated them to become more involved.[28]

STUDIES OF PROFESSIONAL DEVELOPMENT IN THERAPEUTIC RECREATION

Many research studies have been concerned with professional development in the field of therapeutic recreation service. The following are a few illustrations, ranging from relatively simple "head-counting" surveys in the earlier years, to more complex analysis of professional preparation, competencies and functions.

Relative Importance of College Courses in Therapeutic Recreation (1970). This study examined the degree of importance assigned to undergraduate and graduate college courses in nine major categories by a panel of 15 national leaders and 15 educators in therapeutic recreation service. Courses were placed in rank order, and conclusions were drawn that would lead to the improvement of such curricula.[29]

Practitioners' Evaluation of College Curricula in Therapeutic Recreation (1976). Given the lack of uniformity or common agreement about the appropriate course content for undergraduate therapeutic recreation preparation, this study sought to use bachelor-level practitioners to evaluate professional undergraduate courses, required competencies for practice in the field and appropriate functions of professionals on the job. Sixty-five professional undergraduate courses in nine areas, 40 competencies and 27 functions were evaluated and rated in terms of their importance and value.[30]

Analysis of Therapeutic Recreation as a Service (1976). Therapeutic recreation as a service, as conceptualized by a paradigm appearing in the professional literature, was analyzed using the content analysis method. Fifty-three citations drawn from 300 randomly selected references were content analyzed, using the delivery-of-service paradigm, with sub-categories based on specialized knowledge and personnel, primary knowledge base and general and specific target populations.[31]

Employee Commitment in Park and Recreation Agencies (1979). This study examined the degree of commitment of park and recreation supervisors in 49 Illinois agencies to their organization, profession and community. While it did not deal with therapeutic recreation departments as such, many of its findings and recommendations are relevant to that field.[32]

---

[28]S. Harold Smith and John E. Gelvin, Jr.: "A Survey of Therapeutic Recreation Provision in the State of Oregon." *Therapeutic Recreation Journal*, Third Quarter, 1981, pp. 41–46.
[29]Donald Lindley: "Relative Importance of College Courses in Therapeutic Recreation." *Therapeutic Recreation Journal*, Second Quarter, 1970, pp. 8–12.
[30]S. Harold Smith: "Practitioners' Evaluation of College Courses, Competencies and Functions in Therapeutic Recreation." *Therapeutic Recreation Journal*, Fourth Quarter, 1976, pp. 152–156.
[31]John H. Lewko: "An Analysis of Therapeutic Recreation as a Service." *Therapeutic Recreation Journal*, First Quarter, 1976, pp. 35–48.
[32]Manuel London and Gary Howat: "Employee Commitment in Park and Recreation Agencies." *Journal of Leisure Research*, Third Quarter, 1979, pp. 196–206.

Continuing Education Needs of Therapeutic Recreation Professionals (1981).   As part of the effort to upgrade professional development, this study examined the continuing education needs of therapeutic recreators in Wisconsin. In addition to gathering demographic information about professionals in the state, it ranked needs related to 50 topics, including personnel management, planning, programming, activity analysis, evaluation and leadership methods.[33]

Study of Recreation Personnel in Canadian Mental Health Centers (1981).   This study examined the managerial activities, organizational commitment and job involvement of recreation personnel in 76 mental health centers with inpatient populations of at least 100, identified by the 1976 Statistics Canada Directory. It confirmed a higher degree of commitment and involvement among professionals using participative management styles.[34]

Professional Preparation in Therapeutic Recreation (1981).   An updating and extension of earlier studies of professional preparation in therapeutic recreation, this study examined the current status and major issues in the field by surveying undergraduate and master's degree curricula throughout the United States and Canada. It found a relatively high level of specialized education among faculty members, but concluded that there was still a shortage of individuals holding the doctorate and a lack of adequate staffing within this specialization.[35]

STUDIES OF SPECIAL POPULATIONS

Many research studies have been concerned with the leisure characteristics, values or recreational needs of specific population groups with disabilities. Recent studies have also tended to focus on therapeutic techniques geared to meet the special needs of such client groups.

Recreation, Leisure and the Alcoholic (1969).   This study examined the alcoholic's use of leisure time prior to commitment to an alcoholic rehabilitation center and its relationship to his or her drinking problem. A sample of 129 patients was compared with study data on the use of leisure time by the general population which had been gathered by the Outdoor Recreation Resources Review Commission.[36]

A Computerized Analysis of Characteristics of Down's Syndrome and Normal Children's Free-Play Patterns (1971).   This study examined the free-play patterns of a group of 4- to 8-year-old Down's syndrome (mongoloid) children and four groups of normal children of preschool age. The range in play and the use of special

---

[33]Karla A. Henderson: "Continuing Education Needs of Therapeutic Recreation Professionals." *Therapeutic Recreation Journal*, First Quarter, 1981, pp. 4–10.

[34]George S. Nogradi: "Managerial Activities, Organizational Commitment and Job Involvement: A Study of Recreation Personnel in Mental Health Centres." *Therapeutic Recreation Journal*, First Quarter, 1981, pp. 35–46.

[35]Carol Ann Peterson and Peg Connolly: "Professional Preparation in Therapeutic Recreation." *Therapeutic Recreation Journal*, Second Quarter, 1981, pp. 39–45.

[36]H. Douglas Sessoms and Sidney R. Oakley: "Recreation, Leisure, and the Alcoholic." *Journal of Leisure Research*, Winter 1969, pp. 21–31.

pieces of apparatus were recorded by a ceiling-mounted camera; the data gathered in this way were carefully analyzed by computer.[37]

The Leisure Activities and Social Participation of Mental Patients Prior to Hospitalization (1971). This study used data gathered from interviews of a sample of psychiatric patients at a state mental hospital to determine what the leisure activities and social participation of these patients were before hospitalization. The data were used as a basis for policy-making in the area of hospital and community recreation programs and to initiate conceptualization in certain areas of rehabilitation practice.[38]

Analysis of Recreational Involvement of Parolees from a State Correctional Institution (1972). This study examined the recreational pursuits of 20 parolees from a Pennsylvania state prison at three points: prior to entering prison, while in prison and after release. Its purpose was to ascertain what relationships might exist between patterns of involvement during these three periods and to draw implications either for recreation programming in correctional institutions or for community-based services that might be linked to prison programs.[39]

Patterns of Recreation and Social Interaction among Three Client Populations (1979). This study examined the relationship between recreational involvement and social affiliations and interaction among three client populations [welfare recipient families (Aid to Families with Dependent Children), the blind and physically disabled and the aging] in Fulton County (Atlanta), Georgia. In general, disabled and aged persons were more involved in self-directed activity, while welfare subjects were more active with family, friends and neighbors.[40]

Attitudes of Institutionalized, Elderly Iowans Toward Physical Activity (1981). Given the demonstrated relationship between lifelong physical activity and successful aging, this study examined the attitudes of elderly ambulatory residents in residential care facilities in Iowa. As a group, their attitudes were best characterized by social experience, catharsis, and health and fitness. Other differences were noted according to the age and sex of subjects.[41]

Anti-Psychotic Drug Side Effects and Therapeutic Recreation Programming (1982). This study examined the side effects of various medications commonly used in the management of psychotic and depressive clientele. Physical responses and behavioral effects were identified, and guidelines were presented for anticipating and dealing with these in the selection of activities and group leaders.[42]

---

[37]A. G. Linford, et al.: "A Computerized Analysis of Down's Syndrome and Normal Children's Free Play Patterns." *Journal of Leisure Research,* Winter 1971, pp. 44–52.
[38]Irvin Babow and Sol Simkin: "The Leisure Activities and Social Participation of Mental Patients Prior to Hospitalization." *Therapeutic Recreation Journal,* Fourth Quarter, 1971, pp. 161–167.
[39]Larry W. Williams: "An Analysis of the Recreational Pursuits of Selected Parolees from a State Correctional Institution in Pennsylvania." *Therapeutic Recreation Journal,* Third Quarter, 1972.
[40]F. P. Noe: "Patterns of Informal Recreational Activity and Social Interaction Among the AFDC, Aged and Disabled." *Therapeutic Recreation Journal,* Third Quarter, 1979, pp. 33–43.
[41]Ken Mobily: "Attitudes of Institutionalized, Elderly Iowans Toward Physical Activity." *Therapeutic Recreation Journal,* Third Quarter, 1981, pp. 30–39.
[42]Deborah L. Pakes and Gary E. Pakes: "Anti-Psychotic Drug Side Effects and Therapeutic Recreation Program Considerations." *Therapeutic Recreation Journal,* First Quarter, 1982, pp. 12–19.

Therapeutic Recreation Programming for Autistic Children (1982).   This study documented the typical play behavior of autistic children (uncommunicative, solitary, repetitive) and presented a model for successfully involving and motivating such clients in appropriate, socially acceptable recreation activities.[43]

Sponsorship of Research Proposals

Customarily, research may be carried on by a number of different types of sponsors or investigators. These include the following:

Institutions and Agencies.   Many hospitals, rehabilitation centers and other agencies or departments conduct research studies more or less frequently to determine their own effectiveness, establish needs and outcomes or provide a basis for program development.

Colleges and Universities.   A substantial amount of research is carried out by graduate students working on theses or dissertations and by faculty members with student assistants.

Government Agencies.   Government, on its various levels, is a major sponsor of research. In the field of therapeutic recreation service, this may be carried out in government hospitals or treatment centers or, more commonly, by government funding of research projects that are then carried on by research teams in universities or other settings.

Professional Organizations.   National or state organizations may carry on research, usually directed toward determining needs and trends in the field rather than toward the development or evaluation of existing programs.

Increasingly, research of an interdisciplinary nature is being carried on with the collaboration of two or more such sponsors. For example, in some recent studies, collaboration consists of the government approving and funding a research project that is staffed and carried on by researchers drawn from a university faculty and is actually conducted in an institutional setting. Thus all three sponsors have a part in the research effort. Similarly, although the initiative for such research may come from the therapeutic recreation educators, other faculty personnel or research specialists, such as psychologists, sociologists, physicians or statisticians, might be drawn into the research process.

Attitudes of Practitioners Toward Research

One problem facing those who carry out research in the broad field of leisure studies and services today is the gap that exists between researchers and practitioners. Mobley points out that many professionals working in the field believe that research is of little value; indeed, they often are unable to understand it because of the "jargon" used in presenting its findings. He suggests that in recent years, a firm polarization of viewpoints regarding research has emerged:

---

[43]Aubrey H. Fine, Dorothy Ann Feldis, and Barry E. Lehrer: "Therapeutic Recreation Programming for Autistic Children." *Therapeutic Recreation Journal*, First Quarter, 1982, pp. 6–11.

These viewpoints in the extreme suggest that the researcher and the academician insist upon producing research without regard to its utilitarian value while the practitioner rejects any research program that fails to specifically solve "the problem faced on Tuesday morning." Unfortunately, neither of these attitudes meet the research needs of the profession today. There must be a strong feeling of cooperation between the researcher and practitioners . . . in fact, practitioners must become actively involved in research.[44]

Selection of Research Topics

While no one would dispute the need for theoretical research, it is also important that a high priority be given to selecting studies that support the therapeutic recreation profession—particularly those that help to improve practice and demonstrate positive program outcomes. In considering possible topics for scholarly research in therapeutic recreation, the following kinds of questions should be asked:

"Am I—as the researcher—genuinely interested in the problem and free from strong biases that might imperil my objectivity?"

"Is the problem an important one; is the research likely to be helpful to my institution or program, advance knowledge in the field or be of value to other professionals?"

"Has similar research already been carried on, or will the proposed investigation yield substantially new information?"

"Can the needed administrative support and cooperation be obtained in order to carry out the study successfully?"

"Do I have, as an individual, or does my department or agency have the needed expertise to complete the study? If not, can assistance be obtained?"

"Will access to the needed subjects, informants or other resources be available?"

"Will it be possible to gather sufficient data to validate findings?"

Encouragement Given to Research and Evaluation

Within any major department or large-scale institutional program, both evaluation and research should be consistently supported. Obviously, it must not represent a diversion from the primary objective of providing service. The most meaningful programs, however, are those that are intelligently evaluated; the most successful professions are likely to be those with a solid basis of scientifically gained knowledge. Therefore, therapeutic recreation specialists should be encouraged to

1. Use a scientific and systematic approach at all times in gathering information on program needs and services or solving on-the-spot recreation programs.

---

[44]Tony A. Mobley: "Practitioner, Researcher: A Team." *Parks and Recreation*, April 1980, p. 41.

2. Attempt to gain skill in the application of research instruments and the use of research results.

3. Cooperate with personnel in colleges and universities or in other organizations or depart-ments to carry on jointly sponsored research projects.

4. Be alert to the possibilities for foundation or government-sponsored grants for research or demonstration projects.

5. Assist in identifying problems in the field that require research that might be carried on by professional colleagues or experts in a better position to follow up on them.

6. Press for the allocation of both funds and staff time to carry out research and evaluation.

Examples of Research Efforts within an Agency

As an example of an agency that gives a high priority to generating research, Children's Village, in Dobbs Ferry, New York (see p. 361), had eight different research studies under way during a recent year.[45] Approved by the institution's Research Council and a Technical Research Consultation Committee, the projects included the following: (a) a study of *remediation of language difficulties,* with empha-sis on testing remedial procedures; (b) *decision-making in child welfare,* focusing on the placement policies of the child welfare system; (c) *behavior rating reliability study,* an analysis of the usefulness of the agency's behavior rating scales; (d) *Revere Unit follow-up study,* a study of the community adjustment of discharged boys; (e) *after-care team to facilitate community adjustment of discharged boys,* a proposed expanded team approach to assist in this process; (f) *community volunteer continued care program,* a grant proposal to use community volunteers to assist in the community adjustment process; (g) *learning correlates of behavior problems,* a study clarifying the relationship between boys' behavior and learning disabilities; and (h) *teaching young aggressive boys to cooperate through play,* a grant proposal to develop materials and techniques useful in teaching cooperative behavior.

Obviously, several of these research studies either are directly concerned with recreation and its outcomes or use recreation as a medium to improve other pro-cesses or gather data. Similarly, Children's Village carries out extensive evaluation procedures closely linked to its overall research effort. Behavior assessment, studies of the effectiveness of peer tutoring and special reading programs and evaluations of such special recreation activities as African drumming and dance training, the Annual Children's Circus and a new teen-agers' center are all examples of services that underwent systematic evaluation in a recent year. Evaluation, in turn, is closely linked to staff orientation and training at a number of key points. Its essential pur-pose is to improve *accountability*—to make sure that the agency is accomplishing its stated goals as fully as possible. Elias writes,

---

[45]Howard L. Millman: "Research at C.V." *Children's Village Bulletin,* Dobbs Ferry, New York, June 1976, p. 7.

Institutions are generally hesitant to look closely at themselves. Self-examination often seems threatening and seems likely to disrupt the familiar, secure routines. In recent years new programs at Children's Village have been required to be evaluated to see if they meet their goals. This is an advance many children's facilities have not yet undertaken. But Children's Village must still face difficult questions: how effective is its structure in helping children and their families cope with their lives in the community; what within-institution programs lead to strengths that children maintain; which children are more likely to be helped; and how can effectiveness in preparing boys for a less structured environment be improved? . . . . The idea of evaluating the community effectiveness of Children's Village treatment programs so closely fits in with the concepts of continued care and feedback from the community that such evaluation seems attainable in the very near future.[46]

Other disciplines within the health care and rehabilitation fields typically use research and evaluation to promote their own effectiveness. Therapeutic recreation and activity therapy must also conduct such studies and cooperate in multi-disciplinary research efforts if they are to be full-fledged members of the treatment team.

RESEARCH AND EVALUATION: CONCLUDING STATEMENT

It should be made clear that research does not automatically provide the solution to all problems of professional development or program enrichment in therapeutic recreation service. Although rehabilitation authorities may be convinced of the value of activity therapies in general and although medical practitioners may strongly support therapeutic recreation programs, it may not be possible to derive statistical evidence as to its value in many cases.

This limitation is not peculiar to the field of therapeutic recreation. The author has pointed out elsewhere how major educational programs or experiments in social innovation have yielded disappointing results when carefully evaluated. The value of Head Start, for example, a major federally sponsored educational program designed to counteract the effects of poverty and cultural deprivation for preschool children, which was highly praised in its early stages, has been shown to be only temporary and to have no lasting benefits. Intensive group work therapy programs for teen-agers and casework services for families with multiple problems have shown no measurable benefits. Indeed, in the latter case, it was indicated that the more often a problem family was dealt with by a caseworker, the less progress was shown. A heavily financed program of performance contracting by educational firms that were funded to provide specially designed educational programs in both rural areas and large cities has been shown to be no more effective than traditional classroom instruction.

---

[46]Maurice J. Elias: "From Children's Village to Community—How Effective is Treatment?" *Children's Village Bulletin*, Dobbs Ferry, New York, January 1977, p. 18.

Therefore, it should not be expected that research will automatically yield supportive evidence that will assist therapeutic recreation personnel in developing their programs and that will consistently support their professional status and importance. It is essential nonetheless that every effort be made to explore, as systematically as possible, both the theoretical and practical questions underlying this field.

Dissemination of Research Findings

Finally, it is important that new and more effective means of storing, retrieving and making use of research findings be developed. Linford and Kennedy comment that the researcher is often wrongly accused of failing to communicate his or her results to workers in the field. In their view, this criticism is unjustified:

> . . . the role of the researcher is to solve problems. The transmission of information to others is the role of the teacher and communications expert — not the researcher. While they are perhaps not too well qualified as researchers themselves, any college lecturer should be at least able to read research literature and interpret it for students. The communication and dissemination problem is a major one. . . . [47]

The author agrees and is convinced that college and university educators who write textbooks in the field of professional recreation service have a further responsibility to act as intermediaries between the technical or highly specialized professional journals that report research and the faculty member in programs of professional preparation. In this and other texts, the author has documented all major content areas with significant research and literature references; such references are extremely helpful in pointing the way to college teachers as they read professional literature and prepare lectures. They also encourage students to do additional bibliographical research in appropriate sources.

DATA BANKS AND RETRIEVAL SYSTEMS

Dissemination of research findings has been assisted by national "data banks" and other comprehensive collections of research reports and other forms of professional literature, which can systematically organize findings and make them available to the field. A beginning step was made in this direction by the establishment of TRIC (Therapeutic Recreation Information Center), a literature and document storage and retrieval center for the field of therapeutic recreation service. Founded

---

[47]Anthony G. Linford and Dan W. Kennedy: "Research—the State of the Art in Therapeutic Recreation." *Therapeutic Recreation Journal*, Fourth Quarter, 1971, p. 169.

in 1970 at Teachers College, Columbia University, this valuable project was later moved to the University of Waterloo in Ontario, Canada.

Coordinated by Fred W. Martin, TRIC acquired published and unpublished articles, books, conference proceedings and reports. It abstracted and indexed them for storage in a computer-based information retrieval system. Information requests were accepted from educators, professionals, students and others. TRIC included references gained from such primary sources as *Parks and Recreation; Journal of Health, Physical Education and Recreation; Research Quarterly; Journal of Leisure Research; Recreation for the Ill and Handicapped;* and *Therapeutic Recreation Journal.* Secondary sources, such as *Psychological Abstracts; Sociological Abstracts; Mental Retardation Abstracts; Hospital Abstracts; Education Index; Rehabilitation Literature;* and *Educational Resources Information Center (ERIC),* were also used, along with other information systems, particularly the *Medical Literature Analysis and Retrieval System (MED-LARS).*

TRIC was extremely useful in the preparation of course bibliographies by educators offering courses and students engaged in term projects, as well as for surveys of the literature for master's theses and doctoral dissertations. After Martin's return to the United States, the TRIC service was curtailed and then discontinued. A somewhat similar service has also been provided in recent years by the Information and Research Utilization Center (IRUC) of the AAHPER Unit on Programs for the Handicapped (see p. 90). IRUC has assisted faculty members and practitioners with reprint services of hard-to-find materials, updated resource lists, a mailing list and other customized services such as special searches of titles, library and other sources. It has not thus far, however, developed TRIC's computerized retrieval capability.

A number of other retrieval systems within the fields of medicine, education and the social and behavioral sciences also include substantial numbers of references to programs designed for special populations, including activity therapy and therapeutic recreation service. The Smithsonian Science Information Exchange, Inc. is an excellent source of information about basic and applied research in progress in all areas of the life and physical sciences. Under the heading of "Therapy, Rehabilitation, Counseling," it deals with many forms of treatment for special populations.

In Canada today, the Leisure Studies Data Bank at the University of Waterloo, Ontario, is a nonprofit research facility that provides researchers with ready access to a wide variety of sport, fitness, tourism, outdoor recreation, time use and other leisure-related studies. In addition to acquiring and archiving sets of data, the data bank assists in the design of studies and the analysis and interpretation of data for other agencies or research groups.

In addition to such computerized services, the major professional publications in the field of recreation and leisure service, such as the *Therapeutic Recreation Journal, Recreation Review, Leisurability* and the *Journal of Leisure Research,* publish analyses of research trends, which are useful to both educators and practitioners in therapeutic recreation.[48] Finally, research symposiums are held regularly in connection

---

[48]For examples of such analyses, *see* John Lewko and Rick Crandall: "Research Trends in Leisure and Special Populations," *Journal of Leisure Research,* First Quarter, 1980, pp. 69–79, and David Szymanski: "An Index for Determining Trends in Selected Leisure Journals and Publications," *Therapeutic Recreation Journal,* Third Quarter, 1980, p. 42–51.

with national and regional recreation and park conferences in the United States and Canada. Numerous research studies in therapeutic recreation are presented at these professional meetings.

In Canada, several major Congresses on Leisure Research have been sponsored by the Ontario Research Council on Leisure and other government agencies. Monographs of research abstracts have been published, in addition to the Canadian Catalogue of Leisure Research, to provide a convenient source of leisure research findings for practitioners and scholars in this field.[49]

Programs of this type, which encourage the dissemination of research findings, make a strong contribution to the scientific development of the field of therapeutic recreation service and to the quality of college programs of professional preparation in it. In the years ahead, improved and expanded efforts in both evaluation and research will support and strengthen this field. They deserve to be treated as a priority by all therapeutic agencies and institutions in terms of university curriculum development, government funding and allocation of staff energy and time.

Suggested Topics for Class Discussion, Examination Questions or Student Papers

1. Define and compare the two related processes of evaluation and research, and show how they are vital to upgrading professional practice in therapeutic recreation service. Discuss the growing emphasis on the need for accountability in human-service or rehabilitation programs.

2. Identify and describe several models of evaluation, and show how they may be used in evaluating therapeutic recreation departments or agencies.

3. Develop a statement of a specific problem area in therapeutic recreation service, and carry out a preliminary literature search on it. Then prepare a brief research proposal intended to investigate this problem, including each of the elements or sections that customarily goes into a proposal (statement of the problem, related literature, statement of purposes or hypotheses, definitions and limitations, and research design and methodology).

4. Why is the interdisciplinary cooperation of government, institutions of higher education and agencies serving the disabled necessary to promote effective research in this field? Why is it important in helping to bridge the gap between scholars and practitioners in recreation and leisure studies? Give an example of how such cooperation might be developed.

---

[49]As an example, see *Canadian Catalogue of Leisure Research* and *Abstracts of 101 Papers from Third Canadian Congress on Leisure Research,* both available from Department of Recreation Administration, University of Alberta, Edmonton, Canada, 1978, 1979, 1980.

Appendix A

Selected Films on Recreation and Related Services for the Disabled

A Very Special Dance. (16 mm, Color, Sound.) Award-winning film on creative dance with mentally retarded young adults in Utah. Order from AAHPERD Film Center, 938 K St., N.W., Washington, D.C. 20001.

And So They Move. (16 mm, Black and White, Sound, 19 minutes.) Use of creative play in specially designed environment with physically disabled children. Audio-Visual Center, Michigan State University, East Lansing, Michigan 48824.

Basic Skills for Independent Living. (16 mm, Color, Sound, 10 minutes.) Depicts a special college program for adults with varied physical and mental disabilities; emphasis on recreational and social activities. Continuing Education Division, State University College, Brockport, New York 14420.

Cast No Shadow. (16 mm, Color, Sound, 27 minutes.) Shows wide range of recreation activities for participants with disability at Recreation Center for the Handicapped in San Francisco. Professional Arts, Inc., Box 8484, Universal City, California.

Count Me In. (16 mm, Sound, Color, 17 minutes.) Deals with normalization and mainstreaming of the disabled in society, in varied communities and in residential settings; shows leisure programs. Stanfield House, 900 Euclid Street, Santa Monica, California 90403.

Get It Together. (16 mm, Sound, Color, 20 minutes.) Story of a young paraplegic who lives as a normal person, finishing college, marrying and beginning a career as a recreational therapist. FMS Productions, 1040 North Las Palmas, Los Angeles, California 90038.

John Baker's Last Race. (16 mm, Sound, Color, 34 minutes.) Moving story of a young teacher, a gifted athlete, in his final months with a fatal malignancy. Media Marketing, Brigham Young University, Provo, Utah 84602.

New Concepts in Children's Play Areas. (Filmstrip, 80 frames, Sound, Color, 20 minutes, 33⅓ rpm record.) Shows innovations in playground design to meet children's developmental needs. Associated Film Services, 3419 West Magnolia, Burbank, California 91505.

Paralympics, Israel, 1968. (16 mm, Color, Sound, 14 minutes.) Documentary of international wheelchair athletic competition. U.S. Wheelchair Sports Fund, 40–24 62nd St., Woodside, New York 11377.

Physical Education for Blind Children. (16 mm, Color, Sound, 20 minutes.) Shows visually handicapped school children in varied physical education and recreational sports activities. Charles Buell, 4244 Heather Rd., Long Beach, California 90808.

Recreational Activities for Mentally Retarded Children. (16 mm, Color, Sound, 28 minutes.) Comprehensive summer recreational program, including games, crafts, music, swimming, outings and parties, for mentally retarded. National Association for Retarded Children, 420 Lexington Ave., New York, New York 10017.

Recreation and Occupational Therapy. (16 mm, Black and White, Sound, 13 minutes.) Adapted activities suited for patients with limited mobility or physical disability. Audio-Visual Media Center, Washington State University, Pullman, Washington 99163.

Recreation for the Handicapped. (16 mm, Color, Sound, 23 minutes.) Shows program, over several months, serving varied ages of disabled. Filmed by Stanford University film group. Recreation Center for the Handicapped, Great Highway at Sloat Blvd., San Francisco, California 94132.

Recreation Unlimited. (16 mm, Black and White, Sound, 15 minutes.) Swimming, folk dancing, acting and crafts for mentally retarded children. National Association for Retarded Children, 420 Lexington Ave., New York, New York 10017.

The Shape of a Leaf. (16 mm, Black and White, Color, Sound, 26 minutes.) Creative approach to arts and crafts instruction with retarded children. Perkins School, Lancaster, Massachusetts 01528.

The Therapeutic Community. (16 mm, Color, Sound, 28 minutes.) Milieu therapy approach in hospitalization of geriatric patients. University of Michigan Television Center and Division of Gerontology, Ann Arbor, Michigan.

Therapeutic Camping. (16 mm, Color, Sound, 28 minutes.) Shows multidisciplinary approach of workers with emotionally disturbed adolescents in summer camp. Devereux Schools, Santa Barbara, California 93102.

Therapy Through Play. (16 mm, Color, Sound, 17 minutes.) Adapted sports for physically disabled children. Human Resources Center, Albertson, New York 11507.

To Paint is to Love Again. (16 mm, Color, Sound, 21 minutes.) Art work with retarded children at Exceptional Children's Foundation in Los Angeles. Conrad Films, 6331 Weidlake Drive, Hollywood, California 90028.

To Serve a Purpose. (16 mm, Color, Sound, 15 minutes.) Depicts scope of services and populations served in field of therapeutic recreation. Resource Development Specialist, Therapeutic Recreation Curriculum Development Project, Office of Recreation and Park Resources, University of Illinois, Champaign-Urbana, Illinois.

You're It. (16 mm, Color, Sound, 25 minutes.) Shows role of recreation in educational program for mentally retarded. MacDonald Training Center, 4424 Tampa Bay Boulevard, Tampa, Florida 33614.

1975 International Special Olympics Games. (16 mm, Color, Sound, 23 minutes.) Covers Fourth International Special Olympics held in Michigan, with CBS sports team reporting on mentally retarded athletes competing in eight major sports. Joseph P. Kennedy, Jr. Foundation, 1701 K St., N.W., Suite 205, Washington, D.C. 20006.

Appendix B

List of Organizations*

NATIONAL ORGANIZATIONS ACTIVE IN THE RECREATION FIELD OR WITH A SPECIAL CONCERN WITH DISABILITY

Administration on Aging, 330 C St., S.W., Washington, D.C. 20201

American Art Therapy Association, 6010 Broad Branch Rd., N.W., Washington, D.C. 20015

American Association for Leisure and Recreation, 1900 Association Drive, Reston, Virginia 22091

American Association on Mental Deficiency, 5201 Connecticut Ave., N.W., Washington, D.C. 20015

American Association of Retired Persons, 1225 Connecticut Ave., N.W., Washington, D.C. 20036

American Camping Association, Bradford Woods, Martinsville, Indiana 46151

American Cancer Society, 219 E. 42nd St., New York, New York 10017

American Diabetes Association, 18 E. 48th St., New York, New York 10017

American Foundation for the Blind, 15 W. 16th St., New York, New York 10011

American Heart Association, 44 East 23rd St., New York, New York 10010

American National Red Cross, 17th and D Sts., N.W., Washington, D.C. 20000

American Nursing Home Association, 1346 Connecticut Ave., N.W., Washington, D.C. 20006

American Occupational Therapy Association, 251 Park Ave. So., New York, New York 10010

American Physical Therapy Association, 1156 15th St., N.W., Washington, D.C. 20005

American Psychiatric Association, 1700 18th St., N.W., Washington, D.C. 20000

Arthritis Foundation, 1212 Avenue of the Americas, New York, New York 10036

Asthma and Allergy Foundation of America, 19 W. 44th St., New York, New York 10036

Athletic Institute, 705 Merchandise Mart, Chicago, Illinois 60654

Bureau of Education for the Handicapped, U.S. Office of Education, 400 Maryland Ave., S.W., Washington, D.C. 20202

Canadian Wheelchair Sports Association, 333 River Rd., Ottawa, Ontario, Canada K1L 8B9

Children's Bureau, Office of Child Development, 300 Independence Ave., S.W., Washington, D.C. 20201

Council for Exceptional Children, 1920 Association Drive, Reston, Virginia 22091

Epilepsy Foundation of America, 1828 L St., N.W., Suite 406, Washington, D.C. 20036

International Society for Rehabilitation of the Disabled, 219 E. 44th St., New York, New York 10017

Muscular Dystrophy Association of America, 1790 Broadway, New York, New York 10019

---

*This list consists primarily of organizations in the United States. There are numerous comparable organizations in Canada on the national and provincial levels. The major Canadian organization in the recreation field is the Canadian Parks/Recreation Association, 333 River Rd., Vanier City, Ontario K1L 8B9.

National Association for Mental Health, 10 Columbus Circle, New York, New York 10019
National Association for Music Therapy, P.O. Box 610, Lawrence, Kansas 66044
National Association for Retarded Children, 420 Lexington Ave., New York, New York 10017
National Association of the Deaf, 814 Thayer Ave., Silver Spring, Maryland 20910
National Community Education Association, 1017 Avon St., Flint, Michigan 48503
National Council for Therapy and Rehabilitation through Horticulture, 701 N. St. Asaph St.,
    Alexandria, Virginia 22314
National Council on the Aging, 1828 L St., N.W., Washington, D.C. 20036
National Easter Seal Society for Crippled Children and Adults, 2023 W. Ogden Ave., Chicago,
    Illinois 60612
National Foundation for Neuromuscular Diseases, 250 W. 57th St., New York, New York
    10019
National Institutes of Health, 9000 Rockville Pike, Bethesda, Maryland 20010
National Multiple Sclerosis Society, 257 Park Ave. So., New York, New York 10010
National Paraplegia Foundation, 333 North Michigan Ave., Chicago, Illinois 60601
National Recreation and Park Association/National Therapeutic Recreation Society, 3101
    Park Center Drive, Alexandria, Virginia 22302
National Rehabilitation Association, 1522 K St., N.W., Washington, D.C. 20005
United Cerebral Palsy Association, 66 E. 34th St., New York, New York 10036
Veterans' Administration Central Office, Washington, D.C. 20420
World Leisure and Recreation Association, 345 E. 46th St., New York, New York 10017

OTHER ORGANIZATIONS SERVING
SPECIFIC GROUPS OF DISABLED WITH
SPORTS

American Association for the Deaf, P.O. Box 105, Talladega, Alabama 35160
American Blind Bowling Association, P.O. Box 306, Louisville, Kentucky 40201
American Junior Blind Bowling Association, 4244 Heather Rd., Long Beach, California 90808
American Wheelchair Bowling Association, Route 2, Box 750, Lutz, Florida 33549
National Amputation Foundation (Golf), 12–45 150th St., Whitestone, New York 11357
National Amputee Skiing Association, 3738 Walnut Ave., Carmichael, California 95608
National Track and Field Committee for the Visually Impaired, 4244 Heather Rd., Long
    Beach, California 90808
National Wheelchair Basketball Association, Rehabilitation-Education Center, Oak St. and
    Stadium Dr., University of Illinois, Champaign-Urbana, Illinois 61820
National Wheelchair Athletic Association, 40–24 62nd St., Woodside, New York 11377
Ontario Wheelchair Sport Association, 585 Tretheway Drive, Toronto, Ontario, Canada M6M
    4B8
Special Olympics, Inc., 1701 K. St., N.W. (Joseph P. Kennedy, Jr. Foundation), Washington,
    D.C. 20006

Appendix C

Professional Standards

The following statement of professional standards for practice in therapeutic recreation service was developed by the Program and Personnel Standards Committee of the National Therapeutic Recreation Society. For a summary of the process involved, see Glen E. Van Andel: "Professional Standards: Improving the Quality of Services." *Therapeutic Recreation Journal*, Second Quarter, 1981, pp. 23–26.

STANDARD I.   SCOPE OF SERVICE
Comprehensive therapeutic recreation program services are available to all clients in the agency/facility.
  Criteria
  A.   There are general recreation services which provide a wide range of activities designed to meet the needs, competencies, capabilities and interests of clients during leisure time.
    1. Orientation
      a. Clients are assisted in orienting themselves to the physical surroundings and are helped to achieve maximum mobility and independence.
      b. Clients receive orientation to the available leisure programs, facilities and resources with initial entrance into the program.
    2. Program Development and Implementation
      a. Participant committees, when appropriate, are used in planning and implementing the general recreation program.
      b. There is an established method for assessing the needs, interests, competencies and capabilities of all clients.
      c. Activities take into consideration the cultural, economic, social and educational backgrounds of clients.
      d. The therapeutic recreation program is carefully and consistently integrated with other programs to achieve maximum use of agency/facility resources.
      e. Provision is made for each client to participate at his/her optimal level of functioning and to progress at his/her own speed.
      f. Provision is made for clients to use their own initiative in selecting and participating in recreational activities.
      g. Provision is made for clients to assume leadership responsibilities.
      h. Activities are modified and special aids or adaptive equipment are utilized to assure success experiences and sequential development for each client.
      i. Provision is made for bedside/homebound activities when and where appropriate.
    3. Program Contents
      a. Opportunities are provided for clients to participate in activities which utilize physical behaviors (sensory-motor domain), mental behaviors (cognitive domain) and emotional behaviors (affective domain).
      b. In day and residential facilities, opportunities are provided for clients to participate in daily periods of activity.
      c. Opportunities are provided for individual, small, and large group participation.
      d. The program provides both regularly scheduled activities and special events.

e. The program provides for the utilization of a wide variety of public and private community resources and services.

f. The program provides for various levels of integration of the client population with the general population.

B. Leisure education services are available.
1. Program Development and Implementation
   a. There is an established method for assessing leisure function.
   b. When appropriate, leisure counseling is available for clients and/or families.
   c. There is an established method for referral and follow-up when needed to assist clients make successful adjustment in the use of community leisure resources.
2. Program Content
   a. Opportunities are provided to explore and develop new activity skills that have carry-over value at home and in the community.
   b. Identification and instruction are provided in the use of appropriate leisure resources available in the client's community.
   c. Opportunities are provided for exploration of leisure concepts, attitudes and values.

C. Treatment services are available which are goal oriented and directed toward (re)habilitation, amelioration and/or modification of specific physical, emotional, mental and/or social behaviors.
1. Where interdisciplinary teams are utilized, the therapeutic recreation staff functions as part of that team.
2. The therapeutic recreation staff determines appropriate goals relative to therapeutic recreation and interventions to achieve the goals.
3. There is a written plan for implementing the therapeutic recreation goals.
4. There is periodic evaluation of the therapeutic recreation treatment program plan in accordance with standards of regulatory agencies.
5. The treatment goals and plan are modified according to the results of the evaluation and needs of the client.

STANDARD II.   OBJECTIVES

Specific objectives are stated for each type of therapeutic recreation service based upon the philosophy and goals of the therapeutic recreation unit/agency/department and translated into operational terms.

Criteria

A. The statement of objectives is in writing.
B. The statement is prepared by the therapeutic recreation staff in consultation with appropriate professional staff of the agency/facility (e.g., medical, educational, recreational and/or designated representative of the administration).
C. The statement is reviewed by therapeutic recreation staff at least semiannually.
D. The statement is used as a program planning and evaluation tool.

STANDARD III.   INDIVIDUAL TREATMENT/PROGRAM PLAN

The therapeutic recreation staff develop an individualized treatment/program plan for each client referred to the unit/agency/department.

Criteria

A. The plan is based on complete and relevant diagnostic/assessment data.
1. The plan reflects the client's physical, social, mental, and emotional aptitudes and skills and current level of leisure functioning.
2. The plan indicates precautions, restrictions or limitations related to an individual's participation as determined by the diagnosis/assessment.
B. The plan is stated in behavioral terms that permit the progress of the individual to be assessed.
C. The plan is periodically reviewed, evaluated and modified as necessary to meet the changing needs of the client.
D. The plan differentiates among short-term, long-term and discharge/transition goals.
E. The plan is documented in the personal record of the client.

F. The plan reflects an integrated approach.
    1. The plan is consistent with interdisciplinary treatment goals for the client.
    2. When feasible, the client and/or his/her family assist in developing and implementing the therapeutic recreation treatment plan.
    3. The plan reflects the client's goals and expectation of benefits to be derived from the therapeutic recreation program.

STANDARD IV.   DOCUMENTATION

Therapeutic recreation personnel record specific information on assigned clients for the client/participant's record on a regular basis in accordance with the policies and procedures of the agency.

Criteria

A. The individualized therapeutic recreation treatment/program plan is recorded in the client/participant's record. It should include:
    1. The referral document or reason for referral.
    2. Assessment data.
    3. Identification of client's problem and needs.
    4. Treatment objectives.
    5. Methods and plans for implementation of the therapeutic recreation program.
    6. Methods and plans for evaluation of the objectives.
B. Progress of the individual and his/her reactions to the therapeutic recreation program are systematically recorded in the client/participant's record and reported to all appropriate parties (e.g., interdisciplinary team, parents, etc.).
    1. Subjective interpretation of client progress is supported with concise behavioral observations.
    2. Documentation of progress is directly related to the treatment goals.
C. A discharge/transition plan is included in the personal record and should include:
    1. A summary of the treatment/program implemented and the client's progress.
    2. An assessment of the client's current level of leisure function.
    3. Recommendations for post-discharge/transition planning.
    4. Information regarding appropriate community recreation resources and referral information as indicated.
D. Client records are reviewed regularly by therapeutic recreation staff in accordance with standards of regulatory agencies and documentation of such review is entered in the personal record.

STANDARD V.   SCHEDULING OF SERVICES

Specific times are allocated for therapeutic recreation programs.

Criteria

A. The master schedule is established in cooperation with other programs and services provided for the client.
B. Each client receives a schedule of the comprehensive therapeutic recreation program or has easy access to posted schedules and schedule changes.

STANDARD VI.   ETHICAL PRACTICES

Therapeutic recreation service delivery is designed to respect the personal rights of the individual clients and their families.

Criteria

A. It conforms with the local, state and federal guidelines such as the "Patient's Bill of Rights" and Mental Health/Mental Retardation Act.
B. It conforms with the National Recreation and Park Association/National Therapeutic Recreation Society Code of Ethics.

Appendix D

Equipment and Supply Sources*

This list identifies a number of major manufacturers and distributors of recreation equipment, materials and supplies that may be used directly in community programs, hospitals, special schools, and other institutions serving the disabled, or may be adapted to such use.

Boin Arts and Crafts Company, 87 Morris St., Morristown, New Jersey 07960. Wide range of kits, tools and supplies for varied craft activities useful for all ages.

CEDCO Distributors Corporation, 128 Main St., Hempstead, New York 11550. Useful arts and crafts materials, with projects specially designed for exceptional children and adults, nursing homes and similar settings.

Children's Music Center, 5373 West Pico Blvd., Los Angeles, California 90019. Records, books and instruments for use in programs of music and dance therapy.

Economy Handcrafts, 50–21 69th St., Woodside, New York 11377. Extensive supplies for arts and crafts activities useful for all ages.

Flaghouse, Inc., 18 West 18th St., New York, New York 10010. Distributes full range of athletic, recreational and camping supplies and equipment for schools, colleges, public recreation, institutions and similar agencies.

Game Time, Inc., 6874 Washington Ave., South Eden Prairie, Minnesota 55343. One of the largest manufacturers of playground equipment, such as swings, slides, jungle gyms, and other creative equipment for children's play.

Hoctor Products for Education, Waldwick, New Jersey 07463. Distributes music, instruction, records and related products for varied forms of dance, gymnastics and children's rhythms.

Lansford Publishing Company, P.O. Box 8711, San Jose, California 95155. Manufactures and distributes management aids and audio-visual materials useful in staff development, group dynamics programs and related activities.

Mexico Forge, P.O. Box 565, Reedsville, Pennsylvania 17084. Manufactures heavy-duty recreational equipment, play systems, benches, lockers and related products.

Miracle Recreation Equipment Company, Grinnell, Iowa 50112. Manufactures standard playground equipment, along with creative or theme structures or products, accessories, wood "villages," pools and so on; also provides design service.

J. A. Preston Corporation, 71 Fifth Ave., New York, New York 10003. Manufactures equipment, games, tests, kits and so forth designed to promote perceptual-motor dvelopment for exceptional children and youth.

Theraplay Products (Division of PCA Industries), 2298 Grissom Dr., St. Louis, Missouri 63141. Manufactures rehabilitative play equipment for special populations, such as blind,

---

*Most of these companies will send catalogues on request. They and hundreds of other manufacturers and distributors advertise in professional recreation journals and exhibit their products at recreation and park conferences.

deaf, mentally retarded and so on. Includes safety-designed playground equipment (slides, beams, bridges, bouncers, etc.), manipulative games and equipment geared for use with wheelchairs.

U.S. Games, Inc., 1009 Aurora Rd., Melbourne, Florida 32935. Designs and manufactures standard recreational sports equipment, along with new and improvised game materials for active groups.

World Wide Games, Box 450, Delaware, Ohio 43015. Manufactures unique group of game materials for folk games from many nations, useful with participants of all ages and abilities.

Bibliography

GENERAL REFERENCES ON RECREATION, REHABILITATION AND THERAPEUTIC RECREATION

W. Scott Allan: *Rehabilitation: A Community Challenge.* New York, John Wiley, 1958.

Elliott M. Avedon: *Therapeutic Recreation Service: An Applied Behavioral Science Approach.* Englewood Cliffs, New Jersey, Prentice-Hall, 1974.

Awareness Papers Vol. 1: Report of White House Conference on Handicapped Individuals. Washington, D.C., U.S. Government Printing Office (232-034/6199), May 1977.

Leo Buscaglia: *The Disabled and Their Parents: A Counseling Challenge.* Thorofare, New Jersey, Charles B. Slack, 1975.

Reynold E. Carlson, Janet R. MacLean, Theodore R. Deppe and James R. Peterson: *Recreation and Leisure: The Changing Scene.* Belmont, California, Wadsworth, 1979.

Effie Fairchild and Larry Neal: *Common-Unity in the Community: A Forward-Looking Program of Recreation and Leisure Services for the Handicapped.* Eugene, Oregon, Center for Leisure Studies, 1975.

Virginia Frye and Martha Peters: *Therapeutic Recreation: Its Theory, Philosophy and Practice.* Harrisburg, Pennsylvania, Stackpole, 1972.

Geoffrey Godbey: *Leisure in Your Life: An Exploration.* Philadelphia, Saunders College Publishing, 1980.

Scout Lee Gunn and Carol Ann Peterson: *Therapeutic Recreation Program Design: Principles and Procedures.* Englewood Cliffs, New Jersey, Prentice-Hall, 1978.

Paul Haun: *Recreation: A Medical Viewpoint* (Elliott M. Avedon, ed.). New York, Teachers College, Columbia University, Bureau of Publications, 1965.

Fern Kaufman Ingber: *Issues and Guidelines for Establishing Third Party Reimbursement for Therapeutic Recreation.* (Ray E. West, ed.). Arlington, Virginia, National Therapeutic Recreation Society, July 1978.

Seppo E. Iso-Ahola: *The Social Psychology of Leisure and Recreation.* Dubuque, Iowa, Wm. C. Brown, 1980.

Jerry J. Jordan, William P. Dayton and Kathryn H. Brill: *Theory and Design of Competency-Based Education.* Philadelphia, Proceedings from National Symposium at Temple University, May 1977.

Jerry D. Kelley, ed: *Expanding Horizons in Therapeutic Recreation II.* Urbana-Champaign, University of Illinois, Office of Recreation and Park Resources, 1974.

Richard Kraus: *Recreation and Leisure in Modern Society.* Santa Monica, California, Goodyear, 1978; *Recreation Today: Program Planning and Leadership,* Santa Monica, California, Goodyear, 1977; and (with Barbara Bates and Gay Carpenter) *Recreation Leadership and Supervision.* Philadelphia, Saunders College Publishing, 1981.

Ministry of Culture and Recreation: *Professional Development Planning for Leisure Service Practitioners.* Ontario, Sports and Fitness Branch, 1979.

Susanna Millar: *The Psychology of Play.* Baltimore, Penguin, 1968.

James F. Murphy: *Concepts of Leisure.* Englewood Cliffs, New Jersey, Prentice-Hall, 1980.

National Committee, Arts for the Handicapped: *A Guide to Resources for Program Development in the Field of Arts for Disabled Individuals*. Washington, D.C., 1980.

Gerald S. O'Morrow: *Administration of Activity Therapy*. Springfield, Illinois, Charles C Thomas, 1966; and *Therapeutic Recreation: A Helping Profession*. Reston, Virginia, Reston, 1976.

Robert P. Overs, Elizabeth O'Connor and Barbara De Marco: *Avocational Activities for the Handicapped: A Handbook for Avocational Counseling*. Springfield, Illinois, Charles C Thomas, 1974.

David C. Park, coordinator: *Focus on Research, Recreation for Disabled Individuals*. Washington, D.C., George Washington University, April 1980.

Janet Pomeroy: *Recreation for the Physically Handicapped*. New York, Macmillan, 1964.

Josephine L. Rathbone and Carol Lucas: *Recreation in Total Rehabilitation*. Springfield, Illinois, Charles C Thomas, 1970.

Frank M. Robinson, Jr.: *Therapeutic Recreation: Ideas and Experiences*. Springfield, Illinois, Charles C Thomas, 1974.

H. Douglas Sessoms, Harold D. Meyer and Charles K. Brightbill: *Leisure Services: The Organized Recreation and Park System*. Englewood Cliffs, New Jersey, Prentice-Hall, 1975.

Thomas M. Shea: *Camping for Special Children*. St. Louis, C. V. Mosby, 1977.

Claudine Sherrill: *Adapted Physical Education and Recreation: A Multidisciplinary Approach*. Dubuque, Iowa, Wm. C. Brown, 1981.

Jay S. Shivers and Hollis Fait: *Therapeutic and Adapted Recreational Services*. Philadelphia, Lea and Febiger, 1975.

Thomas Stein and H. Douglas Sessoms: *Recreation and Special Populations*. Boston, Holbrook, 1977.

P. Valletutti and F. Christoplos: *Interdisciplinary Approaches to Human Services*. Baltimore, University Park Press, 1977.

Paul Wehman and Stuart J. Schleien: *Leisure Programs for Handicapped Persons*. Baltimore, University Park Press, 1981.

Jody Witt, Marilyn Campbell and Peter Witt: *A Manual of Therapeutic Group Activities for Leisure Education*. Ottawa, Leisurability, 1975.

RECREATION AND THE MENTALLY RETARDED OR LEARNING DISABLED

Issam B. Amary: *Creative Recreation for the Mentally Retarded*. Springfield, Illinois, Charles C Thomas, 1975.

American Association for Health, Physical Education and Recreation (AAHPER) and Sex Information and Education Council of the United States: *A Resource Guide in Sex Education for the Mentally Retarded*. Washington, D.C., 1971.

Elliott M. Avedon and Frances B. Arje: *Socio-Recreative Planning for the Retarded: A Handbook for Sponsoring Groups*. New York, Teachers College, Columbia University, Bureau of Publications, 1964.

Norman R. Bernstein, ed.: *Diminished People, Problems and Care of the Mentally Retarded*. Boston, Little, Brown, 1970.

La Donna Bogardus: *Camping with Retarded Persons*. Nashville, Tennessee, Cokesbury, 1970.

Bernice Wells Carlson and David R. Ginglend: *Recreation for Retarded Teenagers and Young Adults*. Nashville, Tennessee, Abingdon, 1968.

Philip Chinn, Clifford J. Drew and Don R. Logan: *Mental Retardation, A Life Cycle Approach*. St. Louis, C. V. Mosby, 1975.

Nola R. Colvin and Joan M. Finholt: *Guidelines for Physical Educators of Mentally Handicapped Youth.* Springfield, Illinois, Charles C Thomas, 1981.

Herbert J. Grossman, ed.: *Manual on Terminology and Classification in Mental Retardation.* Washington, D.C., American Association on Mental Deficiency, 1973.

James H. Humphrey and Dorothy D. Sullivan: *Teaching Slow Learners Through Active Games.* Springfield, Illinois, Charles C Thomas, 1970.

Helen Jo Mitchell, et al.: *The Young Retarded Child at Play: A Guide for Pre-School Play Centers.* Washington, D.C., Department of Recreation, 1969.

Larry L. Neal: *Recreation's Role in the Rehabilitation of the Mentally Retarded.* Eugene, University of Oregon, 1970.

President's Committee on Mental Retardation: *MR 72: Islands of Excellence.* Washington, D.C., U.S. Government Printing Office, 1973.

G. Lawrence Rarick, A. Alan Dobbins and Geoffrey D. Broadhead: *The Motor Domain and Its Correlates in Educationally Handicapped Children.* Englewood Cliffs, New Jersey, Prentice-Hall, 1976.

RECREATION AND THE AGED

Nancy N. Anderson: *Senior Centers: Information from a National Survey.* Minneapolis, American Rehabilitation Foundation, 1969.

Alex Comfort: *A Good Age.* New York, Simon and Schuster, 1976.

Gertrude Cross: *Program Ideas for Senior Citizens* and *Senior Citizens Travel Manual.* Flint, Michigan, Recreation and Park Board, 1970.

Joan M. Cutter, Edna B. Russell and Elizabeth A. Stetler: *An Activity Center for Senior Citizens.* Washington, D.C., Administration on Aging, U.S. Dept. of HEW, 1961.

Paula Gross Gray: *Dramatics for the Elderly: A Guide for Residential Care Settings and Senior Centers.* New York, Teachers College, Columbia University Press, 1974.

Tom Hickey: *Health and Aging.* Monterey, California, Brooks/Cole Publishing Co., 1980.

Joe J. Jordan: *Senior Center Facilities: An Architect's Evaluation.* Washington, D.C., National Institute of Senior Centers, National Council on the Aging, 1975.

Max Kaplan: *Leisure: Lifestyle and Lifespan: Perspectives for Gerontology.* Philadelphia, W. B. Saunders, 1980.

Douglas Kimmell: *Adulthood and Aging.* New York, John Wiley, 1974.

Robert Kleemeier: *Aging and Leisure.* New York, Oxford University Press, 1961.

Carol Lucas: *Recreational Activity Development for the Aging in Hospitals and Nursing Homes.* Springfield, Illinois, Charles C Thomas, 1974.

Toni Merrill: *Activities for the Aged and Infirm: A Handbook for the Untrained Worker.* Springfield, Illinois, Charles C Thomas, 1967.

Dorothy G. Mullen: *Recreation in Nursing Homes.* Arlington, Virginia, National Recreation and Park Association Management Aid, No. 88, 1971.

National Institute of Senior Centers: *Senior Center Standards: Guidelines for Practice.* Washington, D.C., National Council on the Aging, 1978.

Public Health Service: *Activity Supervisor's Guide: A Handbook for Activities Supervisors in Long-Term Nursing Care Facilities.* Washington, D.C., U.S. Dept. of HEW, 1969.

Retirement Roles and Activities. Washington, D.C., Report of White House Conference on Aging, 1971.

Jay S. Shivers and Hollis F. Fait: *Recreational Service for the Aging.* Philadelphia, Lea and Febiger, 1980.

Shura Saul: *Aging: An Album of People Growing Old.* New York, John Wiley, 1974.

Annabel Sissons and Debby Vigoda: *Leisure Can Be Pleasure: Changing Roles in Retirement.* Toronto, Ontario Ministry of Culture and Recreation, 1981.

Bernard Stotsky: *The Nursing Home and the Aged Psychiatric Patient.* New York, Appleton-Century-Crofts, 1970.

RECREATION AND PHYSICAL DISABILITY

Ronald C. Adams, Alfred N. Daniel and Lee Rullman: *Games, Sports and Exercises for the Physically Handicapped.* Philadelphia, Lea and Febiger, 1982.

Daniel D. Arnheim, David Auxter and Walter C. Crowe: *Principles and Methods of Adapted Physical Education.* St. Louis, C. V. Mosby, 1973.

Brian Bolton, ed.: *Psychology of Deafness for Rehabilitation Counselors.* Baltimore, University Park Press, 1976.

Charles E. Buell: *Physical Education and Recreation for the Visually Handicapped.* Washington, D.C., AAHPER, 1973.

Barry Corbet: *Options: Spinal Cord Injury and the Future.* Denver, A. B. Hirschfeld Press, 1980.

Dolores Geddes: *Physical Activities for Individuals with Handicapping Conditions.* St. Louis, C. V. Mosby, 1978.

Glorya Hale, ed.: *The Source Book for the Disabled.* New York and London, Paddington Press, 1979.

Sheila Hewett: *The Family and the Handicapped Child: A Study of Cerebral Palsied Children in Their Homes.* Chicago, Aldine, 1970.

Jerry D. Kelley, ed.: *Recreation Programming for Visually Impaired Children and Youth.* New York, American Foundation for the Blind, 1981.

Frank H. Krusen, Frederick J. Kottke and Paul M. Ellwood, eds.: *Handbook of Physical Medicine and Rehabilitation.* Philadelphia, W. B. Saunders, 1971.

Louis A. Michaux: *The Physically Handicapped and the Community.* Springfield, Illinois, Charles C Thomas, 1970.

Muscular Dystrophy—The Facts. New York, Muscular Dystrophy Association of America, 1970.

Multiple Sclerosis: The Crippler of Young Adults. New York, Multiple Sclerosis Society, 1968.

Sylvia B. O'Brien: *More Than Fun: A Handbook of Recreational Programming for Children and Adults with Cerebral Palsy.* New York, United Cerebral Palsy Association, n.d.

Frank L. Porter, ed.: *The Diabetic at Work and Play.* Springfield, Illinois, Charles C Thomas, 1971.

Howard Rusk: *Rehabilitation Medicine: A Textbook on Rehabilitation Medicine.* St. Louis, C. V. Mosby, 1971.

Hilder K. Waldron: *Rehabilitation of the Physically Handicapped Adolescent.* New York, John Day, 1972.

Ruth Hook Wheeler and Agnes M. Hooley: *Physical Education for the Handicapped.* Philadelphia, Lea and Febiger, 1976.

MENTAL ILLNESS AND SOCIAL DEVIANCE

AAHPER: *Physical Education, Recreation, and Related Programs for Autistic and Emotionally Disturbed.* Washington, D.C., American Alliance for Health, Physical Education and Recreation, 1976.

Ruth Cavan, ed.: *Readings in Juvenile Delinquency.* Philadelphia, J. B. Lippincott, 1969.

Carl Delacato: *The Ultimate Stranger: The Autistic Child.* Garden City, New York, Doubleday, 1976.

Marshall Edelson: *Sociotherapy and Psychotherapy.* Chicago, University of Chicago Press, 1970.

Joan M. Erikson: *Activity, Recovery, Growth: The Communal Role of Planned Activities.* New York, W. W. Norton, 1976.

Kurt Freeman and Ronald R. Koegler: *From Skid Row to the Olympics.* Castaic, California, Institute of Creative Leisure, 1978.

Patricia Gallagher: *Teaching Students with Behavior Disorders.* Denver, Love Publishing Company, 1979.

Don C. Gibbons: *Delinquent Behavior.* Englewood Cliffs, New Jersey, Prentice-Hall, 1970.

William Glasser: *Reality Therapy: A New Approach to Psychiatry.* New York, Harper and Row, 1965.

Malcolm W. Klein: *Street Gangs and Street Workers.* Englewood Cliffs, New Jersey, Prentice-Hall, 1971.

Thomas P. Lowry, ed.: *Camping Therapy: Its Uses in Psychiatry and Rehabilitation.* Springfield, Illinois, Charles C Thomas, 1974.

Jerrold S. Maxmen, Gary J. Tucker and Michael LeBow: *Rational Hospital Psychiatry: The Reactive Environment.* New York, Brunner/Mazel, 1974.

Jack Meislin, ed.: *Rehabilitation Medicine and Psychiatry.* Springfield, Illinois, Charles C Thomas, 1976.

Theodore Rothman, ed.: *Changing Patterns in Psychiatric Care.* New York, Crown, 1970.

H. Lee Swanson and Henry Reinert: *Teaching Strategies for Children in Conflict.* St. Louis, C. V. Mosby, 1979.

PROFESSIONAL PUBLICATIONS WITH ARTICLES OR RESEARCH RELATED TO THERAPEUTIC RECREATION

Journal of Leisure Research. Published quarterly by the National Recreation and Park Association, 3101 Park Center Drive, Alexandria, Virginia 22302.

Journal of Physical Education, Recreation and Dance. Published monthly by the American Alliance for Health, Physical Education, Recreation and Dance, except for July and August, with November and December issues combined, 1900 Association Drive, Reston, Virginia 22091.

Parks and Recreation. Published monthly by the National Recreation and Park Association (address above).

Recreation Canada. Published monthly by the Canadian Parks/Recreation Association, 333 River Road, Vanier City, Ontario K1L 8B9.

Recreation Review. Published quarterly by the Ontario Research Council on Leisure, 400 University Avenue, Toronto, Ontario M7A 1H9.

Research Quarterly for Exercise and Sport. Published quarterly by the American Alliance for Health, Physical Education, Recreation and Dance (address above).

Therapeutic Recreation Journal. Published quarterly by the National Therapeutic Recreation Society/National Recreation and Park Association (address above).

Other professional journals related to specific areas of disability, such as mental retardation or geriatrics, are cited throughout the text. The American Alliance for Health, Physical Education, Recreation and Dance publishes an extensive list of manuals, bibliographies, and pamphlets for those working with the handicapped.

Author Index

Subject Index